Fourth Edition

Tableting Specification Manual

(Previously referred to as the *IPT Standard Specifications for Tableting Tools*)

CW00952874

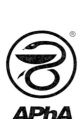

APhA

Published by
American Pharmaceutical Association
2215 Constitution Avenue, NW
Washington, DC 20037-2985

Linda L. Young
Managing Editor

Mary Jane Hickey
Graphic Design and Production

**Glen Ebey, Trevor Higgins, Bill Hnatuk,
Richard Kirk, Dale Natoli, Paul Schaa**
C.A.D. Illustrations and Tables

Michael J. Gerrior
C.A.D. Editor

Julian I. Graubart
Director, Special Projects Department

James P. Caro
Senior Director
Division of Programming and Publications

Library of Congress Catalog Card Number: 81-67973
ISBN: 0-917330-67-6

©Copyright 1995 American Pharmaceutical Association
©Copyright 1990, 1981, 1971

Notice of Copyright: This publication, including all portions hereof, is copyrighted by the American Pharmaceutical Association (APhA) and is protected by the copyright laws of the United States and other laws respecting proprietary rights. No part of this publication, including any portion herein, may be reproduced, transmitted, or redistributed in any form, or by any means, electronic or mechanical or otherwise, including photocopying, recording, or use in any information storage and retrieval system, without written permission from the publisher, APhA (with the exception of certain forms on which permission to copy is stated thereon). Such unauthorized reproduction, transfer, and/or use may be a violation of criminal and civil law.

Requests to reproduce, transmit, and/or transfer this publication, including any portion herein, may be sent to *Tableting Specification Manual*; American Pharmaceutical Association; 2215 Constitution Avenue, NW; Washington, DC 20037. A nominal fee may be assessed for processing such requests.

Notice of Liability: The publisher, APhA, and the Tableting Specification Steering Committee have made every effort to ensure the accuracy and completeness of the information presented in this publication. However, the publisher, Steering Committee members, editors, contributors, and reviewers cannot be held responsible for the continued currency of the information, any inadvertent errors or omissions, or the application of this information. Therefore, the named parties shall have no liability to any person or entity with regard to claims, loss, or damage caused or alleged to be caused, directly or indirectly, by the use of information contained herein.

Contents

© American Pharmaceutical Association

List of Figures

List of Tables

© American Pharmaceutical Association

Acknowledgments

e American Pharmaceutical Association wishes to acknowledge the individuals listed below for their assistance in ducing this book. We thank the Committee Guests for sharing specific information about their tooling or presses, and contributing their expertise to the discussions of tooling specifications.

hough space limitations prevent our listing each person's specific contribution, we also thank the Reviewers and ntributors for suggesting topics to discuss in the fourth edition, providing information for selected topics, and/or cri-uing the preliminary copy.

.r deepest gratitude is reserved for the Steering Committee, whose twelve members developed the updated specifica-ns; wrote new guidelines; prepared C.A.D. illustrations and tables; and reviewed and revised materials numerous les. We could not have produced such a comprehensive revision of the *Manual* without their dedication and generous ntributions of time, knowledge, and materials.

bleting Specification eering Committee Members

bert Andrew
axo Inc.
bulon, North Carolina

en C. Ebey
omas Engineering Inc.
ffman Estates, Illinois

l Froat
hering Plough Corporation
nilworth, New Jersey

evor M. Higgins
Holland Limited
ttingham, England

l Hnatuk, *Committee Chairman*
atuk Associates (Consulting)
erck & Co., Inc. (Retired)
aple Glen, Pennsylvania

chard Kirk
izabeth Carbide Die Co. Inc.
cKeesport, Pennsylvania

le Natoli
toli Engineering Co., Inc.
esterfield, Missouri

rry F. Odar
e Upjohn Company
alamazoo, Michigan

Paul E. Schaa
A.C. Compacting Presses
North Brunswick, New Jersey

Sean Scully
Fette America
Rockaway, New Jersey

Linda K. Stanfill
Marion Merrell Dow
Kansas City, Missouri

William D. Supplee
McNeil Consumer Products
Company
Fort Washington, Pennsylvania

Committee Guests

Norbert Friedrichs
Kilian & Co., Inc.
Horsham, Pennsylvania

Jack McGinley
Holland McGinley
Malvern, Pennsylvania

John Malfettano
United Chemical Machinery Inc.
Toms River, New Jersey

Bill Mohn
Key International, Inc.
Englishtown, New Jersey

Reviewers and Contributors

Joseph P. Estwin, Sr.
Parke Davis Division
Warner Lambert Co. Inc.
Moris Plains, New Jersey

Francis R. Donchez
Francis R. Donchez Consulting Co.
Bethlehem, Pennsylvania

Joachim Reinders
Horn + Noack Pharmatechnik
GmbH
Worms, Germany

Suzette Schultz
Zeneca Pharmaceuticals
Newark, Delaware

Naresh Singhania
Pharmachine Manufacturing
Company
Bombay, India

Rick Stager
Wyeth-Ayerst
Philadelphia, Pennsylvania

Preface

Since the publication of the third edition of the *Tableting Specification Manual* (TSM) in June 1990, the technologies associated with tablet manufacturing have continued their rapid advancement. To keep abreast of the dynamic changes in the industry, the American Pharmaceutical Association (APhA) invited six representatives from tablet press and tooling manufacturers and six representatives from pharmaceutical manufacturers to serve on the Tableting Specification Steering Committee for the fourth edition of the *Manual*.

The Steering Committee's main goals were to update the material in the third edition and to suggest topics that would broaden the *Manual*'s scope and serve numerous other industry needs. To this end, all manufacturers of tablet presses and/or tooling, as well as manufacturing personnel at 24 pharmaceutical companies, were asked to offer suggestions for updating the *Manual*. Those persons or companies that offered material for consideration and/or attended planning meetings are listed in the "Acknowledgments."

At its first planning meeting, the Steering Committee reviewed these suggestions to identify (1) specifications that had become outdated, (2) industry needs for training material, and (3) other areas of tablet manufacturing for which the industry needed or wanted guidelines. At two subsequent meetings, the Steering Committee and guest representatives from tablet press manufacturers reviewed materials prepared by Steering Committee volunteers and identified additional, supporting information for inclusion in the fourth edition. As the final stage of the review process, the compiled material was sent to all tablet press and/or tooling manufacturers and to numerous pharmaceutical companies for evaluation.

As a result of this broad-based input, the Steering Committee established new specifications, suggested changes to some of the specifications listed in the third edition, and developed information and/or guidelines for several new topics. The "Introduction" provides an overview of the updated specifications and the new topics in each section; Section 2 contains the specific information about the updated specifications, including the rationale for their development or revision.

The *Tableting Specification Manual* continues to be the only established standards in the world for tablet design and tablet tooling manufacturing. The Steering Committee and the American Pharmaceutical Association wish to thank publicly everyone who offered information for updating the *Manual*. Your contributions helped us produce specifications that will further standardize U.S. tablet tooling . . . and compile guidelines for tablet design and tooling maintenance that have universal application.

— The Tableting Specification Steering Committee

© American Pharmaceutical Association

Introduction

Special Notice to Readers: Unless otherwise indicated, figures and text illustrations in the *Manual* are not drawn to scale. Further, unless otherwise indicated, the dimensions listed in figures and tables are given first in inches, followed by the equivalent millimeters in brackets.

The first edition of the *Tableting Specification Manual*, published in 1971, offered the first industry-wide specifications for tablet tooling. The specifications, which were developed under the direction of the Industrial Pharmaceutical Technology (IPT) section of APhA's Academy of Pharmaceutical Sciences, are often referred to as the "IPT standards." Because the IPT section no longer exists, APhA and the Steering Committee are introducing a new catchphrase: "TSM standards." Linking the catchphrase with the abbreviation of the *Tableting Specification Manual,* rather than a specialty group, should provide a more stable point of reference.

Objectives

The fourth edition of the *Manual* continues to provide comprehensive information on specifications and quality control programs for tablet tooling. After evaluating each dimensional and tolerance specification published in the third edition, the Steering Committee revised existing specifications for a few dimensions and tolerances of commonly used tablet tooling, and also suggested some new specifications. The changes to existing specifications, as well as development of new specifications, were based on making the tablet tooling more compatible with today's high-speed presses.

The scope of the fourth edition has been broadened to offer basic information on tablet tooling and presses, guidelines on tablet design, more tooling design options, more information on tool steels, step-by-step instructions for inspecting and maintaining tablet tooling, and comprehensive troubleshooting tables for production problems with tablets and tooling.

The information in this edition should aid all personnel involved in tablet design, tablet manufacturing, tooling manufacturing, and press manufacturing to:

- Communicate clearly about the basic and special features of production tooling, as well as the basic components and operations of a tablet press
- Communicate clearly about the basic configurations and design considerations of tablets
- Understand the advantages of using presses that are compatible with TSM specifications
- Implement methods to ensure standardization of tooling

Depending on their information needs, purchasers of the fourth edition also have ready access to guidelines that will help them to:

- Understand tooling dimensions, including tolerances and clearances, and the purpose of tooling specifications
- Understand the factors that affect tablet design and how to use this knowledge to create optimal tablet designs
- Understand the properties of the various types of tool steels and how the compression forces to which they are subjected affect the life cycle of tooling
- Determine the maximum punch tip forces for capsule, oval, and compound-cup oval tooling
- Lengthen the service life of tooling by reducing premature wear and excessive breakage
- Determine the causes of common tablet and tooling problems, and implement methods to reduce or eliminate the problems by selecting the appropriate tooling options
- Interchange tooling appropriately between different makes and models of tablet presses
- Order tooling from multiple suppliers
- Avoid the costly work stoppages and poor-quality tablets that can result from using poor-quality punches or misusing good-quality tooling

New Topics and Guidelines

The new topics in this edition offer basic information for personnel new to the industry, technical information on tablet design and tool steels, and detailed information on procuring and maintaining tooling. A summary of the new topics in each section is presented here so that readers can quickly identify their areas of interest.

Section 1: "Guidelines for Using This Manual"

Section 1 provides basic information about tablet manufacturing, tablet tooling, and tooling specifications, including the rationale for standardization of tools. Specifically, these guidelines:

- Provide definitions of tooling terminology
- Discuss the punches and dies commonly used in production presses
- Compare round and shaped tablet tooling
- Explain the functions of the various positions on a rotary press
- Explain the concepts of clearances, tolerances, and reference dimensions
- Explain how to interpret specification drawings
- Compare U.S. and international tablet tooling specifications
- Explain the advantages of standardizing tooling
- Explain the problems associated with nonconformance of tooling to TSM specifications

Section 2: "TSM Tooling Specifications and Design Options"

Section 2 discusses the updated—revised and new—specifications and contains the specification drawings for punches and dies. Revised tooling specifications include:

- Length of upper punch tips
- Tolerances for tip lengths of lower punches
- Tip straights of lower punches
- Stem-to-barrel radius

- Updated tooling interchangeability tables
- Punch tip tabulations for some cup depths (see Section 3)

New TSM specifications include:

- Maximum stem length
- Minimum and maximum key extensions for presses with upper punch seals
- Size of optional barrel chamfer
- A tolerance for shaped punch tips
- Standard clearances for shaped punch tips
- Optional punch tip designs
- Optional die designs
- Maximum tablet sizes for standard dies
- Minimum land widths (see Section 3)

Deleted specifications include the British "M" ranges for concave punch tip tabulations. The Steering Committee opted not to include this information because the European metric values are in a state of change. Hopefully, standards for international tooling and presses will be developed in the near future by the appropriate parties.

Section 3: "Tablet Design"

Section 3 is the first section on tablet design to appear in the *Tableting Specification Manual*. This section identifies the factors that affect tablet design and provides guidelines for optimal tablet design that take these factors into consideration. Specific information includes:

- The effects of bad tablet design
- Definitions of tablet terminology with supporting illustrations
- The tablet identification processes and guidelines for optimal tablet identification design
- An expanded illustration of bisect types, as well as standard bisect specifications
- Sample designs for bold and narrow letters and numerals (characters)
- Guidelines for tablet printing
- Punch tip tabulations
- Guidelines for producing detailed tablet drawings
- Guidelines for applying land to tablet designs

© American Pharmaceutical Association

Section 4: "Tool Steels, Compression Forces, and Fatigue Failure"

In section 4, information on tool steels and the compression forces they can withstand has been greatly expanded. New topics in this section include:

- The types of tool steels and their uses
- The effect of chemical elements on steel and the chemical composition of tool steels
- Punch tip forces for round tooling, based on finite element analyses
- A calculation method for determining punch tip forces for shaped tooling
- Typical hardness ranges of tool steels
- Fatigue failure of punch tips, supported by a fatigue curve

Section 5: "Tooling Procurement, Inspection, and Maintenance"

Section 5 provides typical information that a company would need to procure, inspect, disburse, and maintain tablet tooling. New material and supporting illustrations include:

- A model for a standard operating procedures program that can be customized for a particular company's operations
- Instructions for setting up a tablet and tooling directory
- Forms for obtaining approval of tooling drawings

- Forms for ordering, inspecting, and disbursing and repairing tooling
- Comprehensive guidelines for the maintenance of tools

Section 6: "Troubleshooting Tablet Production Problems"

Section 6 is the most comprehensive troubleshooting guide to tablet compressing problems that is available to tablet manufacturers. The preventative and corrective measures presented in this section include:

- Basic rules for avoiding production problems
- Factors that affect punch life
- The possible causes and corrective actions for common tablet problems
- The possible causes and corrective actions for common tooling problems
- A method of determining wear of turret guideways by measuring punch tip deflection

Despite the impressive addition of information to this edition of the *Tableting Specification Manual*, the American Pharmaceutical Association and the Steering Committee will continue to track technological advances in the tablet manufacturing industry and identify emerging topics of interest. Readers are also invited to participate in this quest to identify new information needs. Suggested topics should be sent to the *Tableting Specification Manual*; Special Projects Department; American Pharmaceutical Association; 2215 Constitution Avenue, NW; Washington, DC 20037.

Guidelines for Using This Manual

The first step in learning any industry is mastering its terminology. With this in mind, the Steering Committee has adopted a list of standard, industry-accepted terms for tablet manufacturing. An understanding of these terms will provide a foundation on which persons new to the industry can build a working knowledge of the basic tablet categories, tooling types, press operations, and tooling specification drawings. For those who have industry experience, the information in this section could be a useful reference for ensuring clear communication between production staff, tablet designers, tooling suppliers, and press manufacturers.

Tooling Terminology

The following definitions of the standard terminology for tooling (punches and dies) are illustrated in Figure 1 on page 3.

Punch Terminology

Head: The end of the punch that guides it through the press's cam track.

Head Flat (Dwell Flat): The flat area of the head that receives the full force of the compression rollers when the tablet is being formed.

Outside Head Angle/Radius: The area of the head that is in contact with the press cams and has the initial contact with pressure rollers.

Inside Head Angle: The area of the head that is in contact with the "pull-down" cam (lower punches) and "lifting" cam (upper punches).

Head O.D.: The outside diameter (O.D.) of the punch head extends the effective area of contact between the

cam and both the inside head angle and outside head angle/radius.

Neck: The relieved area between the head and barrel, which provides clearance for the cams.

Barrel (Shank): The area between the neck and stem; the barrel's surface is controlled by the turret punch guides to ensure the punch's alignment with the die.

Stem: The area of the punch opposite the head, beginning at the tip and extending to the point where the full diameter of the barrel begins. If a chamfer is present (see definition for *barrel-to-stem chamfer*), the barrel usually reaches its full diameter just above the chamfer.

Tip: The end of the punch that is compatible with the die bore. The tip determines the size, shape, profile, and identification of the tablet.

Cup: The depression or cavity in the tip. Its depth measurement does not include identification embossing or debossing.

Land: The area between the edge of the punch cup and the outside diameter of the punch tip.

Tip Straight: The area of the tip length that extends from the end of the tip to the tip relief.

Tip Length: The straight portion of the stem that is effective inside the die bore. On lower punches, the tip length allows vertical movement within the die bore for the metering and compression of granulation, and ejection of the tablet.

Barrel-to-Stem Radius: The area at the junction of the barrel and stem, which provides a smooth transition from the tip length to the barrel.

Barrel-to-Stem Chamfer: The beveled area located between the barrel and barrel-to-stem radius. The chamfer allows the punches to be inserted through turret guide seals.

© American Pharmaceutical Association

Relief (Undercut): The area of increased mechanical clearance between the stem and the die bore. The sharp edge between the tip straight and the undercut area acts to clean the die.

Working Length: The length of the punch from the bottom of the cup to the head flat. The working lengths of the upper and lower punches control tablet thickness and weight.

Overall Length: The total punch length as measured from the head flat to the end of the tip.

Key: A structure that projects above the barrel's surface and prevents rotational movement of the punches, thus ensuring their alignment to shaped or multi-bored dies.

Keying Angle: The relationship of the punch key to the tablet shape. The key's position is influenced by the tablet shape, take-off angle, and turret rotation.

Die Terminology

Die O.D.: The outside diameter of the die, which is compatible with the die pockets in the press.

Die Height (Depth): The overall height of the die.

Die Bore: The cavity where the tablet is made. The cavity's shape and size determine the same for the tablet.

Chamfer: Entry angle on the die bore.

Taper: A gradual increase in the size of the die bore that extends from the point of compaction to the mouth of the bore. Tapering of the bore assists in ejecting the tablets (see Figure 17, page 31).

Die Groove: The groove around the periphery of the die, which allows the die to be fixed in the press.

Die Protection Shoulder or Radius: The undercut or rounded area, respectively, between the die groove and O.D. Either of these features can be added to prevent damage to die pockets during installation of dies in the press.

Lined (Insert) Dies: Dies fitted with a liner or insert made from a much harder, more wear-resistant material such as tungsten carbide or a ceramic (see Figure 18, page 32).

General Tooling Terminology

Tooling: A collective term that refers to an upper punch, a lower punch, and a die as a unit. For example, the term *tooling maintenance* means the concept pertains to all three tools.

Dwell Time: The length of time the head flat is in contact with the main compression roller. During this interval, the tablet is undergoing full compression.

Tolerance: The authorized deviation from a tooling dimension measurement. The deviation allows for practicality of manufacture.

T.I.R.: The total indicator reading obtained when measuring certain tooling dimensions with a comparator. The T.I.R. is the difference between the highest and lowest readings noted on the indicator dial during one complete rotation of the punch or die.

Clearance: The difference in size between interacting parts, which creates a working space between the parts and allows for their correct and free movement.

Abrasion: The premature wear of contact surfaces.

Corrosion: A chemical reaction of contact surfaces, which causes pitting and discoloration.

Hardening: A process of heating steel at high temperatures to transform it from a soft (annealed) condition to a hard condition.

Tempering: A process of reheating and cooling steel that follows the hardening process. Tempering toughens the steel and *reduces* its hardness.

Rockwell Hardness: A measurement of the hardness of steel. The Rockwell C scale is customarily used for measuring tool steels.

© American Pharmaceutical Association

FIGURE 1. PUNCH AND DIE TERMINOLOGY

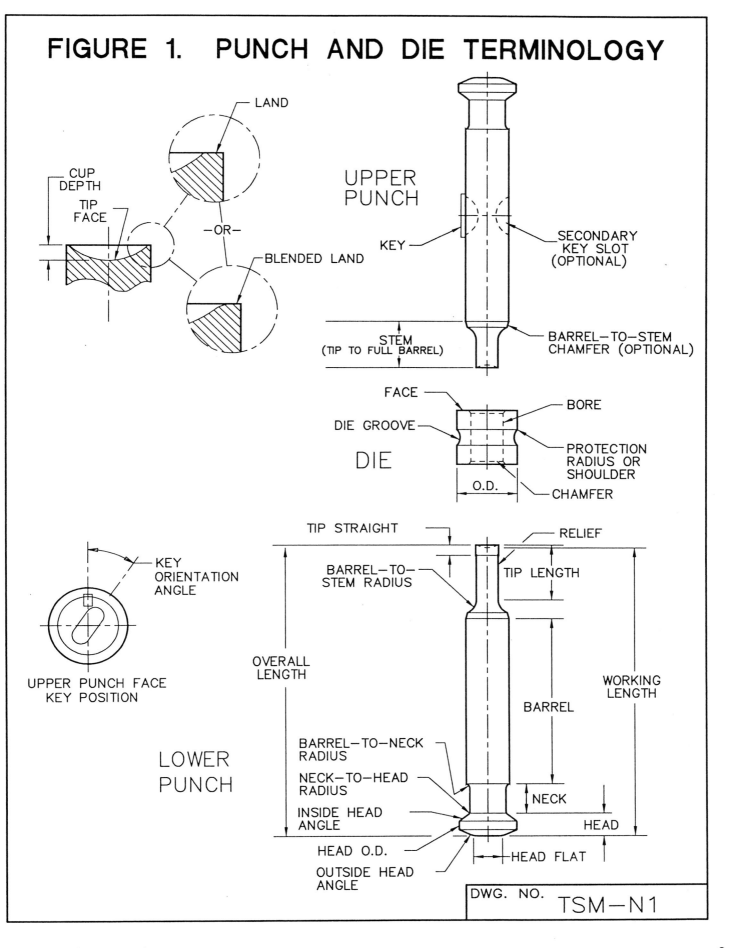

UPPER PUNCH

LAND

—OR—

BLENDED LAND

CUP DEPTH

TIP FACE

KEY

STEM (TIP TO FULL BARREL)

SECONDARY KEY SLOT (OPTIONAL)

BARREL-TO-STEM CHAMFER (OPTIONAL)

FACE

DIE GROOVE

DIE

O.D.

BORE

PROTECTION RADIUS OR SHOULDER

CHAMFER

KEY ORIENTATION ANGLE

UPPER PUNCH FACE KEY POSITION

LOWER PUNCH

TIP STRAIGHT

BARREL-TO-STEM RADIUS

OVERALL LENGTH

BARREL-TO-NECK RADIUS

NECK-TO-HEAD RADIUS

INSIDE HEAD ANGLE

HEAD O.D.

OUTSIDE HEAD ANGLE

RELIEF

TIP LENGTH

BARREL

WORKING LENGTH

NECK

HEAD

HEAD FLAT

DWG. NO. TSM—N1

© American Pharmaceutical Association

3

Tablet Manufacturing

Producing a tablet with a unique design often increases a product's recognition among consumers. Although tablets can be produced in a variety of shapes and sizes, limitations as to their configuration do exist. The limiting factors are usually related to characteristics of the tooling and the press used to produce the tablets. Some categories of tablets are easier to manufacture and comprise the majority of tablets on store shelves.

Tablet Categories

The definitions of tablet terminology, which are based on the geometric properties of the most common tablet shapes, are placed in Section 3, "Tablet Design," for that reason. For the scope of this section, the reader needs only to know that tablets are broadly categorized as either "rounds" or "shapes." To provide illustrative examples of the tablet categories, figures in Section 3 are cross-referenced in the following text.

Round Tablets

Round tablets include primarily convex and flat-faced tablets (see Figure 22, page 46). Frequently, industry people use the term *concave* to describe both the concave surface of a punch cup and the surface of the tablet produced. Technically, the punch cup is usually a concavity and therefore produces a tablet with a convex surface; however, convex cups that produce concave tablets do exist.

Convex tablets can be further categorized according to their cup depth. Figure 24 on page 49 shows convex tablets with shallow, standard, deep, extra-deep, and modified-ball cup depths. Flat-faced tablets can be further categorized as flat-faced plain, flat-faced bevel-edged, and flat-faced radius-edged (see Figure 25, page 51).

Shaped Tablets

Tablets that have geometric configurations other than those listed for rounds are referred to as shapes (see Figure 25). Figure 23 on page 47 uses three common geometric configurations to illustrate the terminology for shaped tablets. To produce a tablet with a particular configuration, the tablet shape is reproduced in the tooling used to manufacture the tablets. Before the method of reproduction can be discussed, a thorough understanding of tablet tooling is required.

Modern Tablet Tooling

The function of tablet tooling is to produce tablets with predetermined physical characteristics, such as shape, thickness, weight, and hardness. To achieve this, the die cavity, or bore, is filled with a granulation or powder to a depth that is determined by the position of the lower punch. The lower punch's position determines the amount of granulation used in each tablet. The upper punch tip is then guided into the bore and force is applied to the punch heads, thereby compressing the material into a tablet. The tablet's shape is determined by the configuration of the die bore and the punch tips. The tablet's thickness and hardness are determined by the amount of compression force applied to the punch heads, whereas its weight is determined by the amount of granulation loaded into the die before compression.

The basic design of tablet punches and dies used in rotary tablet presses has changed very little since these presses were first marketed in the late 1800's. Only minor changes, such as refinements to the head and tip radius, tighter tolerances, and higher surface finishes, have been made. In the U.S. tablet industry, three types of punches and three types of dies are used predominantly in production presses to produce large quantities of tablets for market distribution.

Punches

Punches are classified according to their overall length, barrel diameter, and the O.D. of the punch head. These dimensions, as well as the other specifications for tablet tooling, are nominal: that is, each dimension has a specified measurement, but its actual measurement after the tool is produced may vary from its specification. The allowable variance from a nominal dimension, called its tolerance range, is discussed later in this section under "Tooling Specifications."

© American Pharmaceutical Association

The measurements for specifications discussed in this section are given only in inches so that the reader may more easily grasp the concept under discussion. The equivalent metric measurements are shown in the cross-referenced figures and tables.

The punches most commonly used in production presses are the B-type and D-type punches (see Figure 2, page 6). B2-type punches are used predominantly in a few older models of presses that are no longer being manufactured. During the research stage of a new tablet design, F-type punches and dies (not pictured) and a single-station laboratory press are used to determine the approximate amount of compression force and granulation needed to produce a tablet with the desired physical characteristics.

B-Type Punches have a reference overall length of 5.250 inches and a head O.D. of 1 inch. These dimensions are the same for the upper and lower punches. Although the barrel diameter of a B-type punch is often said to be 3/4 inch, the upper punch has a specified barrel diameter of .7480 inch; the lower punch has a specified value of .7450 inch.

B2-Type Punches also have a barrel diameter of approximately 3/4 inch and a head O.D. of 1 inch; however, the overall lengths of the upper and lower punches differ. The upper punch is 5.250 inches long, whereas the lower punch is 3.562 inches long.

D-Type Punches have the same reference overall length as B-type punches (5.250 inch), but the head O.D. of D-type punches is 1.250 inches. Again, D-type punches are often said to have a barrel diameter of 1 inch; however, the specified barrel diameters are .9980 inch for the upper punches and .9950 inch for the lower punches.

Dies

Dies are classified according to their outside diameters (see Figure 2).

The .945 Die, as the name indicates, has an O.D. of .945 inch. This size die can be used with B- and B2-type punches.

The 1 3/16 Die has an O.D. of 1.1875 inches and can also be used with B- and B2-type punches.

The "D" Die, which has an O.D. of 1.500 inches, is used with D-type punches.

Comparison of Shaped and Round Tooling

Not surprisingly, punches and dies used to manufacture round tablets are often called "round tooling," and punches and dies used to manufacture shaped tablets are called "shaped tooling." After the geometric configuration of a tablet has been determined by the designer, the desired configuration is reproduced in the punch tips and die bores.

The upper punch for a shaped tablet has a device called a key that is inserted into a slot in the barrel and projects above the barrel's surface (see Figure 1). The key prevents the punch from rotating as it is lifted vertically from the die bore so that the punch can re-enter the die bore at the proper alignment. Because round configurations are usually unaffected by rotation of the upper punches, round punches seldom require a key. However, if a round lower punch is embossed, a key is sometimes used to prevent punch rotation and possible distortion of the embossing during tablet ejection.

Regardless of the tablet shape and the type of tooling used, the basic press operations are the same.

Rotary Tablet Presses

Major advancements in the tablet industry have occurred with new models of rotary tablet presses: their speed has increased; a precompression stage has been added to the production cycle; and, in some presses, computer technology automatically adjusts the powder fill mechanism for lower punches to maintain the proper tablet weight. The engineering of these presses was designed around the basic configuration of IPT (now referred to as TSM) tooling to ensure that tablet manufacturers could continue to use their existing inventory of tooling. All presses have designated positions at which certain steps in the production of a tablet occur. The following description of these positions is supported by Figures 3 and 4 on pages 8 and 9.

FIGURE 2. TSM PRODUCTION TOOLING

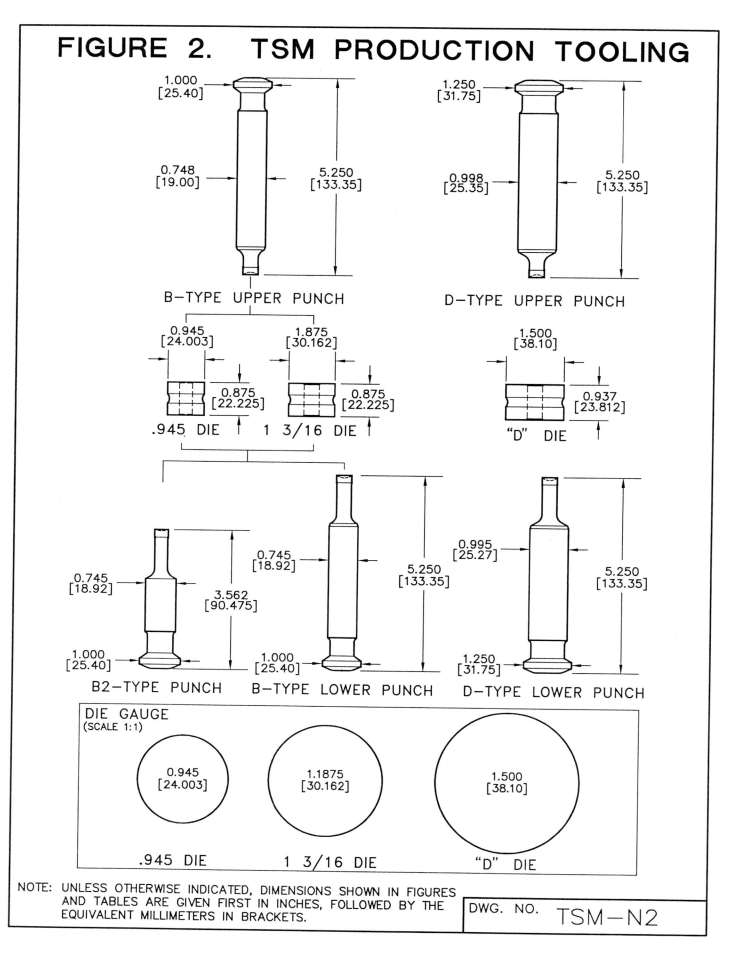

B—TYPE UPPER PUNCH

D—TYPE UPPER PUNCH

.945 DIE   1 3/16 DIE

"D" DIE

B2—TYPE PUNCH   B—TYPE LOWER PUNCH   D—TYPE LOWER PUNCH

DIE GAUGE
(SCALE 1:1)

0.945
[24.003]

1.1875
[30.162]

1.500
[38.10]

.945 DIE   1 3/16 DIE   "D" DIE

NOTE: UNLESS OTHERWISE INDICATED, DIMENSIONS SHOWN IN FIGURES
AND TABLES ARE GIVEN FIRST IN INCHES, FOLLOWED BY THE
EQUIVALENT MILLIMETERS IN BRACKETS.

DWG. NO. TSM—N2

© American Pharmaceutical Association

Fill Position (Die Fill)

At the fill position, the lower punch is pulled down by the fill cam as the die is passing under the feed frame. The pulling down of the lower punch creates a slight vacuum and a void in the die bore. Initially, the combined effect of the vacuum and the void allows loose powder to flow into the die bore. As the die continues its pass under the feed frame, the powder continues to flow into the bore under the force of gravity. The powder can be brought over the die by either a gravity feeder as just described (material flows without a mechanical aid) or by a mechanical feeder (material is actively pushed over the die by rotating paddles).

Typically, the position of the fill cam remains fixed for the entire production run and can only be readjusted or changed manually. Keeping the fill cam at a fixed position allows each die to be filled with the same amount of powder. After the die bore has been filled, the lower punch is transferred to the weight-adjustment cam.

Weight-Adjustment Position

The weight-adjustment cam next raises the lower punch, which pushes excess powder out of the filled die. After the die leaves the area of the feed frame, a spring-loaded, knife-edged blade scrapes the surface of the die and removes any excess powder.

The highest vertical position reached by the weight-adjustment cam regulates the amount of powder expelled and the amount of powder remaining in the die, thus determining the final weight of the tablet. Increasing the highest vertical position of this cam will expel more powder, resulting in a lighter tablet; likewise, decreasing the cam's highest vertical position will expel less powder, resulting in a heavier tablet. On manual presses, a manual handwheel controls the position of the weight adjustment cam; on automated presses, a computer-controlled feedback loop sets the cam's position.

Pull-Down Position

Newer press models have a pull-down position, which allows the lower punch to be pulled down slightly so that the top of the powder column in the die bore is below the surface of the die table. Simultaneously, the upper punch is lowered by the lowering segment of the upper cam track. The lowering of the powder column prevents any powder from being blown out of the die as the upper punch enters the die bore, thus preventing variations in tablet weight. When the upper punch enters the die, precompression begins.

Precompression Position

During precompression, loose powder is consolidated in the die by the removal of any air trapped in the powder column and by the physical orientation of the powder particles. Typically, precompression forces tend to be less than the main compression forces. In presses where the fill cam can be automatically adjusted, the precompression position can be monitored for automatic control of tablet weight. The "tablet" formed at this step is now ready for main compression.

Main Compression Position

The main compression step gives a tablet its final characteristics. The final tablet thickness is determined by the distance between the punch rollers, which determines the distance between the punch tips. Again, in some presses, the main compression position can be monitored for automatic weight control.

Tablet Ejection and Take-Off Position

Before reaching the full ejection position, the upper punch is lifted out of the die bore while the lower punch is being pushed up by the ejection cam, thereby pushing the tablet out of the die. At the full ejection position, a tablet take-off bar located above the die table guides the tablet off the table.

The successful completion of each stage of tablet production depends on how well the tablet tools work with each other and within the tablet press. Making sure that tooling and presses conform to TSM specifications can eliminate many production problems. Understanding specification drawings is critical in determining if a tool conforms to TSM specifications.

FIGURE 3. ROTARY TABLET PRESS CYCLE

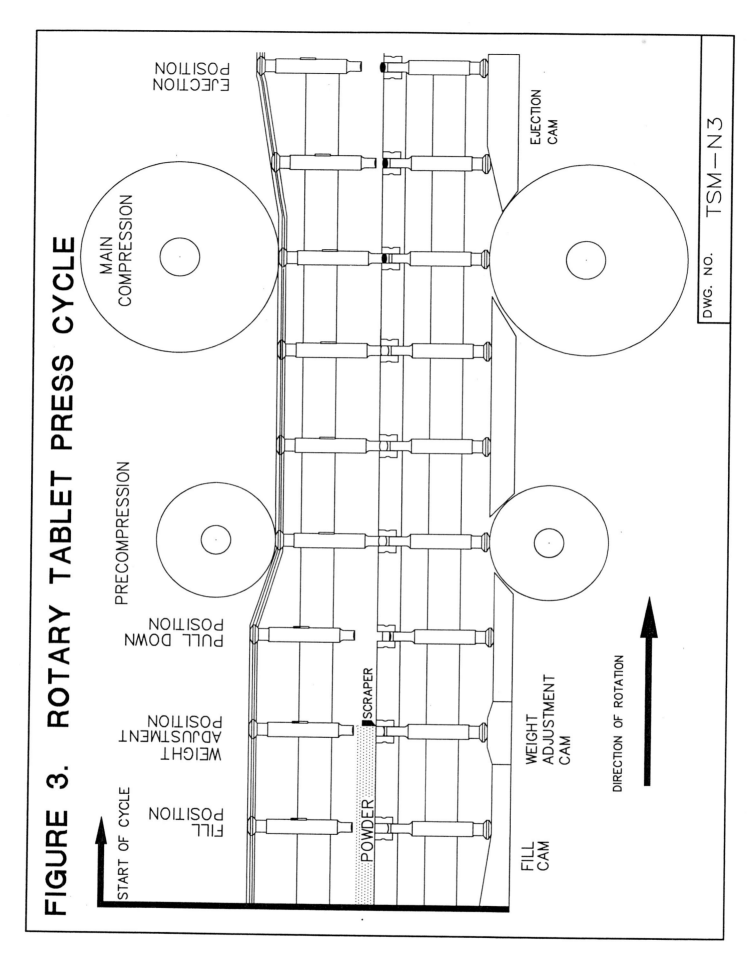

© American Pharmaceutical Association

8

FIGURE 4. TOP VIEW OF TABLET PRESS CYCLE

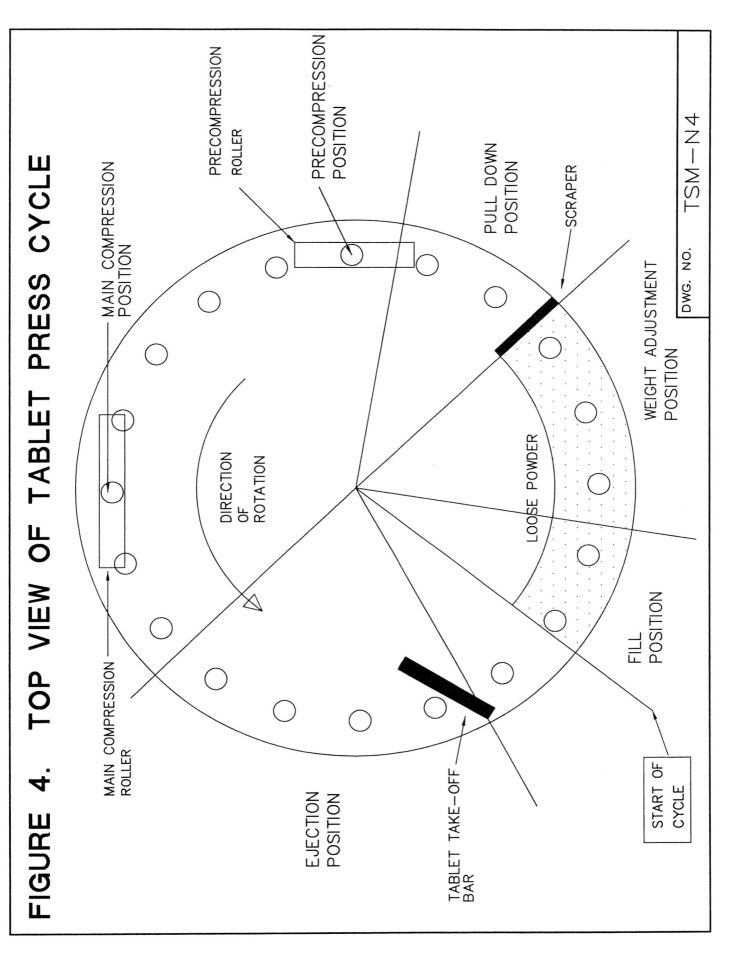

© American Pharmaceutical Association

Tooling Specifications

A tool that conforms to specifications has been machined to meet specific dimensions within a designated range called a tolerance range. Dimensions have been specified for all components of the punches and dies shown in Figure 1. The specifications drawings for standard punches and dies (Figures 8–11 and 14–16; pages 22–25, 28–30) list these dimensions first in inches, followed by the equivalent millimeters placed in brackets. For specifications of radii, an *R* follows the measurement. If the specification is a reference dimension, the abbreviation *REF.* follows the measurement. An explanation of reference dimensions follows the discussions of tolerances and clearances—two other dimensional specifications that affect the proper manufacturing and operation of tablet tooling.

Clearances

If tablet tools are to work properly, there must be enough space between interacting parts to allow them to function without making forced contact. This working space is called clearance. For example, punch tips must be allowed to enter and leave the die bore without making forced contact with the die bore wall. The amount of clearance between interacting parts is affected by the tolerance range of tooling dimensions.

Tolerances

Producing tooling that match specifications exactly would be accomplished only at great expense to tooling manufacturers and ultimately to the companies that purchase the tooling. For that reason, tolerances, or allowable deviations, have been established for tooling specifications. These permissible deviations from specified dimensions, established in cooperation with leading tooling and press manufacturers, ensure that tools can be purchased at a reasonable price and that they will operate properly in the press to produce good-quality tablets.

Specifically, a tolerance is given as a range with an upper limit that determines how much a dimension can be exceeded and a lower limit that determines how much a dimension can be reduced. For example, a tooling dimension that has the specification 1 1/32 inches ±1/32 inch can vary from a high value of 1 1/16 inches to a low value of 1 inch and still be considered to meet specifications.

The tolerance range for a particular specification immediately follows the dimensional value. The range is given either as a number preceded by a plus and minus sign (±) or a set of numbers, one of which is preceded by a plus sign, the other by a minus sign. If a tolerance range is not listed next to the dimensional value, the appropriate tolerances can be found in the block located in the lower right corner of each specification drawing. For dimensions given as a fraction, the appropriate tolerance range is the value labeled as "fractional." The same rule applies to dimensions given as decimals and angles.

The tolerance block also lists the acceptable tolerances for concentricity of die bores, punch tips, and punch heads. Concentricity refers to the placement of one tooling element in the center of another larger element (i.e., the two tooling elements share the same axis). The tolerance is given as a T.I.R., or total indicator reading. Indicator readings measure the form or location of one surface with respect to another. The surface relationships of concern here are the die bore to the O.D.; the punch head to the barrel; and the punch tip to the barrel. The instrument used to measure concentricity, called a comparator, has a readout dial that indicates any deviations in concentricity as measured by a pointer attached to the dial. The T.I.R. is the difference between the highest and lowest readings recorded during one complete rotation of a punch or die.

Reference Dimension

A reference dimension is derived from, or is the result of, other toleranced dimensions that are machined first. For example, the die groove diameter for a .945-inch die is given as a reference value of 27/32 inch ±.015 inch (see Figure 14, page 28). When making this die, the die groove width (1/4 inch ±.015 inch) and the protection radius (3/16 inch ±.015 inch) are machined, or

© American Pharmaceutical Association

"worked to," first. When these dimensions have been achieved within their specified tolerance ranges, the resultant die groove diameter should fall near its reference dimension.

Comparison of U.S. and International Tooling Specifications

Presently, there are three major "standards" of tooling on the international market: the U.S. TSM, the Euro-Standard, and the Japan Norm. As shown in Figure 21 on page 43, the most significant differences in punch specifications are those for barrel diameter, overall punch length, shape of the top of the punch head (domed versus angled), and inner head angle. Also shown for the three standards of B-type tools are the correlating differences in die specifications.

Figures 6 and 7 on pages 20 and 21 give detailed illustrations of the dimensional and configurational differences of angled and domed punch heads. Angled punch heads have an outside head angle, whereas domed heads have a radius. Domed heads, which were developed by European tooling manufacturers, increase the dwell time during the tablet compression stage.

Standardization—Its Purpose and Advantages

Since the first edition of the *Tableting Specification Manual* was published almost a quarter of a century ago, many U.S. tablet press manufacturers have voluntarily redesigned their presses to conform with the specifications. International press manufacturers are also realizing the economic advantages of making their presses compatible with TSM tooling. Tablet manufacturers, especially those with international production facilities, have compelling reasons for preferring presses that meet TSM standards.

Advantages of Standardized Tooling

Standardizing tablet tooling offers the following economic and procedural advantages:

- A uniform quality of tooling can be achieved.
- Tooling suppliers can produce tooling more economically by standardizing their fabrication equipment and manufacturing procedures, and by producing batch quantities of frequently ordered tooling.
- Tooling suppliers can fulfill orders faster by carrying an inventory of standard sizes of round tooling.
- Procedures for purchasing tooling can be simplified.
- Tablet manufacturers can use tooling interchangeably in presses purchased from different manufacturers.
- Tablet manufacturers can reduce their tooling inventory.
- Tablet manufacturers can use standard inspection equipment and validation procedures.
- Multinational pharmaceutical companies can interchange tools and discuss tooling technicalities on the same level.
- Press manufacturers can be sure that their machines will perform well with standard TSM tooling.

Problems of Nonconformance to Specifications

Using tools that do not conform to dimensional specifications can affect tablet quality, press performance, and tablet production rate. Nonconformance of tooling to specifications can also (1) reduce the life of punches, (2) impair the efficient operation of machinery, and (3) cause severe damage to tools and presses.

The remaining sections of this *Manual* provide the necessary information to determine whether a new tool conforms to TSM specifications. The reader will also find detailed guidelines on tablet design, standard operating procedures for procuring and inspecting tooling, and step-by-step instructions for maintaining tools—an important function in protecting tooling *and* presses.

Notes:

© American Pharmaceutical Association

TSM Tooling Specifications and Design Options

e detailed drawings of punches and dies contained in s section represent the bulk of the TSM specifications. Although the nominal dimensions shown on these awings have remained basically unchanged over the ars, the tolerances for these dimensions and surface ishes of the tooling have changed, to some degree, as e equipment used to manufacture the tooling has proved. In some cases, the tolerances are based strict-on what is reasonably achievable using the existing uipment. In most cases, however, the tolerances are e result of careful consideration of what limits provide users with satisfactory tooling performance *and* o allow suppliers to provide tooling at a reasonable st.

ffect of Tooling Dimensions n Tablet Manufacturing

e proper interaction between tools and the presses on ich they are installed is the crux of determining the propriate dimensions and tolerances for tablet tool-. Understanding how individual tooling dimensions ect the tablet manufacturing process is essential to reciating the need for standardized dimensions and erances.

orking Length

e working length, or "length from head flat to bottom cup (LBC)," is the most critical dimension of a nch (see Figure 5, page 14). Variations in working gth of lower punches translate directly into varia-ns in tablet weight. The effect of the tolerance range working length (±.001 inch [±.025 millimeter]) on iations in tablet weight can be as little as a fraction a percent for large tablets and as large as 2% for very all tablets.

In presses that compress tablets to a constant thickness, variations in working length will also cause proportionate variations in tablet thickness. Electronic weight-monitoring devices (force and thickness types) are affected by punch length; the effect is more pronounced when the device is used to reject individual tablets of nonuniform weight than when used for actual weight control.

The working length of a *new* punch is measured directly, using a pointed indicator tip that is positioned as closely to the center of the punch cup as possible. As long as the variation in length throughout the set is within the tolerance range, the working length need not be measured at the exact center of the punch cup. If embossing or a bisect is present, the indicator tip is positioned between the embossing characters or beside the bisect; the working length for *each* punch should be measured at the *same location* on the individual punch cups.

The common practice of reworking head flats on punches throughout the useful life of a set of tooling can result in working lengths that vary considerably from the tooling's initial values. Aside from having to change the height of the tablet ejection cam, a decrease in working length is of little consequence, as long as the variation in length throughout the set remains within the tolerance range.

Cup Depth and Overall Length

Variations in cup depth have very little effect on tablet weight or hardness. However, small deviations in cup depth can cause considerable changes in land width for some cup configurations. The effect is most pronounced on shallow concave and flat-faced bevel-edged (F.F.B.E.) tooling. Reducing the land width decreases the strength of the punch tip edge.

The cup depth dimension for punches has a tolerance of ±.003 inch [±.076 millimeter]. This dimension is rarely

FIGURE 5. OVERALL AND WORKING LENGTHS

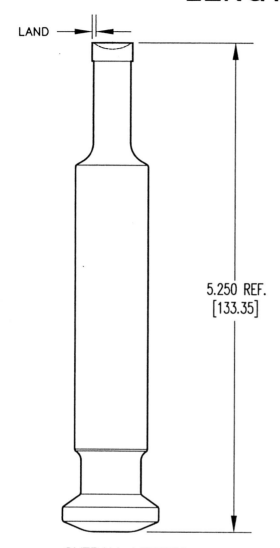

LAND

5.250 REF.
[133.35]

OVERALL LENGTH

EQUALS REFERENCE LENGTH 5.250
[133.35] AFTER APPLICATION OF A LAND

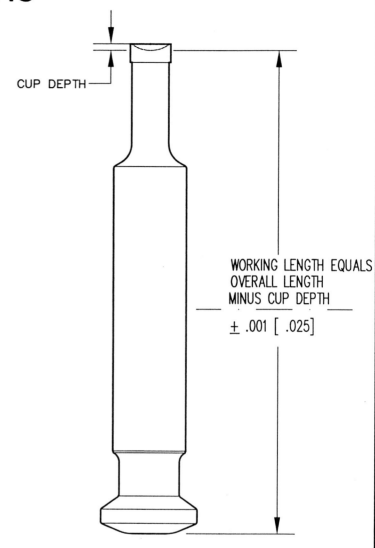

CUP DEPTH

WORKING LENGTH EQUALS
OVERALL LENGTH
MINUS CUP DEPTH

± .001 [.025]

WORKING LENGTH

EQUALS OVERALL LENGTH MINUS NOMINAL CUP DEPTH
± .001 [.025]

OR

ONE PUNCH IN A SET SERVES AS A DATUM. THE
VARIATION WITHIN THE COMPLETE SET FROM THE
DATUM'S WORKING LENGTH SHOULD NOT EXCEED A
RANGE OF .002 [.05] T.I.R. (I.E., ± .001 [.025]).

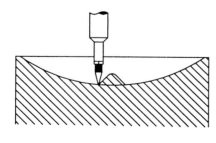

IN CASE OF EMBOSSING, BISECTS, ETC., THE WORKING
LENGTH SHOULD BE MEASURED AS CLOSELY AS POSSIBLE
TO THE CENTER OF THE TIP FACE.

DWG. NO. TSM—N5

© American Pharmaceutical Association

measured directly because different indicator tips are needed to locate the land and the bottom of the cup. Instead, the cup depth is obtained by subtracting the working length from the overall length.

On reworked tooling, overall length and cup depth may vary significantly from the tooling's initial measured values. Again, the variation in overall length within the set is more important than the average value.

Head Thickness

On many tablet presses, the thickness of lower punch heads plays an important role in maintaining consistent tablet weight and/or limiting the upward flight of the punches at the point of final weight adjustment and tablet ejection.

Although the tolerance on punch head thickness is ±.010 inch [±.25 millimeter], the deviation throughout a new set of tooling is usually much less than the tolerance range. Punch heads, particularly the inside head angles, are the most commonly reworked area on tablet tooling. When punch heads are reworked, maintaining a uniform punch head thickness throughout the set should be the primary concern.

Head Flat Diameter

The diameter of the punch head flat and the turret speed of the press determine the amount of time the tablet material undergoes maximum compression. The time of maximum compression, often referred to as *dwell time*, directly affects the tablet hardness.

The TSM specifications for the head flats of B- and D-type tooling are .500 inch [12.70 millimeters] and .750 inch [19.05 millimeters], respectively. These dimensions refer to the head flat diameter before the 5/16-inch [7.94-millimeter] blend radius is added between the outside head angle and the head flat. The specification is based on the "preblended" dimension, rather than the actual finished dimension, because of the difficulty in measuring exactly where the blend radius ends and the head flat starts. These preblended dimensions are often designated as "over sharp corners (OSC)."

For B-type punches, the head flat is approximately .367 inch [9.3 millimeters] after the blend radius is applied

(see Figure 6, page 20). Similarly, for a D-type punch, the head flat is approximately .611 inch [15.52 millimeters] after the blend radius is applied (see Figure 7, page 21).

Tip Straight

Tip straights, a standard feature on lower punches, can also be applied to upper punches. This relieved area at the tip of the punch guides the punch in the die, and provides a tight fit between the punch and die to prevent the loss of fine granulation particles from the die bore.

Punch Tip Undercut

The stem area of lower punches is usually undercut to allow free movement of the punch tip in the die bore; the undercut reduces the chance of a punch tip binding in the die bore. The undercut, or relief, forms a sharp corner at the back edge of the tip straight; this corner can scrape film off the die wall as the lower punch moves up and down in the die. An undercut can also be added to upper punches to improve retention of dust cups.

The specifications for several of the dimensions just discussed have been revised. The specific changes and the rationale for them are discussed in the following paragraphs.

Updated Specifications

During the development of the fourth edition specifications, the Steering Committee took every precaution to ensure that existing tooling would not be adversely affected by the revised or new specifications, *and* that new tooling produced according to these specifications would perform in all presses that existed at the time of publication of the fourth edition.

Revised Specifications

A few of the changes to the third edition specifications were necessary to accommodate a new dimension: the maximum stem length. This new dimension and its purpose are explained later in the discussion of "New Specifications." Most of the remaining revised specifications are related to changes in tolerances.

Head Flat Tolerance

The tolerance for the head flat diameter on B-type and D-type punches has been changed to +.000, –.030 inch [+.00, –.76 millimeter] (see Figures 8–11, pages 22–25). The previous tolerance range was +.000, –.015 inch [+.00, –.38 millimeter]. The head flat tolerance was changed to make it more consistent with allowable tolerance buildup from the other punch head dimensions.

Punch Tip Lengths

The length of upper punch tips for B- and D-type tooling was changed to a 5/16 inch [7.94 millimeters] minimum to lengthen the punch barrels for use in presses with upper punch seals (see Figures 8 and 10). The previous specification was 1/2 inch ±.015 [12.70 millimeters ±.38]. The revised tip length will accommodate the maximum upper punch entry of .315 inch [8 millimeters] offered by press manufacturers, while also allowing room for a dust cup.

Tip Length Tolerances

The tolerance for tip lengths of *B-type* lower punches was changed to +.060, –.031 inch [+1.52, –.79 millimeter] (see Figure 9). The previous specification was ±.015 inch [±.38 millimeter].

The tolerance for tip lengths of *D-type* lower punches was changed to +.060, –.015 inch [+1.52, –.38 millimeter] (see Figure 11). The previous specification was ±.015 inch [±.38 millimeter].

Punch Tip Undercut

An undercut diameter of .020-inch [.51-millimeter] reduction is specified for all sizes of tip straights; however, shal-

lower undercuts may be considered for extremely small tablets. A surface finish of 125 microinches is specified for the undercut (see Figure 12, page 26).

Barrel-to-Stem Radius

The barrel-to-stem radius on upper and lower punches was changed to 3/16 inch +1/8, –1/16 [4.76 millimeters +3.18, –1.59] to accommodate the shorter overall tip length required by some presses with upper punch seals (see Figures 8–11). The previous specification was 1/4 inch ±.015 [6.35 millimeter ±.38].

Tooling Interchangeability Tables

Based on feedback from tablet press manufacturers, new press models were added, corrections to third edition information were made, and some press models were deleted from the tooling interchangeability tables (see Tables 4–7, pages 38–42). To be listed, a press manufacturer must have had a significant number of operating presses in the United States; no new manufacturers were added.

Concave Punch Tip Tabulations

The changes in the table below labeled as *New Cup Depth* have been incorporated in Table 10, "Punch Tip Tabulations," on page 68.

Corrections, rather than revisions, were made to the specifications listed in the third edition for domed punch heads, the head flat of D-type punches, and surface finishes.

Revised Punch Tip Tabulations

Concavity Type	Punch Tip Size	New Cup Depth	Old Cup Depth
Standard	1/4 [6.350]	.031 [.787]	.033 [.838]
Deep	9/32 [7.142]	.046 [1.168]	.047 [1.194]
Extra-Deep	1/8 [3.175]	.030 [.762]	.024 [.610]
Extra-Deep	5/32 [3.970]	.036 [.914]	.030 [.762]
Extra-Deep	3/16 [4.763]	.042 [1.067]	.036 [.914]
Extra-Deep	7/32 [5.555]	.048 [1.219]	.042 [1.067]
Extra-Deep	1/4 [6.350]	.050 [1.270]	.048 [1.219]

© American Pharmaceutical Association

Domed Punch Heads

The head flat dimension for B-type, TSM (IPT) and European domed head punches was changed to .375 inch [9.53 millimeters] (see Figure 6). The third edition incorrectly showed a .250-inch [6.35-millimeter] head flat for the European and TSM domed heads.

Head Flat Dimension

In specification drawings of D-type punches, the third edition listed a head flat dimension of .714 inch [18.14 millimeter], which is actually the head flat size derived from blending a head flat of .750 inch [19.05 millimeters] with the 5/16-inch [7.94 millimeter] radius. To be consistent with the specification drawings of B-type punches, the head flat dimension for D-type punches was changed to the preblended value of .750 inch [19.05 millimeters] (see Figures 10 and 11).

Surface Finish Note

The metric conversion measurement of the surface finish specification (see Note 2 on Figures 8–11, 14–16) was changed to read .508 microns ±.127. The third edition listed these values as 508 microns ±127.

New Specifications

New specifications in this edition span a wide range of tooling concerns. Punch dimensions that accommodate the increased use of upper punch seals were established, along with tolerances and clearances for shaped punch tips, tooling design options, maximum tablet sizes, and new methods of determining maximum compression forces.

Shaped Punch Tip Tolerance

Although the tip tolerance of –.0005 inch [–.013 millimeter] was developed for round punch tips, tooling users have come to accept this tolerance as a standard for shaped punch tips as well. Because shaped tips are more difficult to machine and their dimensions are also more difficult to measure, the TSM Committee has adopted –.0008 inch [–.020 millimeter] as the first standard tolerance for shaped punch tips (see Figures 8–11).

Tooling Design Options

Specifications for the punch tip options–undercuts and Bakelite relief–are given in Figures 12 and 13 on pages 26 and 27. Specifications for the die options–tapered dies and die groove reliefs–are given in Figures 17 and 18 on pages 31 and 32.

Maximum Tablet Sizes

Table 1 on page 33 lists the recommended maximum sizes of round and shaped tablets for standard dies.

Shaped Punch Tip Clearances

A nominal clearance of .0017 inch [.043 millimeter] is specified for all sizes of shaped *upper* punch tips; the clearance range for upper shaped tips is .0017/.0030 inch [.043/.076 millimeter]. For shaped *lower* punch tips of all sizes, a nominal clearance of .0012 inch [.030 millimeter] is specified; the clearance range for lower shaped tips is .0012/.0025 inch [.030/.064 millimeter]. (See Figure 19 and boxed text on page 33.)

Clearances for round punch tips are listed in Table 2 on pages 34 and 35.

Maximum Stem Length

Tablet presses with optional upper punch seals are becoming more common. To provide a barrel length that is useable with virtually all press makes and models, a maximum stem length of .730 inch [18.54 millimeters] was established (see Figures 8–11). The stem length is measured from the end of the tip to the point where the barrel reaches its full diameter.

Some presses with upper punch seals may require a stem length that is much less than the .730-inch [18.54-millimeter] dimension to avoid damaging the seal or affecting its performance (see Tables 3A and B, page 37). In such cases, the tooling or press supplier should be consulted.

Available Key Space

Based on information received from tablet press manufacturers, a *minimum* extension dimension of the key relative to the head flat (distance from the head flat to the beginning of the key) was established for each manufacturer's presses that require upper punch seals. A *maximum* extension dimension of the key relative to the head flat (distance from the head flat to the end of the key) was also established for these manufacturer's presses (see Tables 3A and B). These dimensions indicate the *maximum space available* on a punch for placement of a key, which will not cause damage to cams and punch seals.

The dimensions from the head flat to the *center* of the key shown in Figure 20 on page 36 apply to presses that do not require seals on upper punches. The minimum and maximum extension dimensions replace the dimension to the center of the key for presses that require upper punch seals. When dealing with presses from the *same manufacturer*, punches designed for presses with upper punch seals will also work in the manufacturer's presses that do *not* have the seals; the reverse may not be true.

Size of Optional Barrel Chamfer

The dimension for a barrel chamfer is noted on the specification drawings as "Variable" because it is difficult to grind a chamfer of uniform size around the barrel of a shaped punch (see Figures 8–11). An .08-inch [2-millimeter] chamfer is recognized as the maximum chamfer size; however, .02 inch [.5 millimeter] is a more realistic size. A small chamfer can be used to help tooling manufacturers meet the new maximum stem length by leaving more space for the tolerances. For some presses with upper punch seals, the standard "Break Sharp Edge" may be adequate. The tooling supplier should be consulted if the appropriate chamfer size is in question.

Minimum Land Widths

Minimum land widths for concave and F.F.B.E. punch tips are listed in Table 9 on page 67. Each value is based on the width of the land before the sharp corner

is blended. Use of the recommended minimum land will strengthen tip edges.

Tool Steels

Table 12 on page 72 lists the typical hardness range of tool steels. This new table replaces the third edition table that gave values for the toughness and wear resistance of tool steels.

Punch Tip Compression Forces

Punch tip forces for round tooling based on finite element analysis (FEA) are listed in Table 13 on page 74. For shaped tooling, a calculation method of determining punch tip forces is presented on pages 73–77. The calculation method yields more accurate punch tip forces for shaped punches than do data derived from a table alone.

TSM Compatibility of International Presses

The attempts of press manufacturers in Japan, European countries, and other countries to make their newer press models compatible with TSM tooling have not always been successful. Some of the newer international presses advertised as being compatible with TSM tooling *can* operate with this tooling in place, but *not* at the maximum efficiency rate achieved in U.S. presses. Figure 21 on page 43 shows the differences in specifications for TSM, European, and Japanese tooling.

During its review of the third edition specifications, the Steering Committee realized the need to inform international press manufacturers of the standard TSM configurations (with some options) that, if included in their press designs, would allow their presses to provide maximum tablet output and trouble-free operation while using TSM tooling.

© *American Pharmaceutical Association*

Section 2: Tooling Specification Figures and Tables

FIGURE 6. COMMON HEAD CONFIGURATIONS OF B-TYPE PUNCHES
(3/4" [19 mm] DIAMETER BARREL)

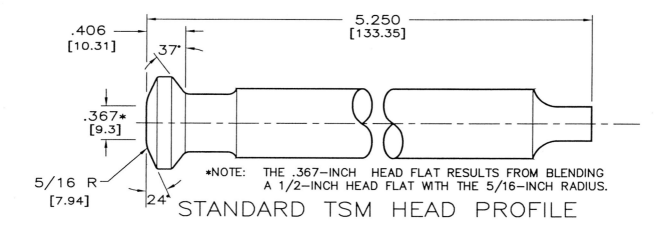

.406 [10.31]
37°
5.250 [133.35]
.367* [9.3]
5/16 R [7.94]
24°

*NOTE: THE .367-INCH HEAD FLAT RESULTS FROM BLENDING A 1/2-INCH HEAD FLAT WITH THE 5/16-INCH RADIUS.

STANDARD TSM HEAD PROFILE

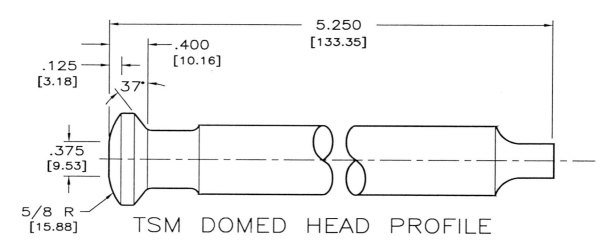

.125 [3.18]
37°
.400 [10.16]
5.250 [133.35]
.375 [9.53]
5/8 R [15.88]

TSM DOMED HEAD PROFILE

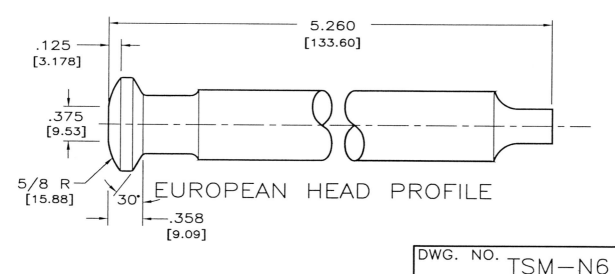

.125 [3.178]
5.260 [133.60]
.375 [9.53]
5/8 R [15.88]
30°
.358 [9.09]

EUROPEAN HEAD PROFILE

DWG. NO. TSM—N6

© American Pharmaceutical Association

FIGURE 7. COMMON HEAD CONFIGURATIONS OF D-TYPE PUNCHES
(1" [25.4 mm] DIAMETER BARREL)

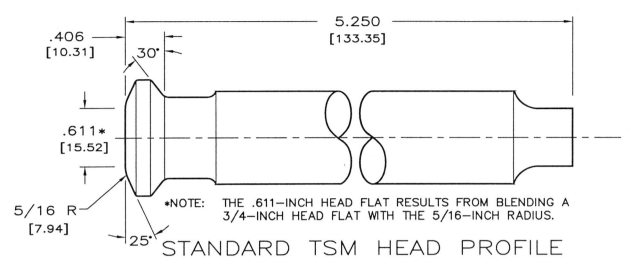

5.250
[133.35]

.406
[10.31]

30°

.611*
[15.52]

5/16 R
[7.94]

25°

*NOTE: THE .611-INCH HEAD FLAT RESULTS FROM BLENDING A
3/4-INCH HEAD FLAT WITH THE 5/16-INCH RADIUS.

STANDARD TSM HEAD PROFILE

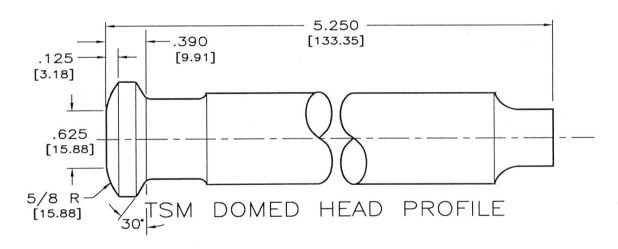

5.250
[133.35]

.390
[9.91]

.125
[3.18]

.625
[15.88]

5/8 R
[15.88]

30°

TSM DOMED HEAD PROFILE

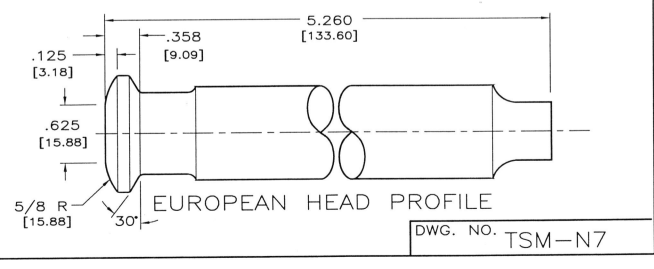

5.260
[133.60]

.358
[9.09]

.125
[3.18]

.625
[15.88]

5/8 R
[15.88]

30°

EUROPEAN HEAD PROFILE

DWG. NO. TSM-N7

© American Pharmaceutical Association

FIGURE 8. STANDARD B-TYPE UPPER PUNCH
(3/4" [19 mm] DIAMETER BARREL)

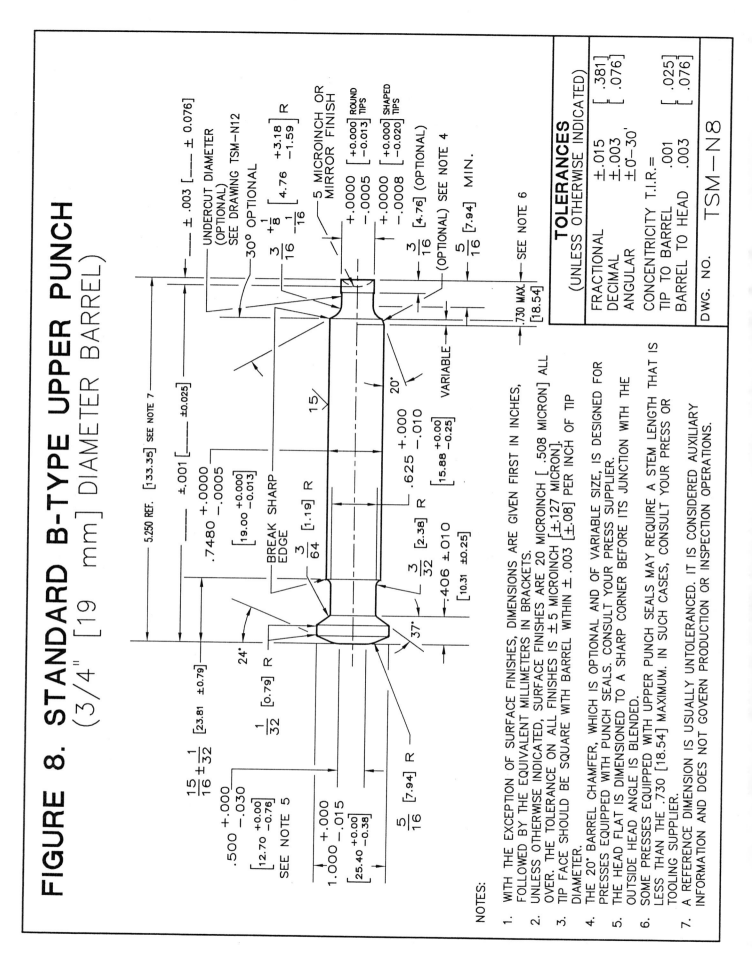

NOTES:

1. WITH THE EXCEPTION OF SURFACE FINISHES, DIMENSIONS ARE GIVEN FIRST IN INCHES, FOLLOWED BY THE EQUIVALENT MILLIMETERS IN BRACKETS.

2. UNLESS OTHERWISE INDICATED, SURFACE FINISHES ARE 20 MICROINCH [.508 MICRON] ALL OVER. THE TOLERANCE ON ALL FINISHES IS ±5 MICROINCH [±.127 MICRON].

3. TIP FACE SHOULD BE SQUARE WITH BARREL WITHIN ± .003 [±.08] PER INCH OF TIP DIAMETER.

4. THE 20° BARREL CHAMFER, WHICH IS OPTIONAL AND OF VARIABLE SIZE, IS DESIGNED FOR PRESSES EQUIPPED WITH PUNCH SEALS. CONSULT YOUR PRESS SUPPLIER.

5. THE HEAD FLAT IS DIMENSIONED TO A SHARP CORNER BEFORE ITS JUNCTION WITH THE OUTSIDE HEAD ANGLE IS BLENDED.

6. SOME PRESSES EQUIPPED WITH UPPER PUNCH SEALS MAY REQUIRE A STEM LENGTH THAT IS LESS THAN THE .730 [18.54] MAXIMUM. IN SUCH CASES, CONSULT YOUR PRESS OR TOOLING SUPPLIER.

7. A REFERENCE DIMENSION IS USUALLY UNTOLERANCED. IT IS CONSIDERED AUXILIARY INFORMATION AND DOES NOT GOVERN PRODUCTION OR INSPECTION OPERATIONS.

TOLERANCES
(UNLESS OTHERWISE INDICATED)

FRACTIONAL	±.015	[.381]
DECIMAL	±.003	[.076]
ANGULAR	±0-30'	
CONCENTRICITY T.I.R.=		
TIP TO BARREL	.001	[.025]
BARREL TO HEAD	.003	[.076]

DWG. NO.   TSM-N8

© American Pharmaceutical Association

FIGURE 9. STANDARD B-TYPE LOWER PUNCH
(3/4" [19 mm] DIAMETER BARREL)

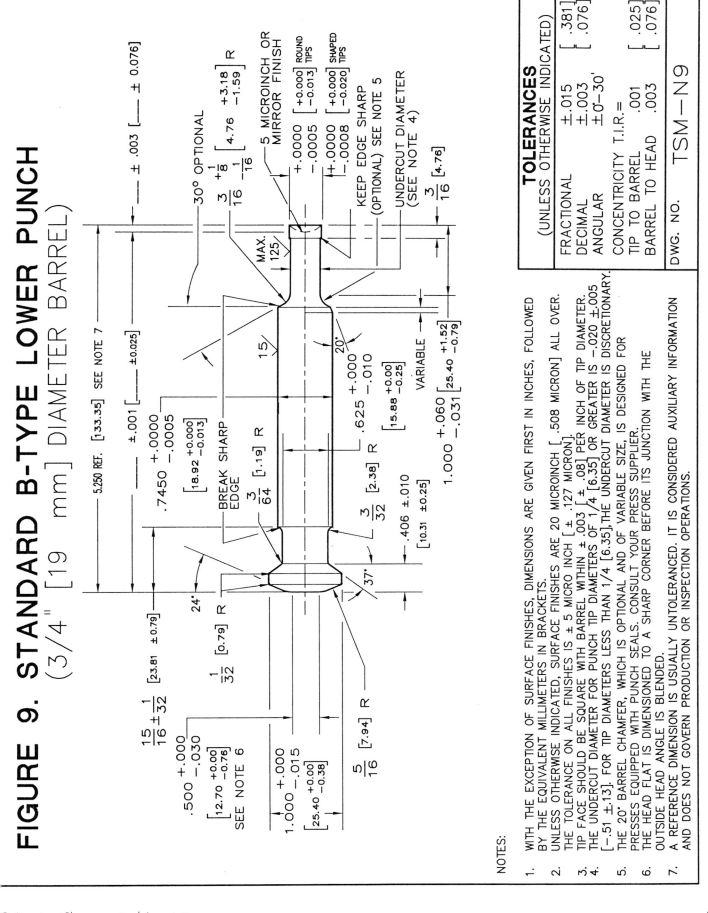

NOTES:

1. WITH THE EXCEPTION OF SURFACE FINISHES, DIMENSIONS ARE GIVEN FIRST IN INCHES, FOLLOWED BY THE EQUIVALENT MILLIMETERS IN BRACKETS.
2. UNLESS OTHERWISE INDICATED, SURFACE FINISHES ARE 20 MICROINCH [.508 MICRON] ALL OVER. THE TOLERANCE ON ALL FINISHES IS ± 5 MICRO INCH [± .127 MICRON].
3. TIP FACE SHOULD BE SQUARE WITH BARREL WITHIN ±.003 [±.08] PER INCH OF TIP DIAMETER.
4. THE UNDERCUT DIAMETER FOR PUNCH TIP DIAMETERS OF 1/4 [6.35] OR GREATER IS −.020 ±.005 [−.51 ±.13]. FOR TIP DIAMETERS LESS THAN 1/4 [6.35], THE UNDERCUT DIAMETER IS DISCRETIONARY.
5. THE 20° BARREL CHAMFER, WHICH IS OPTIONAL AND OF VARIABLE SIZE, IS DESIGNED FOR PRESSES EQUIPPED WITH PUNCH SEALS. CONSULT YOUR PRESS SUPPLIER.
6. THE HEAD FLAT IS DIMENSIONED TO A SHARP CORNER BEFORE ITS JUNCTION WITH THE OUTSIDE HEAD ANGLE IS BLENDED.
7. A REFERENCE DIMENSION IS USUALLY UNTOLERANCED. IT IS CONSIDERED AUXILIARY INFORMATION AND DOES NOT GOVERN PRODUCTION OR INSPECTION OPERATIONS.

TOLERANCES
(UNLESS OTHERWISE INDICATED)

FRACTIONAL	±.015 [.381]
DECIMAL	±.003 [.076]
ANGULAR	±0°−30'
CONCENTRICITY T.I.R.=	
TIP TO BARREL	.001 [.025]
BARREL TO HEAD	.003 [.076]

DWG. NO. TSM−N9

© American Pharmaceutical Association

23

FIGURE 10. STANDARD D-TYPE UPPER PUNCH
(1" [25.4 mm] DIAMETER BARREL)

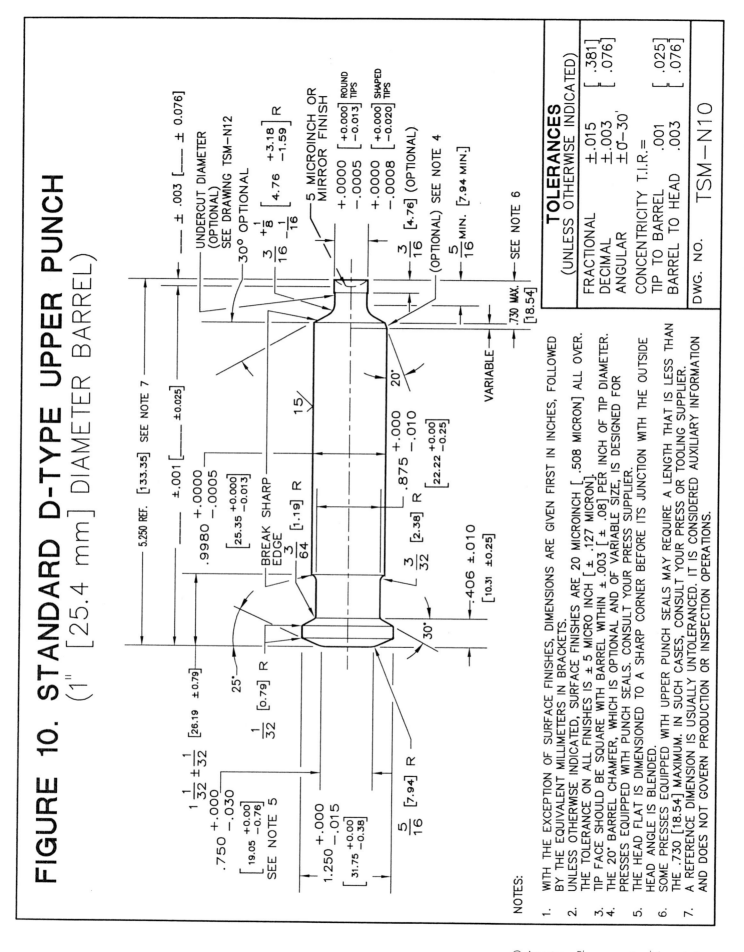

NOTES:

1. WITH THE EXCEPTION OF SURFACE FINISHES, DIMENSIONS ARE GIVEN FIRST IN INCHES, FOLLOWED BY THE EQUIVALENT MILLIMETERS IN BRACKETS.

2. UNLESS OTHERWISE INDICATED, SURFACE FINISHES ARE 20 MICROINCH [.508 MICRON] ALL OVER. THE TOLERANCE ON ALL FINISHES IS ±5 MICRO INCH [±.127 MICRON].

3. TIP FACE SHOULD BE SQUARE WITH BARREL WITHIN ±.003 [±.08] PER INCH OF TIP DIAMETER.

4. THE 20° BARREL CHAMFER, WHICH IS OPTIONAL AND OF VARIABLE SIZE, IS DESIGNED FOR PRESSES EQUIPPED WITH PUNCH SEALS. CONSULT YOUR PRESS SUPPLIER.

5. THE HEAD FLAT IS DIMENSIONED TO A SHARP CORNER BEFORE ITS JUNCTION WITH THE OUTSIDE HEAD ANGLE IS BLENDED.

6. SOME PRESSES EQUIPPED WITH UPPER PUNCH SEALS MAY REQUIRE A LENGTH THAT IS LESS THAN THE .730 [18.54] MAXIMUM. IN SUCH CASES, CONSULT YOUR PRESS OR TOOLING SUPPLIER.

7. A REFERENCE DIMENSION IS USUALLY UNTOLERANCED. IT IS CONSIDERED AUXILIARY INFORMATION AND DOES NOT GOVERN PRODUCTION OR INSPECTION OPERATIONS.

TOLERANCES
(UNLESS OTHERWISE INDICATED)

FRACTIONAL	±.015	[.381]
DECIMAL	±.003	[.076]
ANGULAR	±0°-30'	
CONCENTRICITY T.I.R.=		
TIP TO BARREL	.001	[.025]
BARREL TO HEAD	.003	[.076]

DWG. NO.   TSM-N10

© American Pharmaceutical Association

FIGURE 11. STANDARD D-TYPE LOWER PUNCH
(1" [25.4 mm] DIAMETER BARREL)

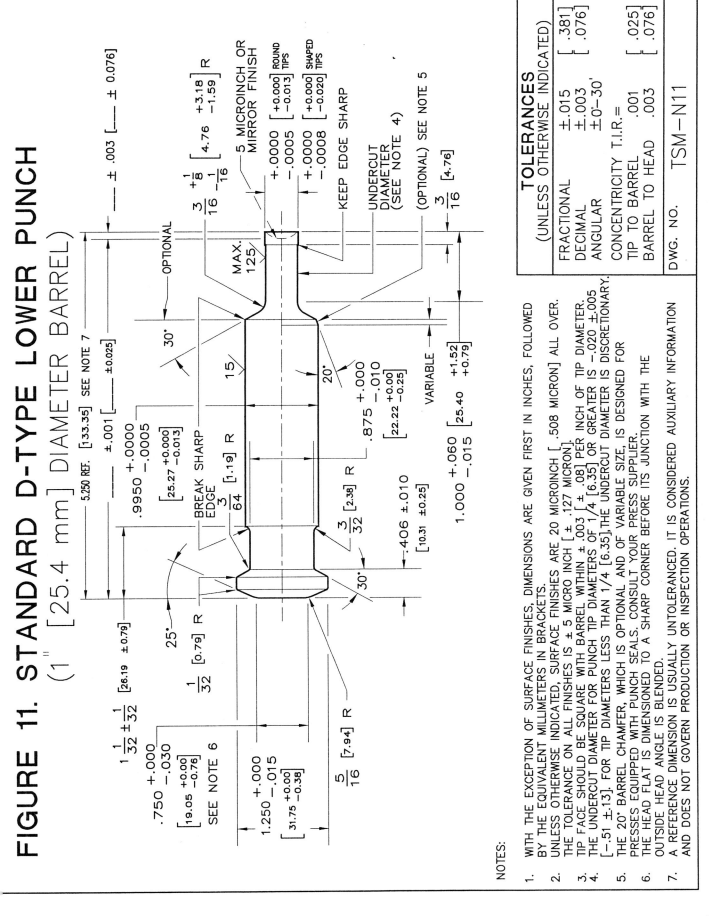

TOLERANCES (UNLESS OTHERWISE INDICATED)		
FRACTIONAL	±.015	[.381]
DECIMAL	±.003	[.076]
ANGULAR	±0°-30'	
CONCENTRICITY T.I.R.=		
TIP TO BARREL	.001	[.025]
BARREL TO HEAD	.003	[.076]
DWG. NO. TSM—N11		

NOTES:

1. WITH THE EXCEPTION OF SURFACE FINISHES, DIMENSIONS ARE GIVEN FIRST IN INCHES, FOLLOWED BY THE EQUIVALENT MILLIMETERS IN BRACKETS.
2. UNLESS OTHERWISE INDICATED, SURFACE FINISHES ARE 20 MICROINCH [.508 MICRON] ALL OVER. THE TOLERANCE ON ALL FINISHES IS ± 5 MICRO INCH [± .127 MICRON].
3. TIP FACE SHOULD BE SQUARE WITH BARREL WITHIN ±.003 [± .08] PER INCH OF TIP DIAMETER.
4. THE UNDERCUT DIAMETER FOR PUNCH TIP DIAMETERS OF 1/4 [6.35] OR GREATER IS −.020 ±.005 [−.51 ±.13]. FOR TIP DIAMETERS LESS THAN 1/4 [6.35], THE UNDERCUT DIAMETER IS DISCRETIONARY.
5. THE 20° BARREL CHAMFER, WHICH IS OPTIONAL AND OF VARIABLE SIZE, IS DESIGNED FOR PRESSES EQUIPPED WITH PUNCH SEALS. CONSULT YOUR PRESS SUPPLIER.
6. THE HEAD FLAT IS DIMENSIONED TO A SHARP CORNER BEFORE ITS JUNCTION WITH THE OUTSIDE HEAD ANGLE IS BLENDED.
7. A REFERENCE DIMENSION IS USUALLY UNTOLERANCED. IT IS CONSIDERED AUXILIARY INFORMATION AND DOES NOT GOVERN PRODUCTION OR INSPECTION OPERATIONS.

© American Pharmaceutical Association

FIGURE 12. SPECIAL PUNCH TIP OPTIONS

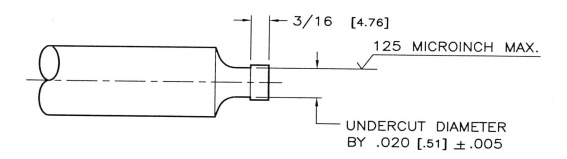

— 3/16 [4.76]

125 MICROINCH MAX.

UNDERCUT DIAMETER
BY .020 [.51] ±.005

UNDERCUT UPPER PUNCH TIP

UPPER PUNCH TIPS CAN BE MANUFACTURED TO INCLUDE THE SAME TYPE OF UNDERCUT FOUND ON LOWER PUNCHES. UPPER PUNCH UNDERCUTS PROVIDE A LIP FOR BETTER RETENTION OF DUST CUPS.

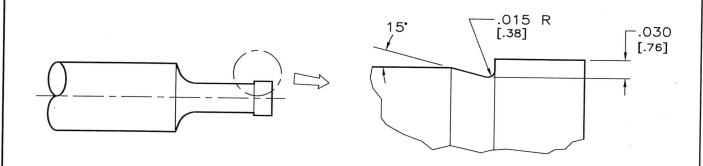

15°   .015 R
         [.38]

.030
[.76]

BAKELITE RELIEF

SOME MATERIALS TEND TO LEAVE A THIN FILM ON DIE BORE SURFACES. THIS FILM CAN BUILD UP TO A POINT WHERE BINDING OCCURS BETWEEN THE LOWER PUNCH TIPS AND DIE WALLS. BAKELITE RELIEFS PROVIDE A DEEPER, SHARPER RELIEF THAN A STANDARD UNDERCUT, AS WELL AS AN ANGULAR BACKDRAFT THAT HELPS KEEP DIE WALLS CLEAN.

DWG. NO. TSM—N12

© American Pharmaceutical Association

FIGURE 13. SPECIAL PUNCH BARREL OPTIONS

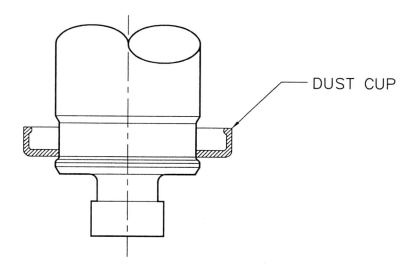

DUST CUP

EUROPEAN DUST CUP RELIEF
(SEAL GROOVE)

A REUSABLE AND INTERCHANGEABLE DUST CUP, WHICH FITS IN A SPECIAL GROOVE MACHINED IN UPPER PUNCH BARRELS, CAN BE SUPPLIED. THIS DUST CUP HAS A CIRCULAR HOLE SIZED TO MATCH THE GROOVE DIAMETER, THUS ELIMINATING THE NEED TO PUNCH HOLES IN THE DUST CUPS.

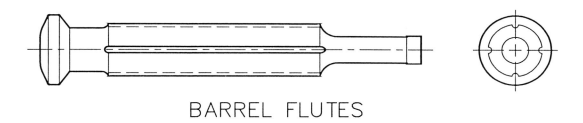

BARREL FLUTES

UPPER AND LOWER PUNCHES WITH RADIUSED GROOVES ON THE BARREL CAN BE SUPPLIED. THE GROOVES AID IN KEEPING THE PUNCH GUIDEWAYS CLEAN. LOWER PUNCH RESTRAINING PLUGS CANNOT BE USED WITH FLUTED LOWER PUNCHES.

DWG. NO.	TSM—N13

© American Pharmaceutical Association

FIGURE 14. STANDARD .945 DIE
(.945" [24.0 mm] DIAMETER)

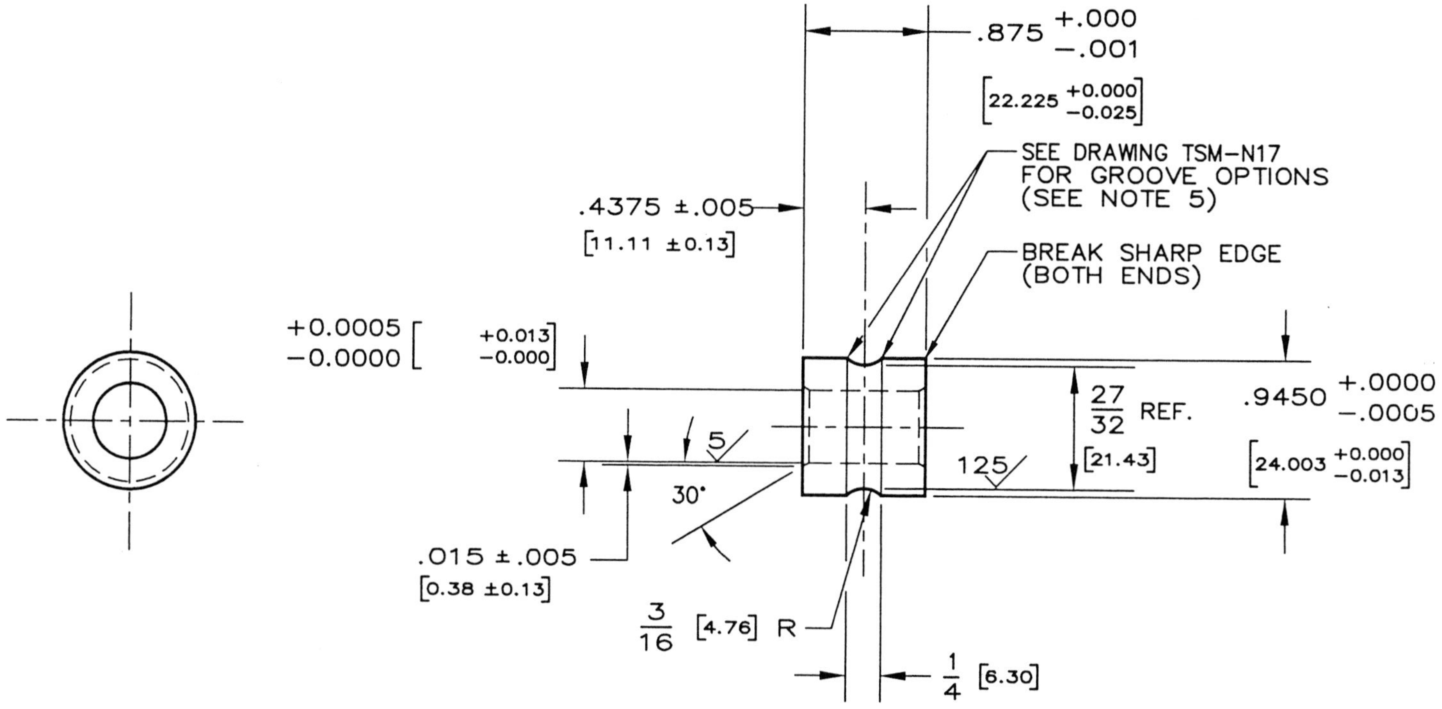

.875 +.000 −.001
[22.225 +0.000 −0.025]

SEE DRAWING TSM–N17
FOR GROOVE OPTIONS
(SEE NOTE 5)

BREAK SHARP EDGE
(BOTH ENDS)

.9450 +.0000 −.0005
[24.003 +0.000 −0.013]

27/32 REF.
[21.43]

125/

1/4 [6.30]

.4375 ±.005
[11.11 ±0.13]

5/

30°

3/16 [4.76] R

+0.0005 [+0.013 −0.0000 [−0.000]

.015 ±.005
[0.38 ±0.13]

TOLERANCES
(UNLESS OTHERWISE INDICATED)

FRACTIONAL	±.015	[.381]
DECIMAL	±.003	[.076]
ANGULAR	±0–30'	
CONCENTRICITY T.I.R.=		
BORE TO O.D.	.001	[.025]

DWG. NO. TSM–N14

NOTES:

1. WITH THE EXCEPTION OF SURFACE FINISHES, DIMENSIONS ARE GIVEN
   FIRST IN INCHES, FOLLOWED BY THE EQUIVALENT MILLIMETERS IN
   BRACKETS.
2. UNLESS OTHERWISE INDICATED, SURFACE FINISHES ARE 20 MICROINCH
   [.508 MICRON] ALL OVER. THE TOLERANCE ON ALL FINISHES IS ±5 MICRO–
   INCH [± .127 MICRON].
3. DIE FACES SHOULD BE SQUARE WITH O.D. WITHIN .001 [.025] T.I.R.
4. BARREL–SHAPED BORES ARE NOT RECOMMENDED.
5. DIE GROOVE OPTIONS ARE DESIGNED TO REDUCE THE OCCURRENCE
   OF BURRS LEFT BY RETAINING SCREWS.
6. A REFERENCE DIMENSION IS USUALLY UNTOLERANCED. IT IS CONSIDERED AUXILIARY
   INFORMATION AND DOES NOT GOVERN PRODUCTION OR INSPECTION OPERATIONS.

© American Pharmaceutical Association

FIGURE 15. STANDARD 1 3/16 DIE
(1.1875" [30.162 mm] DIAMETER)

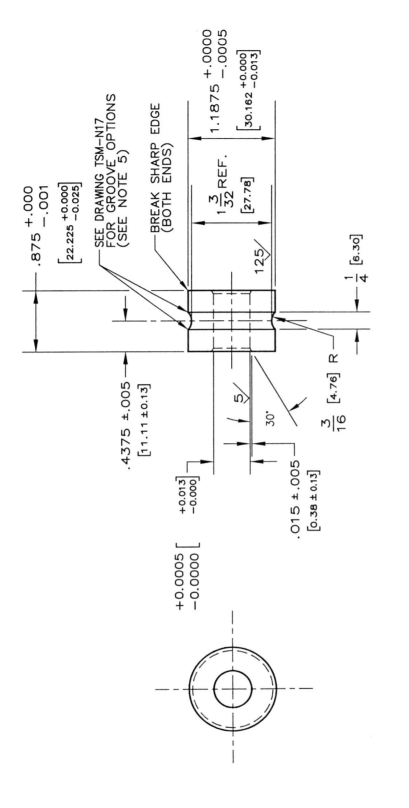

TOLERANCES (UNLESS OTHERWISE INDICATED)		
FRACTIONAL	±.015	[.381]
DECIMAL	±.003	[.076]
ANGULAR	±0'-30'	
CONCENTRICITY T.I.R.=		
BORE TO O.D.	.001	[.025]

DWG. NO. TSM–N15

NOTES:

1. WITH THE EXCEPTION OF SURFACE FINISHES, DIMENSIONS ARE GIVEN FIRST IN INCHES, FOLLOWED BY THE EQUIVALENT MILLIMETERS IN BRACKETS.

2. UNLESS OTHERWISE INDICATED, SURFACE FINISHES ARE 20 MICROINCH [.508 MICRON] ALL OVER. THE TOLERANCE ON ALL FINISHES IS ±5 MICRO–INCH [±.127 MICRON].

3. DIE FACES SHOULD BE SQUARE WITH O.D. WITHIN .001 [.025] T.I.R.

4. BARREL–SHAPED BORES ARE NOT RECOMMENDED.

5. DIE GROOVE OPTIONS ARE DESIGNED TO REDUCE THE OCCURRENCE OF BURRS LEFT BY RETAINING SCREWS.

6. A REFERENCE DIMENSION IS USUALLY UNTOLERANCED. IT IS CONSIDERED AUXILIARY INFORMATION AND DOES NOT GOVERN PRODUCTION OR INSPECTION OPERATIONS.

© American Pharmaceutical Association

29

FIGURE 16. STANDARD "D" DIE
(1.500" [38.1 mm] DIAMETER)

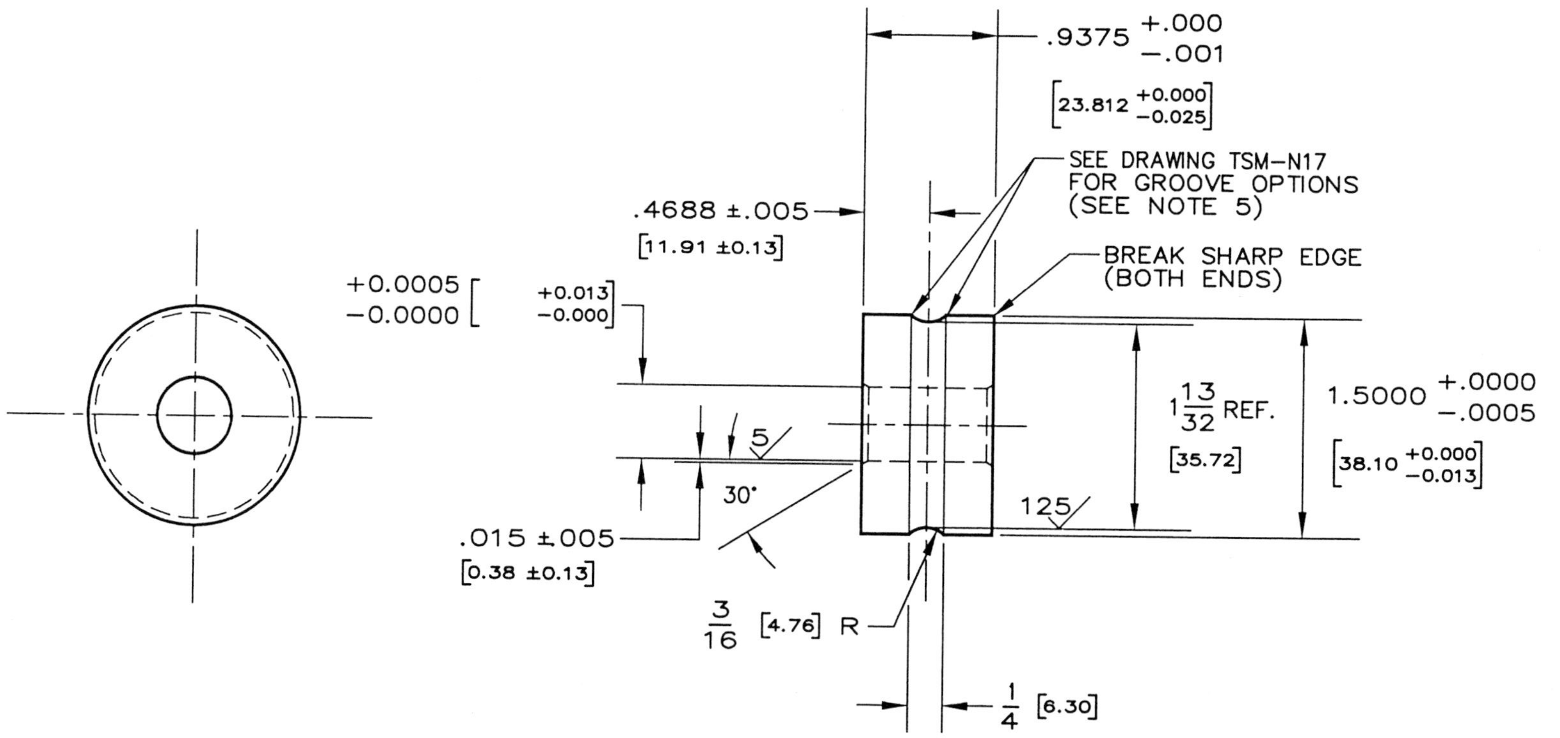

.9375 +.000 −.001 [23.812 +0.000 −0.025]

1.5000 +.0000 −.0005 [38.10 +0.000 −0.013]

1 13/32 REF. [35.72]

SEE DRAWING TSM−N17 FOR GROOVE OPTIONS (SEE NOTE 5)

BREAK SHARP EDGE (BOTH ENDS)

125

1/4 [6.30]

.4688 ±.005 [11.91 ±0.13]

+0.0005 −0.0000 [+0.013 −0.000]

.015 ±.005 [0.38 ±0.13]

5

30°

3/16 [4.76] R

TOLERANCES
(UNLESS OTHERWISE INDICATED)

FRACTIONAL	±.015	[.381]
DECIMAL	±.003	[.076]
ANGULAR	±0−30'	
CONCENTRICITY T.I.R.=		
BORE TO O.D.	.001	[.025]

DWG. NO.   TSM−N16

NOTES:

1. WITH THE EXCEPTION OF SURFACE FINISHES, DIMENSIONS ARE GIVEN FIRST IN INCHES, FOLLOWED BY THE EQUIVALENT MILLIMETERS IN BRACKETS.

2. UNLESS OTHERWISE INDICATED, SURFACE FINISHES ARE 20 MICROINCH [.508 MICRON] ALL OVER. THE TOLERANCE ON ALL FINISHES IS ±5 MICRO−INCH [±.127 MICRON].

3. DIE FACES SHOULD BE SQUARE WITH O.D. WITHIN .001 [.025] T.I.R.

4. BARREL−SHAPED BORES ARE NOT RECOMMENDED.

5. DIE GROOVE OPTIONS ARE DESIGNED TO REDUCE THE OCCURRENCE OF BURRS LEFT BY RETAINING SCREWS.

6. A REFERENCE DIMENSION IS USUALLY UNTOLERANCED. IT IS CONSIDERED AUXILIARY INFORMATION AND DOES NOT GOVERN PRODUCTION OR INSPECTION OPERATIONS.

© American Pharmaceutical Association

FIGURE 17. TAPERED DIES AND DIE GROOVE RELIEFS

(SPECIAL DIE OPTIONS)

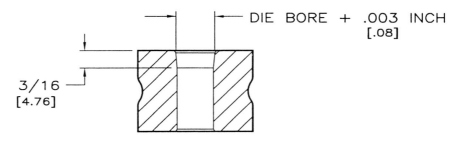

DIE BORE + .003 INCH
[.08]

3/16
[4.76]

TAPERED DIES

DIES WITH A TAPERED BORE ON ONE OR BOTH ENDS CAN BE SUPPLIED.
TAPERED BORES REDUCE THE FORCE WITH WHICH TABLETS ARE EJECTED. THEY
CAN ALSO PROVIDE A GRADUAL RELEASE OF INTERNAL STRESSES THAT CAN
CAUSE CAPPING OF TABLETS.

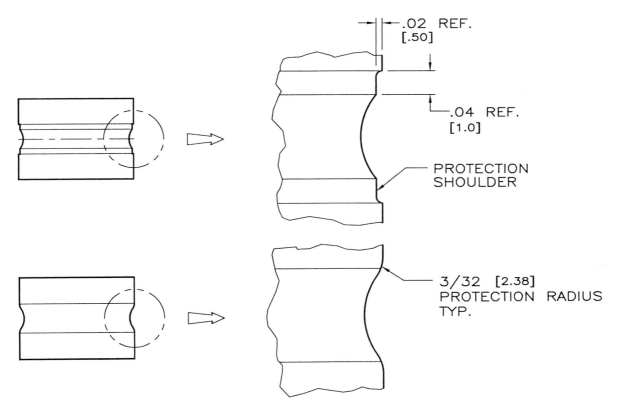

.02 REF.
[.50]

.04 REF.
[1.0]

PROTECTION
SHOULDER

3/32 [2.38]
PROTECTION RADIUS
TYP.

DIE GROOVE RELIEFS

PROTECTION SHOULDERS OR RADII CAN BE ADDED TO DIE GROOVES TO
PREVENT SCORING OF DIE POCKETS CAUSED BY BURRS OR SHARP EDGES ON
THE DIE O.D.

DWG. NO. TSM—N17

© American Pharmaceutical Association

FIGURE 18. LINED DIES
(SPECIAL DIE OPTIONS)

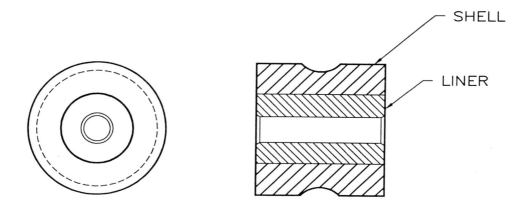

LINED DIES

LINED DIES, COMMONLY CALLED INSERT DIES, ARE USED PRIMARILY TO
COMPRESS ABRASIVE AND/OR CORROSIVE MATERIALS. ALTHOUGH LINED DIES
COST MORE, THEIR LONGER WORKING LIFE IS USUALLY WELL WORTH THE
ADDED COST.

LINED DIES CONSIST OF AN OUTER SHELL AND A LINER. THE MOST COMMON
LINING MATERIALS ARE TUNGSTEN CARBIDE AND INDUSTRIAL CERAMICS SUCH
AS ALUMINA AND PARTIALLY STABILIZED ZIRCONIA (PSZ).

THE OUTER SHELL PROTECTS THE HARDER, MORE BRITTLE LINER FROM
POSSIBLE FAILURE RELATED TO PRESSURE FROM THE DIE-LOCKING SCREW.

INSERT DIES MAY ALSO BE USED IN SITUATIONS WHERE DIE CRACKING
RESULTS FROM POINTED TABLET SHAPES. BECAUSE THE SHELL IS A HEAT-
SHRINK FIT OVER THE LINER, THE LINER IS PRESTRESSED IN COMPRESSION.
THIS PRECOMPRESSIVE STATE REDUCES THE LIKELIHOOD OF THE DIE
CRACKING DURING TABLET PRODUCTION.

DWG. NO. TSM-N18

© American Pharmaceutical Association

FIGURE 19. PUNCH AND DIE CLEARANCES

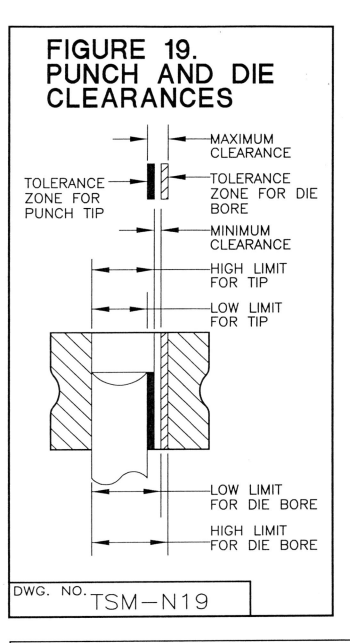

- MAXIMUM CLEARANCE
- TOLERANCE ZONE FOR PUNCH TIP
- TOLERANCE ZONE FOR DIE BORE
- MINIMUM CLEARANCE
- HIGH LIMIT FOR TIP
- LOW LIMIT FOR TIP
- LOW LIMIT FOR DIE BORE
- HIGH LIMIT FOR DIE BORE

DWG. NO. TSM—N19

Shaped Punch Tip Clearances

The TSM Committee developed the following standard clearances for upper and lower punch tips of shaped tooling.

Shaped Upper Punch Tip Clearance

A nominal clearance of .0017 inch [.043 millimeter] is recommended for all sizes of upper punch tips on shaped tooling.

Allowing for the die bore tolerance of +.0005 inch [+.013 millimeter] and the shaped punch tip tolerance of –.0008 inch [–.020 millimeter] gives a maximum possible clearance of .0030 inch [.076 millimeter] for shaped upper punch tips. Therefore, the clearance range for upper punch tips is .0017/.0030 inch [.043/.076 millimeter].

Shaped Lower Punch Tip Clearance

A nominal clearance of .0012 inch [.030 millimeter] is recommended for all sizes of lower punch tips on shaped tooling.

Again, allowing for the die bore tolerance of +.0005 inch [+.013 millimeter] and the shaped punch tip tolerance of –.0008 inch [–.020 millimeter] gives a maximum possible clearance of .0025 inch [.064 millimeter] for shaped lower punch tips. Therefore, the clearance range for lower punch tips is .0012/.0025 inch [.030/.064 millimeter].

TABLE 1. MAXIMUM TABLET SIZES FOR STANDARD DIES

DIE SIZE (O.D.)	DIE GROOVE DIAMETER	MAXIMUM TABLET SIZE	
		ROUND TABLETS	SHAPED TABLETS[1]
.945 [24.0]	.835 [21.43]	1/2 [13]	9/16 [14]
1.1875 [30.162]	1.077 [27.78]	5/8 [16]	3/4 [19]
1.500 [38.1]	1.390 [35.72]	1 [25]	1 [25]

1. POINTED TABLET SHAPES SHOULD HAVE A MINIMUM POINT RADIUS OF .04 [1]. (SEE THE DISCUSSION OF LINED DIES IN FIGURE 18.)

2. THE PRESS MANUFACTURER'S RECOMMENDED TORQUE SETTING FOR TIGHTENING DIE LOCK SCREWS SHOULD ALWAYS BE USED.

© American Pharmaceutical Association

TABLE 2. STANDARD CLEARANCES FOR NORMAL APPLICATION OF ROUND TOOLING

NOMINAL TOOL SIZE	UPPER PUNCH			ACTUAL PUNCH TIP DIAMETER[4]		LOWER PUNCH		
	STANDARD CLEARANCE	MINIMUM CLEARANCE	MAXIMUM[3] CLEARANCE	UPPER	LOWER	STANDARD CLEARANCE	MINIMUM CLEARANCE	MAXIMUM[3] CLEARANCE
1/8 [3.175]	.0015 [.038]	.0015 [.038]	.0025 [.064]	.1235 [3.137]	.1240 [3.150]	.0010 [.025]	.0010 [.025]	.0020 [.051]
5/32 [3.970]	.0015 [.038]	.0015 [.038]	.0025 [.064]	.1548 [3.932]	.1553 [3.945]	.0010 [.025]	.0010 [.025]	.0020 [.051]
3/16 [4.763]	.0015 [.038]	.0015 [.038]	.0025 [.064]	.1860 [4.724]	.1865 [4.737]	.0010 [.025]	.0010 [.025]	.0020 [.051]
7/32 [5.555]	.0016 [.041]	.0016 [.041]	.0026 [.066]	.2171 [5.514]	.2177 [5.530]	.0010 [.025]	.0010 [.025]	.0020 [.051]
1/4 [6.350]	.0016 [.041]	.0016 [.041]	.0026 [.066]	.2484 [6.309]	.2489 [6.322]	.0011 [.028]	.0011 [.028]	.0021 [.053]
9/32 [7.142]	.0017 [.043]	.0017 [.043]	.0027 [.069]	.2795 [7.099]	.2801 [7.115]	.0011 [.028]	.0011 [.028]	.0021 [.053]
5/16 [7.938]	.0017 [.043]	.0017 [.043]	.0027 [.069]	.3108 [7.894]	.3114 [7.910]	.0011 [.028]	.0011 [.028]	.0021 [.053]
11/32 [8.730]	.0018 [.046]	.0018 [.046]	.0028 [.071]	.3419 [8.684]	.3425 [8.700]	.0012 [.031]	.0012 [.031]	.0022 [.056]
3/8 [9.525]	.0018 [.046]	.0018 [.046]	.0028 [.071]	.3732 [9.479]	.3738 [9.495]	.0012 [.031]	.0012 [.031]	.0022 [.056]
13/32 [10.318]	.0019 [.048]	.0019 [.048]	.0029 [.074]	.4043 [10.269]	.4050 [10.287]	.0012 [.031]	.0012 [.031]	.0022 [.056]
7/16 [11.113]	.0019 [.048]	.0019 [.048]	.0029 [.074]	.4356 [11.064]	.4362 [11.080]	.0013 [.033]	.0013 [.033]	.0023 [.058]
15/32 [11.905]	.0020 [.051]	.0020 [.051]	.0030 [.076]	.4667 [11.854]	.4674 [11.872]	.0013 [.033]	.0013 [.033]	.0023 [.058]
1/2 [12.700]	.0020 [.051]	.0020 [.051]	.0030 [.076]	.4980 [12.649]	.4987 [12.667]	.0013 [.033]	.0013 [.033]	.0023 [.058]
17/32 [13.493]	.0021 [.053]	.0021 [.053]	.0031 [.079]	.5291 [13.439]	.5298 [13.457]	.0014 [.036]	.0014 [.036]	.0024 [.061]
9/16 [14.288]	.0022 [.056]	.0022 [.056]	.0032 [.081]	.5603 [14.232]	.5611 [14.252]	.0014 [.036]	.0014 [.036]	.0024 [.061]

NOTES:

1. DIMENSIONS ARE GIVEN FIRST IN INCHES, FOLLOWED BY THE EQUIVALENT MILLIMETERS IN BRACKETS.
2. DUE TO METRIC CONVERSIONS, A DISCREPANCY OF .00004 [.001] OCCURS FOR SOME DIMENSIONS.
3. MAXIMUM CLEARANCE OCCURS AT MAXIMUM DIE SIZE AND MINIMUM PUNCH TIP DIAMETER.
4. THE TOLERANCE FOR ROUND PUNCH TIPS IS + .0000, − .0005.

© American Pharmaceutical Association

TABLE 2. STANDARD CLEARANCES FOR NORMAL APPLICATION OF ROUND TOOLING (CONT.)

NOMINAL TOOL SIZE	UPPER PUNCH			ACTUAL PUNCH TIP DIAMETER[4]		LOWER PUNCH		
	STANDARD CLEARANCE	MINIMUM CLEARANCE	MAXIMUM[3] CLEARANCE	UPPER	LOWER	STANDARD CLEARANCE	MINIMUM CLEARANCE	MAXIMUM[3] CLEARANCE
19/32 [15.080]	.0023 [.058]	.0023 [.058]	.0033 [.084]	.5914 [15.022]	.5923 [15.044]	.0014 [.036]	.0014 [.036]	.0024 [.061]
5/8 [15.875]	.0024 [.061]	.0024 [.061]	.0034 [.086]	.6226 [15.814]	.6235 [15.837]	.0015 [.038]	.0015 [.038]	.0025 [.064]
21/32 [16.668]	.0025 [.064]	.0025 [.064]	.0035 [.089]	.6537 [16.604]	.6542 [16.617]	.0020 [.051]	.0020 [.051]	.0030 [.076]
11/16 [17.463]	.0025 [.064]	.0025 [.064]	.0035 [.089]	.6850 [17.399]	.6855 [17.412]	.0020 [.051]	.0020 [.051]	.0030 [.076]
23/32 [18.255]	.0025 [.064]	.0025 [.064]	.0035 [.089]	.7162 [18.192]	.7167 [18.204]	.0020 [.051]	.0020 [.051]	.0030 [.076]
3/4 [19.050]	.0025 [.064]	.0025 [.064]	.0035 [.089]	.7475 [18.987]	.7480 [18.999]	.0020 [.051]	.0020 [.051]	.0030 [.076]
25/32 [19.843]	.0025 [.064]	.0025 [.064]	.0035 [.089]	.7787 [19.779]	.7792 19.792]	.0020 [.051]	.0020 [.051]	.0030 [.076]
13/16 [20.638]	.0025 [.064]	.0025 [.064]	.0035 [.089]	.8100 [20.574]	.8105 [20.587]	.0020 [.051]	.0020 [.051]	.0030 [.076]
27/32 [21.430]	.0025 [.064]	.0025 [.064]	.0035 [.089]	.8412 [21.367]	.8417 [21.379]	.0020 [.051]	.0020 [.051]	.0030 [.076]
7/8 [22.225]	.0025 [.064]	.0025 [.064]	.0035 [.089]	.8725 [22.162]	.8730 [22.174]	.0020 [.051]	.0020 [.051]	.0030 [.076]
29/32 [23.018]	.0025 [.064]	.0025 [.064]	.0035 [.089]	.9037 [22.954]	.9042 [22.967]	.0020 [.051]	.0020 [.051]	.0030 [.076]
15/16 [23.813]	.0025 [.064]	.0025 [.064]	.0035 [.089]	.9350 [23.749]	.9355 [23.762]	.0020 [.051]	.0020 [.051]	.0030 [.076]
31/32 [24.605]	.0025 [.064]	.0025 [.064]	.0035 [.089]	.9662 [24.542]	.9667 [24.554]	.0020 [.051]	.0020 [.051]	.0030 [.076]
1 [25.400]	.0025 [.064]	.0025 [.064]	.0035 [.089]	.9975 [25.337]	.9980 [25.349]	.0020 [.051]	.0020 [.051]	.0030 [.076]

NOTES:

1. DIMENSIONS ARE GIVEN FIRST IN INCHES, FOLLOWED BY THE EQUIVALENT MILLIMETERS IN BRACKETS.
2. DUE TO METRIC CONVERSIONS, A DISCREPANCY OF .00004 [.001] OCCURS FOR SOME DIMENSIONS.
3. MAXIMUM CLEARANCE OCCURS AT MAXIMUM DIE SIZE AND MINIMUM PUNCH TIP DIAMETER.
4. THE TOLERANCE FOR ROUND PUNCH TIPS IS + .0000, − .0005.

© American Pharmaceutical Association

FIGURE 20. COMMON CONFIGURATIONS AND DIMENSIONS FOR PUNCH KEYS

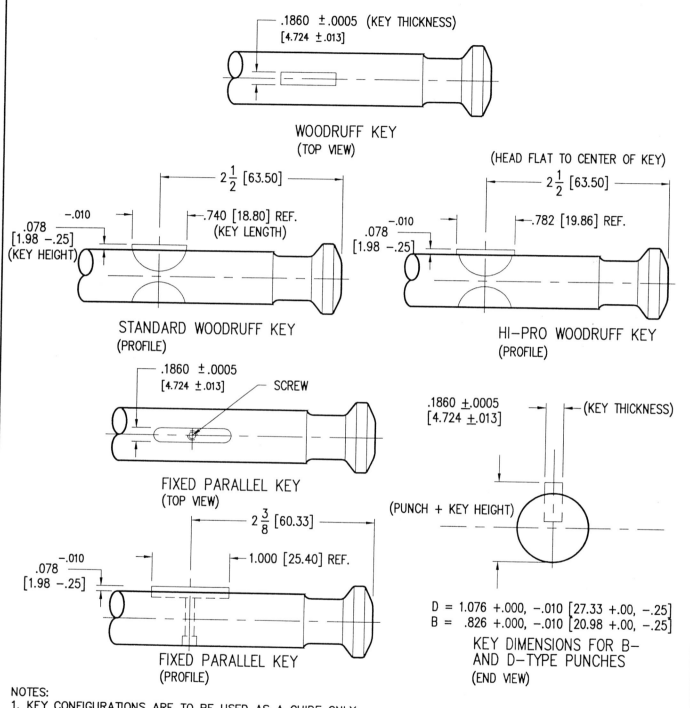

.1860 ±.0005 (KEY THICKNESS)
[4.724 ±.013]

WOODRUFF KEY
(TOP VIEW)

2 1/2 [63.50]

-.010
.078
[1.98 -.25]
(KEY HEIGHT)

.740 [18.80] REF.
(KEY LENGTH)

STANDARD WOODRUFF KEY
(PROFILE)

(HEAD FLAT TO CENTER OF KEY)

2 1/2 [63.50]

-.010
.078
[1.98 -.25]

.782 [19.86] REF.

HI-PRO WOODRUFF KEY
(PROFILE)

.1860 ±.0005
[4.724 ±.013]

SCREW

FIXED PARALLEL KEY
(TOP VIEW)

2 3/8 [60.33]

-.010
.078
[1.98 -.25]

1.000 [25.40] REF.

FIXED PARALLEL KEY
(PROFILE)

.1860 ±.0005
[4.724 ±.013]

(KEY THICKNESS)

(PUNCH + KEY HEIGHT)

D = 1.076 +.000, −.010 [27.33 +.00, −.25]
B = .826 +.000, −.010 [20.98 +.00, −.25]

KEY DIMENSIONS FOR B-
AND D-TYPE PUNCHES
(END VIEW)

NOTES:
1. KEY CONFIGURATIONS ARE TO BE USED AS A GUIDE ONLY.
2. THE DIMENSION FROM HEAD FLAT TO CENTER OF THE KEY APPLIES TO PRESSES THAT DO NOT REQUIRE UPPER PUNCH SEALS. TABLES 3A AND B LIST MAXIMUM KEY EXTENSIONS FOR PRESSES THAT REQUIRE UPPER SEALS.
3. THE FIXED PARALLEL KEY IS HELD IN PLACE BY A SCREW. ALL KEY TYPES CAN BE SUPPLIED WITH THIS FEATURE.

DWG. NO. TSM−N20

© American Pharmaceutical Association

TABLE 3A. AVAILABLE KEY SPACE AND MAXIMUM STEM LENGTHS
(FOR PRESSES WITH UPPER PUNCH SEALS)

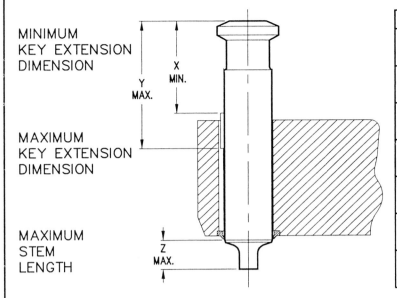

MINIMUM KEY EXTENSION DIMENSION

MAXIMUM KEY EXTENSION DIMENSION

MAXIMUM STEM LENGTH

PRESS TYPE	X MIN.	Y MAX.	Z MAX.
COURTOY	1.800 [45.720]	2.950 [74.930]	.730 [18.542]
HATA	1.712 [43.485]	2.890 [73.406]	.630 [16.002]
FETTE	1.654 [42.000]	2.677 [68.000]	.730 [18.542]
KIKUSUI	N/S	N/S	N/S
KILIAN	1.024 [26.099]	2.402 [61.011]	.730 [18.542]
KORSCH	1.693 [43.002]	2.637 [66.980]	.630 [16.002]
MANESTY	1.687 [42.849]	2.687 [68.250]	.630 [16.002]

1. THE MAXIMUM STEM LENGTH HAS BEEN ADJUSTED −.025 INCH TO ACCOMMODATE REWORKING OF HEAD FLATS DURING MAINTENANCE.
2. PRESSES THAT DO NOT REQUIRE UPPER SEALS ARE CADMACH, STOKES, AND VECTOR.
3. KEY PLACEMENT IS IMPORTANT IN PREVENTING DAMAGE TO SEALS AND CAMS.
4. N/S MEANS MANUFACTURER DID NOT SUPPLY DATA.

TABLE 3B. PUNCH KEY LENGTHS AND AVAILABLE KEY SPACE

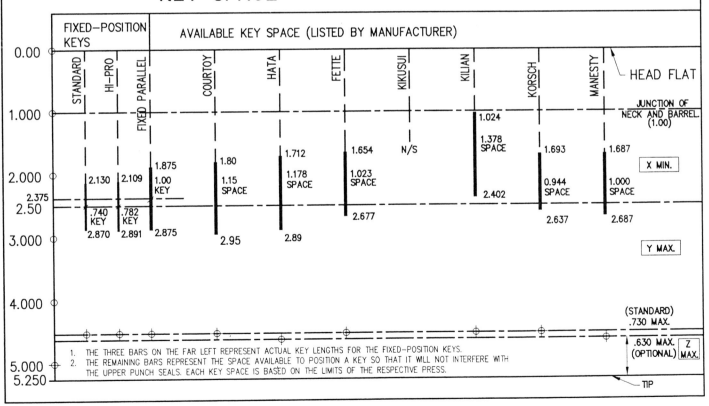

1. THE THREE BARS ON THE FAR LEFT REPRESENT ACTUAL KEY LENGTHS FOR THE FIXED–POSITION KEYS.
2. THE REMAINING BARS REPRESENT THE SPACE AVAILABLE TO POSITION A KEY SO THAT IT WILL NOT INTERFERE WITH THE UPPER PUNCH SEALS. EACH KEY SPACE IS BASED ON THE LIMITS OF THE RESPECTIVE PRESS.

© American Pharmaceutical Association

TABLE 4. INTERCHANGEABLE TOOLING FOR ROTARY TABLET PRESSES
(3/4" PUNCH BARREL AND .945" DIE)

	A	B	C	D	E	F	G	H
INCHES	5.250	.748	³2.500	35°	.945	,875	5.250	.745
MILLIMETERS	133.35	19.00	63.50	35°	24.003	22.225	133.35	18.92

CADMACH	HATA	KIKUSUI	KILIAN	KORSCH	RIVA
BBC−45	HTPAP45−MSU	GEMINI 867−67	T400−67	PH230−20	BB−2−35
BBC4−45	HT−AP65−DU	LIBRA 845−45	RX−67	PH250−30	HIDRO−35
K5500−55	HT−AP71−DU	LIBRA 849−49	T300−40	PH300−43	BB2G−35
K6100−61	HT−AP22−SSU	OCTANS 845−45	TX−40	PH800−77	PRECOM−35
	HT−X71−LDU	VIRGO 524−24	T200−32	REVOLUTION −65	
	HT−X65−LDU		T100−24		
			LX−32		
			RTS−36		

COURTOY	FETTE	MANESTY	STOKES	VECTOR (COLTON)
R1/2LABO−22	P−1000/33	B3B−23	BB−2−33 & 37	MEDALIST− 2400
R090−28	P−1200/30	BB3A/B−33,39 & 45	513−2 (45)	
R090M−28	P−2000/43	BETAPRESS 23	540−41	MAGNA−74
R100−36	P−2080/43	LAYERPRESS 47	551−1 (51)	233−33
R100M−36	P−3000/55	ROTO MI & MII 55	552−1 (51)	241−41
R190−36	P−21/35	ROTO MII 61	¹555−1 PACER	241a−41
R200−65	P−31/51	ROTO MIIA 61	¹560−1 VERSA	242−41
R200M−65	P−3100/55	ROTO MIII 69 & 75	564−1 (45)	243−41
R290−65	PT2100/43	EXPRESS 30	565−1 (65)	244−41
R292−65	PT2090/43	BB4 45	566−3 (45)	246−41
	PT3090/73	UNIPRESS 34	¹580−1 (45)	247−41
		NOVAPRESS 61	586−2 (51)	
		ROTO MIV 69 & 75	593−1 (65)	
		EXCELO 61	610−1 (GTP)	
		ELITE 450−61	¹454−1 (41)	
		ELITE 800−75	454−1−A	
			¹747−1 (65)	

1. THIS PRESS REQUIRES A NECKLESS PUNCH SHANK.
2. A KEY IS USUALLY NOT REQUIRED ON ROUND TOOLING.
3. STOKES PRESSES HAVE A "C" DIMENSION OF 2.750.
4. SOME PRESSES MAY REQUIRE SCREWED−IN FEATHER KEYS. CONTACT PRESS MANUFACTURER FOR RECOMMENDATIONS.
5. "C" AND "D" DIMENSIONS MAY NOT APPLY TO VECTOR (COLTON) PRESSES.
6. "B" AND "H" DIMENSIONS ARE ENGINEERED WITH THE TURRET BORE SIZE SET AT .7500 [19.50].

© American Pharmaceutical Association

TABLE 5. INTERCHANGEABLE TOOLING FOR ROTARY TABLET PRESSES
(3/4" PUNCH BARREL AND 1.1875" DIE)

	A	B	C	D	E	F	G	H
INCHES	5.250	.748	^{3}2.500	35°	1.1875	,875	5.250	.745
MILLIMETERS	133.35	19.00	63.50	35°	30.162	22.225	133.35	18.92

CADMACH	HATA	KIKUSUI		KILIAN	KORSCH	RIVA
BBC–27	HT–AP18–SSU	GEMINI 855–55		T400–55	PH100–3	BB–2–27
BBC–35	HT–AP38–MSU	LIBRA 836–36		RX–55	PH100–6	BB2–33
BBC4–35	HT–AP55–DU	VIRGO 519–19		T300–32	PH230–17	HIDRO–27
K4500–45	HT–X55–LDU	OCTANS 836–36		TX–32	PH250–25	HIDRO–33
DB–16	HT–X38–LDU	VIRGO 512–12		T200–23	PH300–36	
	HT–55–3LS			LX–23	PH800–65	
				T100–18	REVOLUTION –55	
				RTS–26		
				RL–15		

COURTOY	FETTE	MANESTY	STOKES	VECTOR (COLTON)
R1/2LABO–18	P–1000/28	B3A–16, B3B–16	BB–2 (27)	MEDALIST– 1800
R090–23	P–1200/24	BB3A/B 27 & 35	513–3 (35)	
R090M–23	P–2000/36	BETAPRESS 16	540–35	MAGNA–66
R100–30	P–3000/45	LAYERPRESS 39	540–1 (41)	227–27
R100M–30	P–21/30	ROTO MI, MII & MIIA–45	522–2 (41)	232–33
R190–30	P–2100/36		^{1}555–2 PACER	233A–33
R200–55	P–3100/45	ROTO MIII 55	^{1}560–2 VERSA	242–33
R200M–55	PT3090/61	EXPRESS 25	564–2 (35)	24 –43
R290–55	PT2090/36	BB4–27 & 35	565–2 (53)	243–33
R292–55	PT2080/36	UNIPRESS 27	566–2 (27)	242–43
		NOVAPRESS 45	566–102 (35)	244–33
		ROTO MIV 55	^{1}580–2 (35)	247–33
		B4–16 & 25	585–1 (41)	280–65
		EXCELOPRESS 45	593–2 (53)	2216
		ELITE 450–45	690–2 (53)	2247–33
		ELITE 800–55	^{1}454–2 (35)	1800
			^{1}747–2 (53)	246–33
			454–2–A	
			610–2 GTP	

5. "C" AND "D" DIMENSIONS MAY NOT APPLY TO VECTOR (COLTON) PRESSES.
6. "B" AND "H" DIMENSIONS ARE ENGINEERED WITH THE TURRET BORE SIZE SET AT .7500 [19.50].

1. THIS PRESS REQUIRES A NECKLESS PUNCH SHANK.
2. A KEY IS USUALLY NOT REQUIRED ON ROUND TOOLING.
3. STOKES PRESSES HAVE A "C" DIMENSION OF 2.750.
4. SOME PRESSES MAY REQUIRE SCREWED–IN FEATHER KEYS. CONTACT PRESS MANUFACTURER FOR RECOMMENDATIONS.

TABLE 7. INTERCHANGEABLE TOOLING FOR SPECIAL ROTARY TABLET PRESSES (CONT.)

| PRESS MODELS | | | | | | | | | | | |
KILIAN	MANESTY	STOKES	VECTOR (COLTON)	A	B	C	D	E	F	G	H
		DD-2(31)		6.812	0.998	3.000	35°	1.500	1.250	8.812	0.995
		[3]328-4		6.062	1.123	3.000	35°	1.312	1.500	6.250	1.120
		[3]533-45									
		[3]533-4(45)									
		[3]328-125		6.062	1.248	3.000	35°	1.625	1.500	6.250	1.245
		[3]533-124(33)									
		[3]515-3		5.125	1.248	2.750	35°	2.000	1.687	5.375	1.245
	D3B-23			5.250	0.998	2.750	35°	1.1875	0.9375	5.250	0.995
	[7]Drycota 700&900			5.260	0.998	2.125	45°CW	1.1875	0.9375	5.260	0.995
	[7]Bicota 900-23			5.260	0.998	2.125	45°CW	1.1875	0.9375	5.260	0.995
		550-2		5.250	0.998	2.750	35°	1.500	0.9375	5.250	0.995
	Deltapress 23			5.250	0.998	*	35°	1.1875	0.875	5.250	0.995
Prescoter				5.9055	1.2598	3.7795	35°	1.3780	0.9921	6.1811	0.9843
IV											
RU-ZS											
RU-ZS-H											
RU-3S			280-53	5.250	0.9980	*	*	1.500	0.875	5.250	0.9960

1. UNLESS OTHERWISE INDICATED, DIMENSIONS ARE GIVEN IN INCHES.
2. THIS PRESS REQUIRES A DIE WITH A PROTECTIVE SHOULDER.
3. THIS PRESS REQUIRES A NECKLESS PUNCH SHANK
4. A KEY IS USUALLY NOT REQUIRED ON ROUND TOOLING.
5. SOME PRESSES MAY REQUIRE SCREWED-IN FEATHER KEYS. CONTACT PRESS MANUFACTURER FOR RECOMMENDATIONS.
6. "C" AND "D" DIMENSIONS MAY NOT APPLY TO VECTOR (COLTON) PRESSES.
7. THIS PRESS USES EUROPEAN TOOLING.
* INFORMATION NOT SUPPLIED BY MANUFACTURER.

© American Pharmaceutical Association

FIGURE 21. COMPARISON OF TSM AND INTERNATIONAL B-TYPE TOOLING

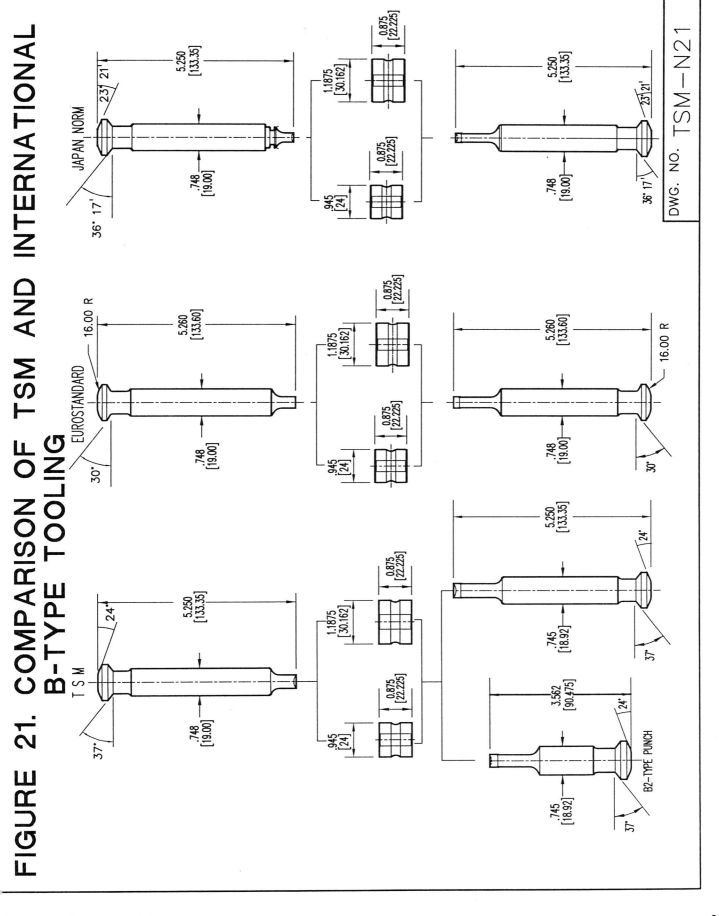

Notes:

© American Pharmaceutical Association

Tablet Design

oducing a tablet that has a unique shape and/or tablet ce design can significantly enhance a product's recogtion. The "uniqueness" of any design is limited by the mpression force required to produce the tablet, the rmulation's characteristics, the design's impact on oling performance, and the tablet's ability to withand packaging and shipping processes. Although blet shape is not the only factor to consider in the esign of a new tablet, the choice of geometric configuation can affect the output of the tablet press and, with me sharp-angled tablet configurations, possibly cause mages to the punches, dies, and cams. Some other fects of poor tablet design include the following:

- Product becomes contaminated with metal from broken punch tips.
- Broken punch tips produce deformed tablets, which could be rejected by Quality Control.
- Costly reworking of tablets occurs (tablets are ground up and reprocessed).
- Higher quantities of broken tablets are present in waste output of sorter (tablets are not reprocessed). Filled bottles contain broken tablets, which could be rejected by Quality Control or, if distributed, diminish corporate image.
- Labor costs are increased, which could result in higher prices to users and affect the product's competitive position in the marketplace.
- Time is lost in distributing the product, which could delay introducing a new product or cause a purchaser to run out of an existing product.
- Some shaped tablets break easily when fed through the printer, sorter, and/or tablet filler.

ablet Terminology

he basic construction of a round or shaped tablet is the me; therefore, many of the terms used in describing blets apply to both tablet categories. Definitions for eneral terminology are presented first, followed by the rms specific to round or shaped tablets.

General Terminology

Figures 22 and 23 on pages 46 and 47 illustrate the general terminology as it pertains to round and shaped tablets, respectively.

Tablet Face: The area within the tablet's periphery.

Band: The area between the opposing cup profiles. The die wall forms the tablet band.

Cup: The depression, or concavity, at the end of a punch tip.

Cup Depth: The distance from the tablet's band to the highest point, or apex, of the cup's radius, or three-dimensional contour.

Cup Radius: A single arc generated from the tablet's centerline (midpoint) across the tablet's diameter, minor axis, or major axis. The cup radius forms the cup's profile. Round convex tablets usually have a single cup radius.

Compound Cup: A cup design in which multiple radii (arcs) are generated from the tablet's centerline across the tablet's diameter, minor axis, or major axis. This configuration, which increases the cup volume by maintaining a required cup depth and reducing the band thickness, is used for round and shaped tablets (see Figure 22, Illus. B; and Figure 23, Illus. C.)

Land: A narrow plane perpendicular to the tablet's band, which creates a junction between the band and the cup radius.

Tablet Thickness: The combined height of the two cups and the band determines the total thickness of a tablet.

Tablet Identification: Any logo, product or company name, identification code, or three-dimensional character contours applied to a tablet's face by means of debossing or embossing. (See the discussion of "Tablet Identification" on pages 50–59 for more information.)

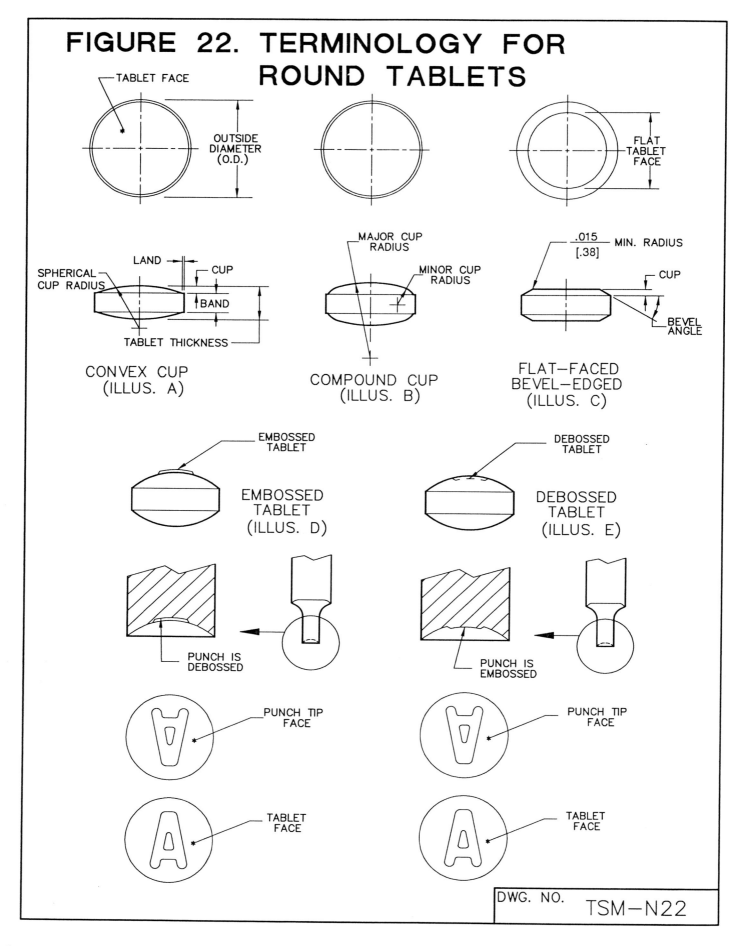

FIGURE 22. TERMINOLOGY FOR ROUND TABLETS

TABLET FACE

OUTSIDE DIAMETER (O.D.)

FLAT TABLET FACE

LAND
CUP
SPHERICAL CUP RADIUS
BAND
TABLET THICKNESS

CONVEX CUP (ILLUS. A)

MAJOR CUP RADIUS
MINOR CUP RADIUS

COMPOUND CUP (ILLUS. B)

.015 [.38] MIN. RADIUS
CUP
BEVEL ANGLE

FLAT-FACED BEVEL-EDGED (ILLUS. C)

EMBOSSED TABLET

EMBOSSED TABLET (ILLUS. D)

DEBOSSED TABLET

DEBOSSED TABLET (ILLUS. E)

PUNCH IS DEBOSSED

PUNCH IS EMBOSSED

PUNCH TIP FACE

PUNCH TIP FACE

TABLET FACE

TABLET FACE

DWG. NO. TSM-N22

© American Pharmaceutical Association

FIGURE 23. TERMINOLOGY FOR SHAPED TABLETS

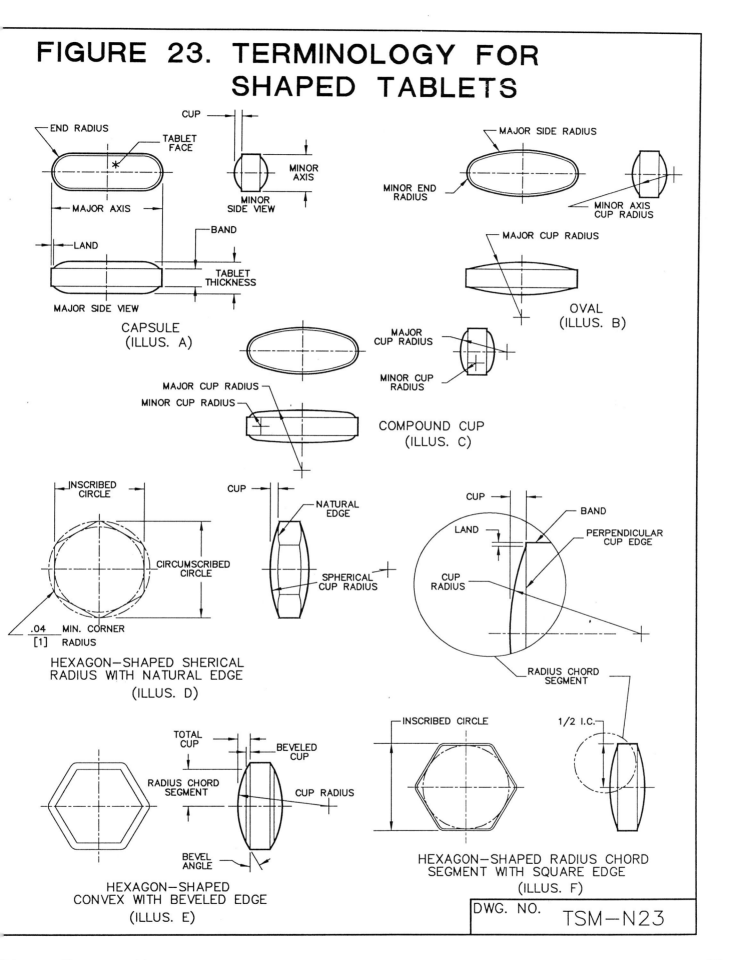

CAPSULE
(ILLUS. A)

OVAL
(ILLUS. B)

COMPOUND CUP
(ILLUS. C)

HEXAGON–SHAPED SHERICAL
RADIUS WITH NATURAL EDGE
(ILLUS. D)

HEXAGON–SHAPED
CONVEX WITH BEVELED EDGE
(ILLUS. E)

HEXAGON–SHAPED RADIUS CHORD
SEGMENT WITH SQUARE EDGE
(ILLUS. F)

DWG. NO. TSM–N23

© American Pharmaceutical Association

Debossed: A tablet identification that is depressed in the tablet's surface, forming a groove or indented pocket. The resultant groove creates a shadowed pocket on the tablet's surface, thus enhancing the tablet identification. The punch tip face that produces a debossed tablet is shown in Figure 22, Illus. D.

Embossed: The protrusion of a tablet identification above the tablet's surface. Due to its exposure above the tablet surface, an embossed identification is susceptible to abrasion and chipping. However, if the embossing is not raised sufficiently above the surface, the identification will lack clarity. The type of punch tip face that produces an embossed tablet is shown in Figure 22, Illus. E.

Tablet Printing: An optional method of applying an identification, in which the identification is mechanically printed on the tablet's surface with a liquid ink. (See the discussion of "Tablet Printing" on pages 59 and 64 for more information.)

Round Tablet Terminology

Outside Diameter (O.D.) with a Spherical Cup Radius: The length of a line segment passing from the centerline to any point on the tablet's periphery. A spherical cup design is merely a chord segment of a spherical ball (see Figure 22, Illus. A).

Flat-Faced Bevel-Edged (F.F.B.E.) Tablet: A tablet configuration consisting of a cup, an *angle* between the cup and tablet face, and, if required, a land. A 30° bevel is preferred to maximize the strength of punch edges. When the bevel is first applied, its contact area with the tablet face is a sharp beveled edge. If the sharp edge remains, a punch tip will fracture at this point. A minimum .015-inch [.38-millimeter] radius is recommended to remove the sharp edge (see Figure 22, Illus. C).

Flat-Faced Radius-Edged (F.F.R.E.) Tablet: A tablet configuration similar to F.F.B.E. consisting of a cup, a *radius* between the cup and tablet face, and, if required, a land. To ensure the strength of punch edges, the radius from the tablet's periphery or land should not exceed the comparable 30° bevel used for the F.F.B.E. design. This limitation on the radius will reduce the flat area on the tablet's face, limiting the surface area available for an identification.

Figure 24 shows the profiles of convex and F.F.B.E. tablets. Although tablets are often referred to as being a shallow concave, standard concave, deep concave, etc., the term *concave* better describes the shape of a punch face. Tablets produced with these punches usually have a *convex* surface.

Shaped Tablet Terminology

Figure 23 provides supporting illustrations for the following terms.

Major Axis: Length of a shaped tablet.

Minor Axis: Width of a shaped tablet.

End Radius: The radius located at either end of a capsule-shaped tablet.

Oval: Although an oval may resemble an elliptical shape, it is formed using only two radii: the major side radius and the minor end radius.

Minor Axis Cup Radius: A single arc generated from the tablet's centerline across the tablet's minor axis. This radius forms the minor axis cup profile.

Major Axis Cup Radius: A single arc generated from the tablet's centerline across the tablet's major axis. This radius forms the major axis cup profile.

> **NOTE:** Geometrically shaped tablets such as triangles, pentagons, octagons, and hexagons have circumscribed and inscribed circles, which determine the tablet's size and configuration.

Circumscribed Circle: The smallest circle that can be drawn around a geometric shape so that it intersects each corner of the inner figure. A circumscribed circle restricts the external boundaries of a given tablet shape.

Inscribed Circle: The largest circle that can be drawn inside a geometric shape so that their boundaries touch at as many points as possible. An inscribed circle restricts the internal boundaries of a given tablet shape.

© American Pharmaceutical Association

FIGURE 24. PROFILES OF CONVEX AND F.F.B.E. TABLETS

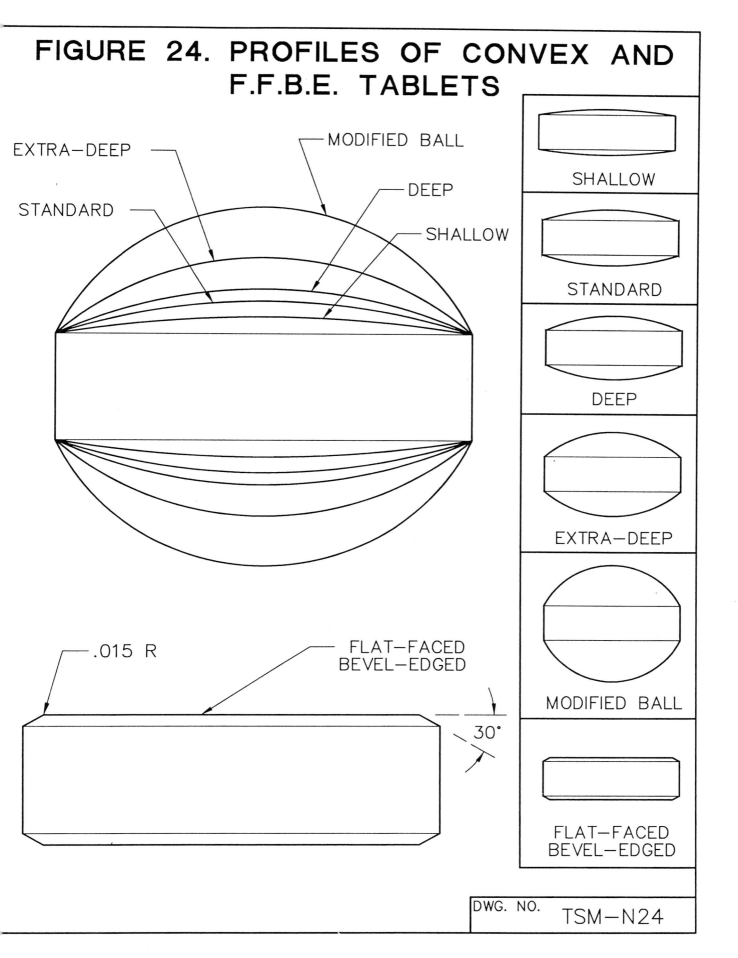

EXTRA—DEEP

STANDARD

MODIFIED BALL

DEEP

SHALLOW

.015 R

FLAT—FACED BEVEL—EDGED

30°

SHALLOW

STANDARD

DEEP

EXTRA—DEEP

MODIFIED BALL

FLAT—FACED BEVEL—EDGED

DWG. NO. TSM—N24

© American Pharmaceutical Association

Corner Radius: The curvature used to eliminate sharp corners on peripheral surfaces where two lines or curves meet. A minimum recommended corner radius is .04 inch [1 millimeter]. (See Figure 23, Illus. D.)

Figure 25 shows the shapes most commonly used in tablet designs.

Tablet Identification

The Food and Drug Administration (FDA) has ruled that all human drug products in solid oral dosage form must bear a code (imprinted or otherwise applied) that identifies the drug product and the holder of the product's approved application for marketing. The manufacturers of pharmaceutical, nonprescription, biological, and homeopathic drugs who are not now in full compliance with this ruling will have until September 13, 1995, to meet all FDA requirements. (For the complete ruling, see the *Federal Register*. Sep. 1993; 58 (175): 47948.)

Before an identification (code) is applied to a tablet's face, the tablet's form (i.e., its geometric shape, contour, and identification) must first be transferred to the punch tip's face. Using the information on a tablet detail drawing, a toolmaker produces a metal fixture called a hob, one end of which contains a reproduction of the tablet detail dimensions. By means of a hydraulic press, the hob is pushed into the soft steel of the punch tip, thereby leaving a duplicate, opposing impression of the tablet's form. Many restrictions on tablet identifications are due to the constraints related to manufacturing a hob.

To deboss or transfer the tablet identification into the hob's surface, the toolmaker uses a tool that cuts a groove or pocket, called a stroke, in the metal (see Figure 26, page 52). Although the cutting tool is not shown on the tablet detail drawing, a cross section of the stroke with dimensional specifications is detailed, allowing the toolmaker to produce the correct cutting tool.

The following factors can affect the optimal design of a tablet identification.

- Tablet coating
- Bisects or scores
- Compressibility of formulations
- Maximum area available for the identification
- Complexity of the identification
- Location of the identification
- Techniques for preventing picking

Tablet Coating
Film-Coated Tablets

Film coating can affect the complexity, font style, and stroke specifications of a tablet identification. As a film coating adheres to a tablet's surface, the coating begins to consume the stroke width and depth, which in turn diminishes the clarity of the identification. The degree to which the clarity is affected depends on the method of application, and the percentage and type of coating applied.

For film-coated tablets the stroke width should equal 22–24% of the font's height. Stroke depths smaller than .007 inch are not recommended unless the tablet manufacturer can verify that smaller stroke depths worked on film-coated tablets produced in the past. Stroke angles can vary from 35–45°, with 35° and a .005- to .007-inch flat in the bottom of the stroke being the optimal design (see Figure 27, page 52). If these parameters cannot be met, the following conditions may exist:

- The designated cup depth is too large.
- The tablet is too small for the number of digits specified for engraving.
- The identification is located outside the maximum identification area of the tablet face.
- The identification is too complex.

Uncoated Tablets

Because design specifications for uncoated tablets are less restrictive, the tablet identification can be more complex. The specifications for uncoated tablets are as follows:
- Stroke width is 18–20% of the font height.
- Stroke depth is 50% of stroke width, or no less than .003 inch.
- Stroke angle is 30–45°.
- The minimum font height is .035 inch with a 30° stroke angle.

© American Pharmaceutical Association

FIGURE 25. COMMON TABLET SHAPES

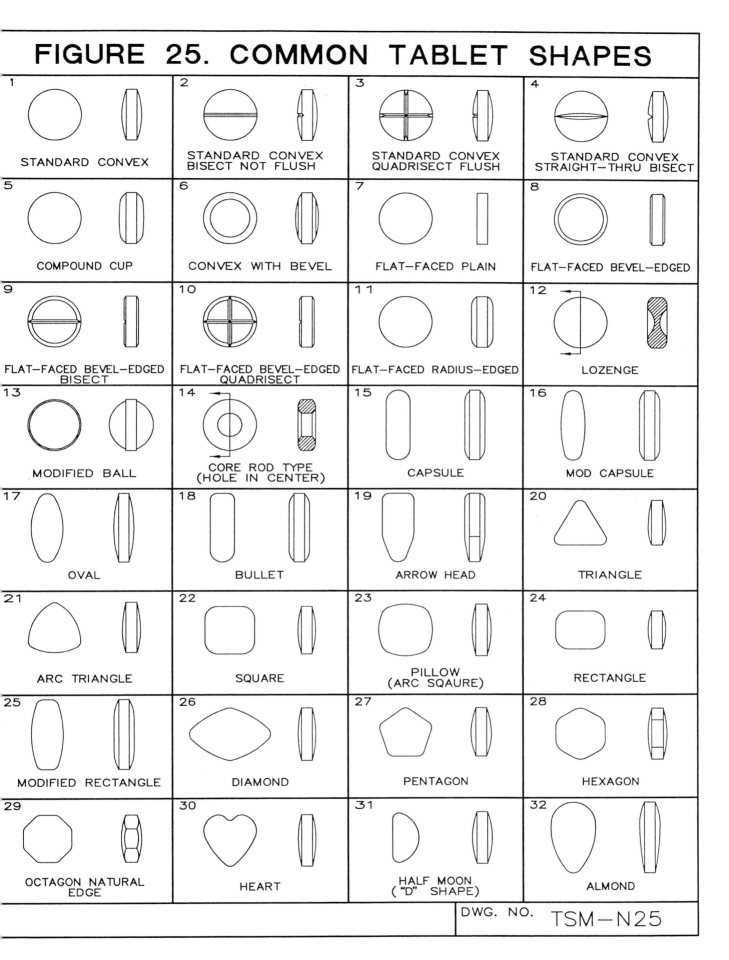

1 STANDARD CONVEX	2 STANDARD CONVEX BISECT NOT FLUSH	3 STANDARD CONVEX QUADRISECT FLUSH	4 STANDARD CONVEX STRAIGHT—THRU BISECT
5 COMPOUND CUP	6 CONVEX WITH BEVEL	7 FLAT—FACED PLAIN	8 FLAT—FACED BEVEL—EDGED
9 FLAT—FACED BEVEL—EDGED BISECT	10 FLAT—FACED BEVEL—EDGED QUADRISECT	11 FLAT—FACED RADIUS—EDGED	12 LOZENGE
13 MODIFIED BALL	14 CORE ROD TYPE (HOLE IN CENTER)	15 CAPSULE	16 MOD CAPSULE
17 OVAL	18 BULLET	19 ARROW HEAD	20 TRIANGLE
21 ARC TRIANGLE	22 SQUARE	23 PILLOW (ARC SQAURE)	24 RECTANGLE
25 MODIFIED RECTANGLE	26 DIAMOND	27 PENTAGON	28 HEXAGON
29 OCTAGON NATURAL EDGE	30 HEART	31 HALF MOON ("D" SHAPE)	32 ALMOND

DWG. NO. TSM—N25

© American Pharmaceutical Association

FIGURE 26. APPLYING TABLET IDENTIFICATION TO PUNCH FACE

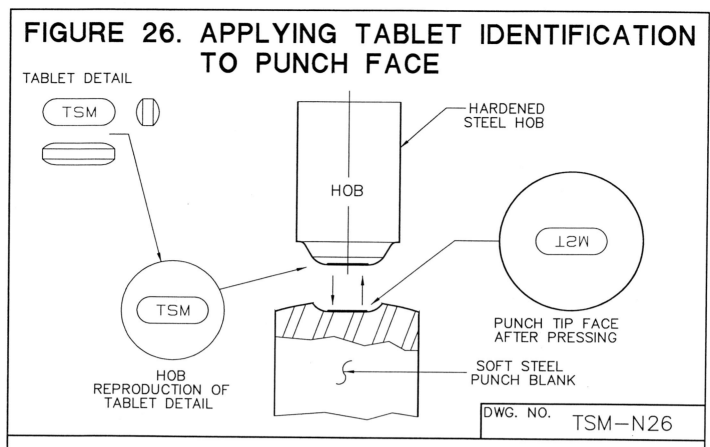

TABLET DETAIL

TSM

HARDENED STEEL HOB

HOB

TSW

PUNCH TIP FACE AFTER PRESSING

TSM

HOB REPRODUCTION OF TABLET DETAIL

SOFT STEEL PUNCH BLANK

DWG. NO. TSM—N26

FIGURE 27. GUIDELINES FOR FILM COATING

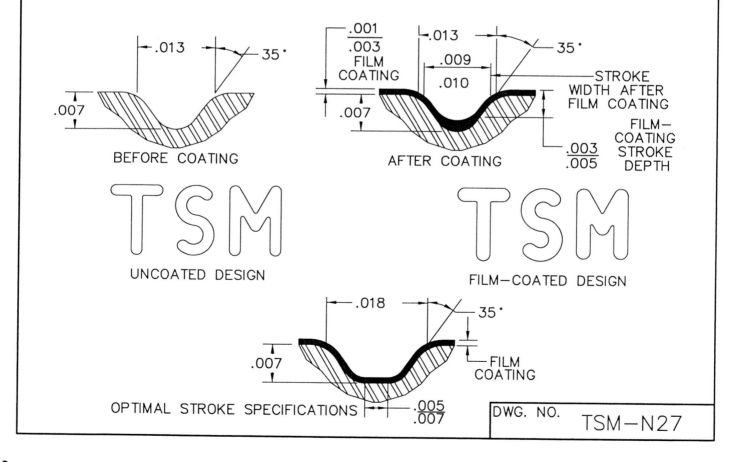

.013
35°
.007
BEFORE COATING

.001 .003 FILM COATING
.013
.009
.010
.007
35°
STROKE WIDTH AFTER FILM COATING
FILM-COATING STROKE DEPTH
.003 .005
AFTER COATING

TSM
UNCOATED DESIGN

TSM
FILM—COATED DESIGN

.018
35°
.007
FILM COATING
OPTIMAL STROKE SPECIFICATIONS
.005 .007

DWG. NO. TSM—N27

© American Pharmaceutical Association

...ects and Scores

...plying a bisect or score to a tablet's surface creates a ...ss line along which the tablet breaks easily, produc-...a partial tablet dosage. The bisect types shown in ...ure 28 on page 54 range from the most functional ...ct (the Type G, or pressure sensitive bisect) to the ...t functional (the Type H, or partial bisect).

...e bisect's purpose—to produce a desired dosage ...ount of a tablet—is affected by the tablet's cup ...th, band thickness, and hardness. Specifications for ...bisect's size are determined by the tablet's size, the ...et identification, and the bisect design. (See Table 8 ...age 55 for the standard bisect specifications.)

...rmulation Compressibility

...ing the compression stage of tablet production, a ...nulation (granulation) may exhibit unusual charac-...stics. Common problems with formulation com-...ssibility include:

...The formulation is hard to compress; a higher ton-nage than normal is required.
...A lower tonnage than normal is required to com-press the formulation.
...The formulation sticks to the punch face.
...Abrasives are higher than normal.

...problems with formulation compressibility should be discussed with the tooling manufacturer.

...nulation characteristics can dictate the (1) stroke ...ifications for the identification and (2) location of ...identification on the tablet face. Taking formulation ...pressibility into consideration at the design stage ...d prevent problems during tablet production.

...ximum Identification Area

...maximum identification area is the percentage of ...ablet face that is available to produce the least dis-...on of the stroke depth. The identification area dic-...s the dimensions of any debossing or embossing ...will be applied to the tablet's surface. Figure 29 on ...e 56 shows the maximum identification area for the ...ous cup depths of round tablets as a circular dashed ...on each tablet's face. As a rule, the identification ...and the dimensions of an identification—in this ...the letter A—decrease as the cup depth increases.

Three factors determine the maximum identification area: (1) the cup radius, (2) stroke specifications, and (3) stroke distortion.

Cup Radius

The cup radius, which is used to generate the tablet's contour, is dictated by the size of the tablet's periphery, cup depth, presence of land, and cup design. As the cup radius increases, the tablet face becomes flatter and the maximum identification area increases.

Stroke Specifications

Stroke specifications consist of the stroke width, depth, and angle, as well as the radius and break radius dimensions (see Figure 30, Illus. A; page 57). A normal stroke results when the cutting tool begins at the apex of the cup radius and cuts a stroke depth and angle that are equal on each side of the stroke width (See Figure 30, Illus. B). The earlier discussion of "Tablet Coating" on page 50 lists the optimal stroke specifications for film-coated and uncoated tablets.

Stroke Distortion

Stroke distortion results when a cut is made at a point on the cup radius that produces a stroke depth and angle that are *not* equal on each side of the stroke width (see Figure 30, Illus. C). As shown in Illustration C, the outside stroke depth is smaller than the inside stroke depth; the amount of stroke distortion equals the nominal inside stroke depth minus the outside stroke depth.

The maximum allowable percentage of distortion equals stroke distortion divided by the required stroke depth multiplied by 100. The size of the identification area should be chosen so that the stroke depth never exceeds 30% of the required stroke depth for film-coated tablet designs, and 35% for uncoated tablets. For shaped tablets, the minor axis cup radius and, when applicable, the major axis cup radius are used to determine the maximum tablet identification area. Exceeding the recommended limits for stroke distortion can adversely affect the clarity of the tablet identification.

On F.F.B.E. tablets, the bevel angle intersects the tablet's face and creates a sharp beveled edge. As shown in Illustration 1 on page 58, an identification

FIGURE 29. MAXIMUM IDENTIFICATION AREA FOR ROUND TABLETS

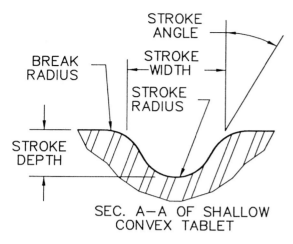

SEC. A–A OF SHALLOW CONVEX TABLET

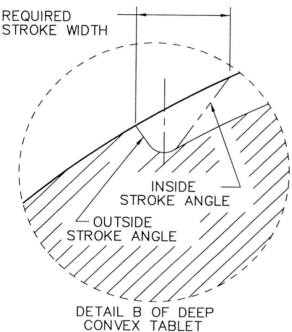

DETAIL B OF DEEP CONVEX TABLET

NOTES:

1. DOTTED LINE ON FACE VIEWS INDICATES USABLE SURFACE AREA FOR TABLET IDENTIFICATION.

2. ALL PERCENTAGES FOR MAXIMUM IDENTIFICATION AREA ARE BASED ON A 30° STROKE ANGLE, .006 INCH STROKE DEPTH, AND NO LAND. INCREASING THE STROKE ANGLE OR DESIGNATING A LAND WILL DECREASE THE PERCENTAGE OF IDENTIFICATION AREA.

3. THE MAX. I.D. AREA FOR A SHALLOW CONVEX TABLET IS SMALLER THAN THAT FOR A STANDARD CONVEX TABLET BECAUSE THE STROKE DEPTH CANNOT EXCEED THE CUP DEPTH AT THE TABLET'S EDGE.

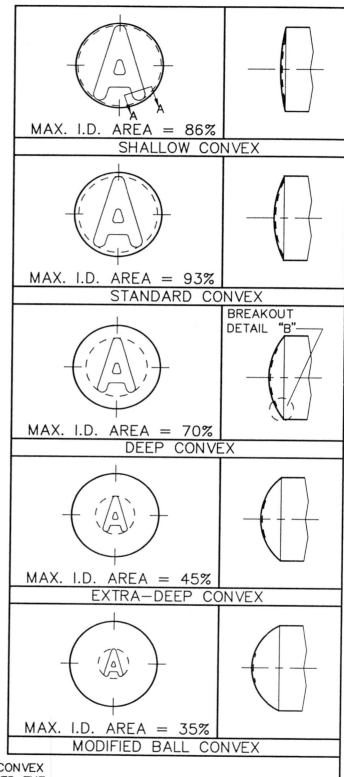

MAX. I.D. AREA = 86%
SHALLOW CONVEX

MAX. I.D. AREA = 93%
STANDARD CONVEX

MAX. I.D. AREA = 70%
DEEP CONVEX

MAX. I.D. AREA = 45%
EXTRA–DEEP CONVEX

MAX. I.D. AREA = 35%
MODIFIED BALL CONVEX

DWG. NO. TSM–N29

© American Pharmaceutical Association

FIGURE 30. STROKE SPECIFICATIONS AND STROKE DISTORTION

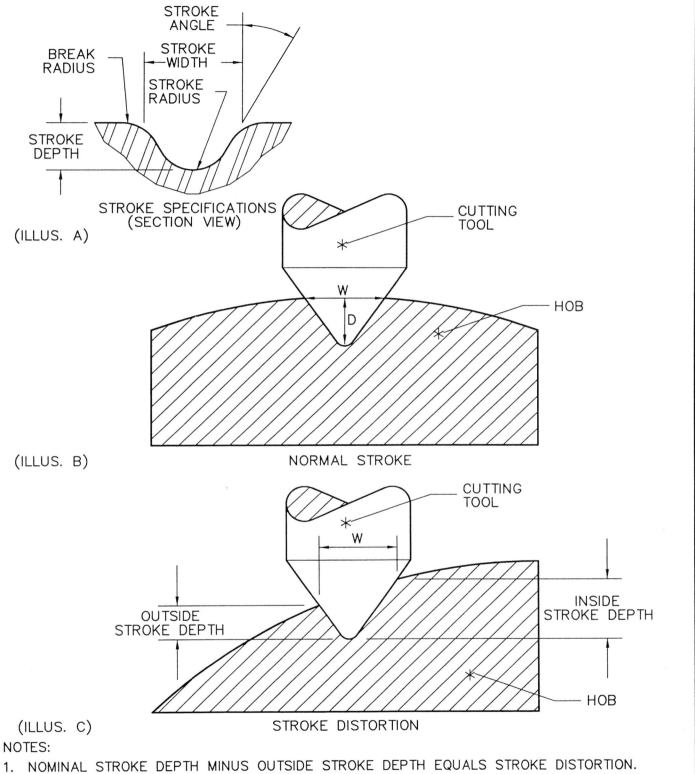

STROKE ANGLE

BREAK RADIUS

STROKE WIDTH

STROKE RADIUS

STROKE DEPTH

STROKE SPECIFICATIONS (SECTION VIEW)

(ILLUS. A)

CUTTING TOOL

W

D

HOB

(ILLUS. B) NORMAL STROKE

CUTTING TOOL

W

OUTSIDE STROKE DEPTH

INSIDE STROKE DEPTH

HOB

(ILLUS. C) STROKE DISTORTION

NOTES:
1. NOMINAL STROKE DEPTH MINUS OUTSIDE STROKE DEPTH EQUALS STROKE DISTORTION.
2. STROKE DISTORTION DIVIDED BY REQUIRED STROKE DEPTH EQUALS MAXIMUM DISTORTION: 30% MAX. DISTORTION FOR FILM–COATED DESIGNS; 35% MAX. DISTORTION FOR UNCOATED DESIGNS.

DWG. NO. TSM–N30

character or symbol should be positioned at least .006 inch plus a stroke width from the beveled edge.

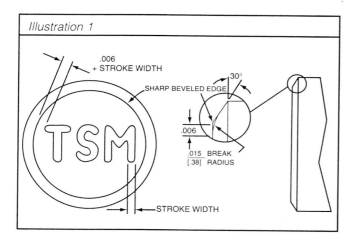

Illustration 1

Complexity of Identification

Unless modified or simplified, an identification designed primarily for advertising copy, letterhead, and packaging may not be practical for tablet designs. The illustrations below show how a design can be simplified by changing the font and applying radii on the corners. A tablet's dosage size and maximum identification area also determine the clarity of the final product's identification.

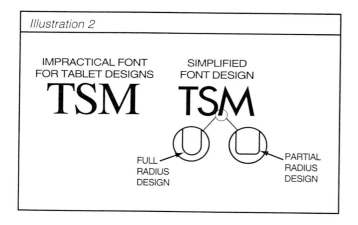

Illustration 2

Location of Identification

After establishing the maximum identification area, the next step is to locate the required tablet identification within the confined area. The number of characters, as well as the cup depth and design, determines the optimal location for the identification. Depending on the number of engraved characters, the identification may be restricted to only one location within the identifica-

tion area. Centering the identification horizontally across the tablet's face can optimize the identification size. Illustration 3, below, shows the largest optimal identification size.

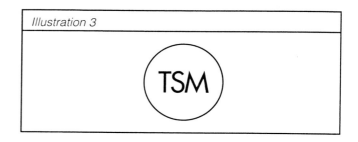

Illustration 3

In some circumstances, characters located in a potentially soft zone of the tablet cup can result in picking or sticking of the formulation to the punch face. When a punch begins compressing a powder into a tablet form, the compression force is initially higher at the land. The dwell time and applied tonnage can affect the equal distribution of the compression force across the entire surface of the cup. If the force is not distributed equally, a soft zone can occur on the face of tablets that have a cup depth category of deep, extra-deep, or modified ball. The soft zone normally appears at the apex of the cup as capping, picking or sticking, or abnormal surface abrasion (see Illustration 4). If reducing the press speed or increasing dwell time does not improve or eliminate the problem, a soft zone is strongly indicated. Reducing the cup depth is the next step in solving the problem; however, if this is not possible, moving the identification away from the cup apex should be considered (see Illustration 5).

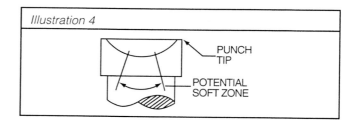

Illustration 4

If design restrictions, such as numerous characters or a cup depth category that provides a small identification area, cannot be changed, the following measures should be considered:

- Use a 35° or greater stroke angle.

8

© American Pharmaceutical Association

- Increase the stroke break radius.
- Use techniques to prevent picking.

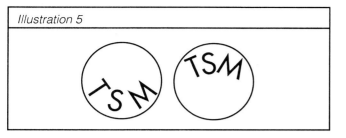

Illustration 5

Techniques To Prevent Picking

Techniques that prevent picking reduce the amount of force needed to compress powder within small confined areas of a tablet identification, referred to as pads or peninsulas. As a result, the incidence of granulation sticking to the punch faces is reduced.

Figure 31 on page 60 shows two techniques to prevent picking in pad areas: (1) increasing the stroke break radius around pads and (2) decreasing the pad depth. If the required cutter depth is *less than .006 inch*, the break radius on the pads can be increased 1.5 to 2 times the outside break radius. If the cutter depth is *.006 inch or greater*, decreasing the depth of pad areas by 25–50% and increasing the break radius can also alleviate picking in pad areas.

Figure 32 on page 61 shows techniques to prevent picking in two other problem areas: peninsulas and corners. Tapering a peninsula by 25–50% of the total cut depth should alleviate picking in this type of confined area. Generating a corner radius in all sharp corners eliminates compound angles, which should alleviate picking in these areas. The minimum value recommended for a corner radius is .002 to .003 inch; the maximum recommended value is .004 to .006 inch.

Although all of these techniques alleviate problems with picking and sticking, the lack of a stroke break radius is a main contributor to the problems. As a rule, the designated stroke break radius should remove approximately one-third of the stroke depth (see Illustration 6).

Figures 33 and 34 on pages 62 and 63 show sample designs of bold and narrow letters and numerals used

by some tooling manufacturers. These and other similar fonts can reduce the incidence of picking and sticking. (See Table 16 on page 106 for other factors that can cause picking and sticking.) If these problems cannot be resolved, printing the identification on the tablet might be an option.

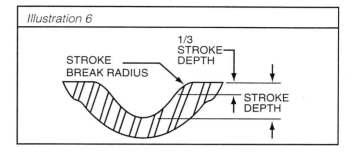

Illustration 6

Tablet Printing

When an identification is mechanically printed on a tablet's surface, the tablet is usually film coated. Of the two types of tablet printing, linear and radial, linear printing is the method used most often.

Radial Printing

Radial printing, also called spin printing, can be used only for caplet shapes that closely approximate the shape of a capsule. In this printing process, the tablet is rotated about its major axis as the characters are applied to the tablet's surface (see Illustration 7). The size and number of characters are determined by the tablet's circumference.

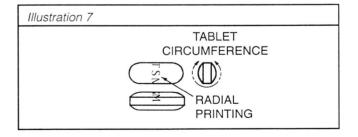

Illustration 7

Linear Printing

In linear printing, the tablet's major axis periphery and minor axis cup are aligned with the printing mechanism. This alignment allows the identification to be

FIGURE 31. TECHNIQUES TO PREVENT PICKING IN PAD AREAS

INCREASE BREAK RADIUS	LOWER PAD AREAS & INCREASE BREAK RADIUS

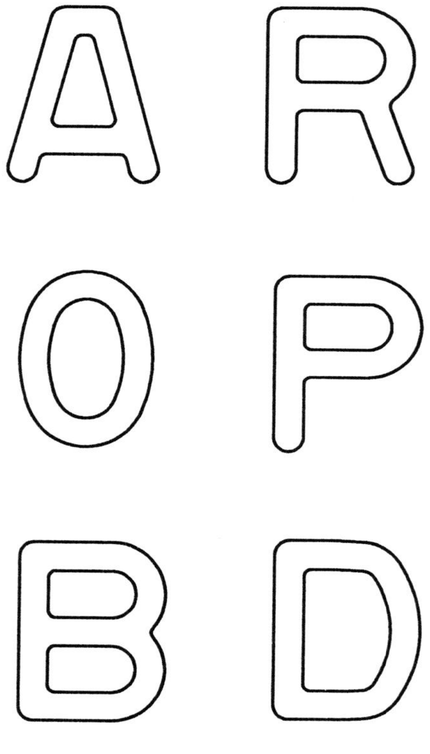

INCREASE BREAK RADIUS ON THE PAD 1.5–2 TIMES THE OUTSIDE BREAK RADIUS

DECREASE DEPTH OF PAD AREAS AND INCREASE BREAK RADIUS

PAD AREAS ARE DECREASED 25–50% OF THE TOTAL DEPTH OF THE CUT

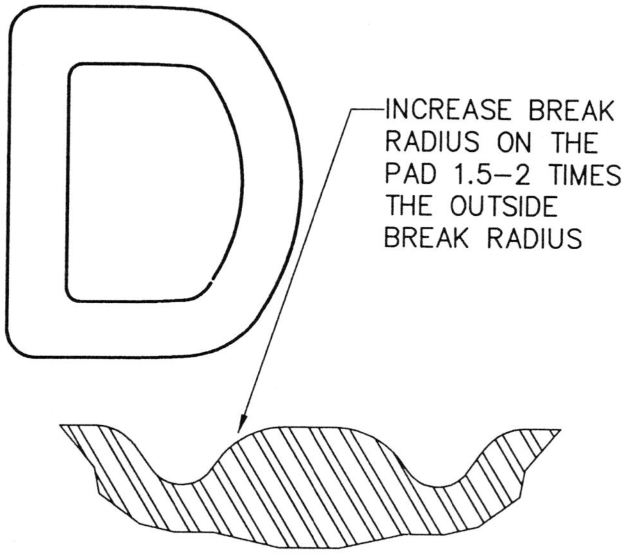

INCREASE THE BREAK RADIUS ON PADS IF THE REQUIRED CUTTER DEPTH IS LESS THAN .006 INCH.

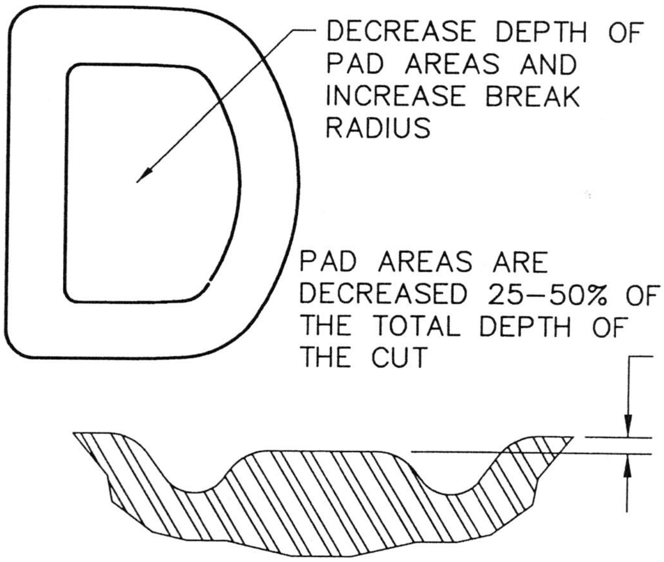

DECREASE DEPTH OF PAD AREAS AND INCREASE BREAK RADIUS IF AND *ONLY IF* THE CUTTER DEPTH IS .006 INCH OR GREATER.

EXAMPLES:

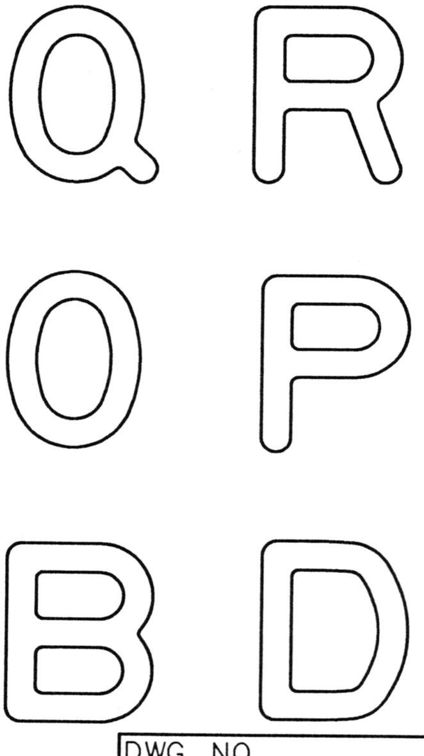

A R

O P

B D

EXAMPLES:

Q R

O P

B D

DWG. NO.	TSM—N31

© American Pharmaceutical Association

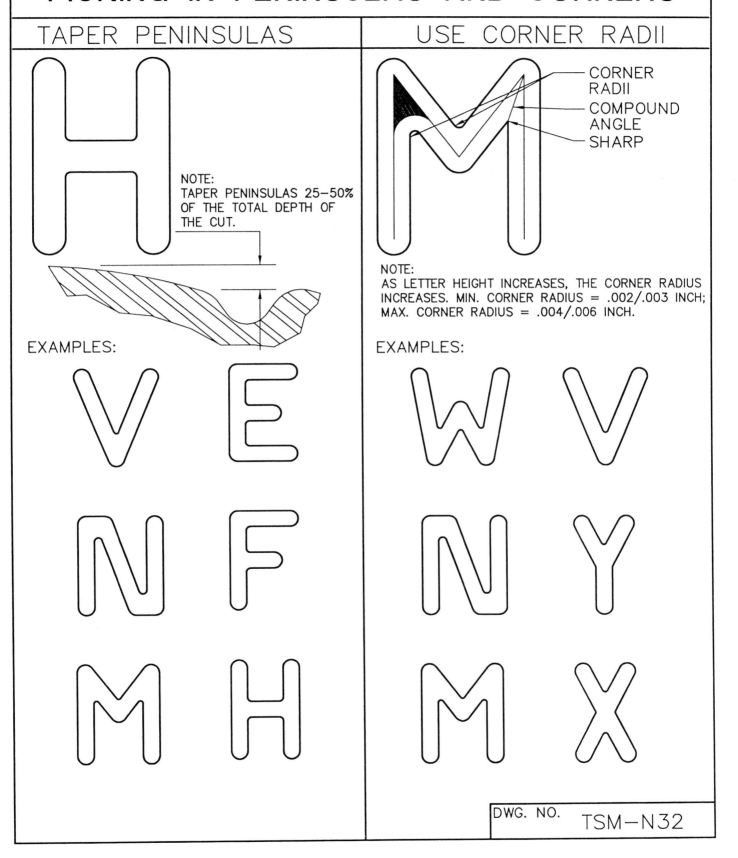

FIGURE 32. TECHNIQUES TO PREVENT PICKING IN PENINSULAS AND CORNERS

TAPER PENINSULAS

NOTE:
TAPER PENINSULAS 25-50% OF THE TOTAL DEPTH OF THE CUT.

EXAMPLES:

USE CORNER RADII

CORNER RADII
COMPOUND ANGLE
SHARP

NOTE:
AS LETTER HEIGHT INCREASES, THE CORNER RADIUS INCREASES. MIN. CORNER RADIUS = .002/.003 INCH; MAX. CORNER RADIUS = .004/.006 INCH.

EXAMPLES:

DWG. NO. TSM-N32

© American Pharmaceutical Association

FIGURE 33. SAMPLE DESIGNS FOR BOLD CHARACTERS

BOLD DESIGN

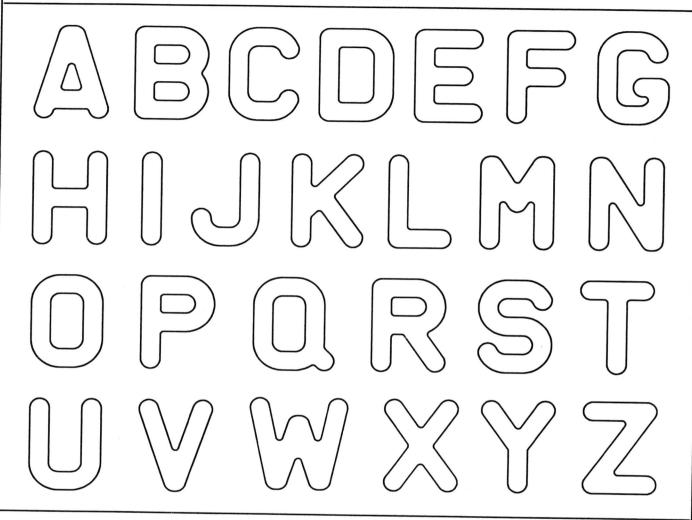

STANDARD DESIGN

DWG. NO. TSM—N33

2

© American Pharmaceutical Association

FIGURE 34. SAMPLE DESIGN FOR NARROW CHARACTERS

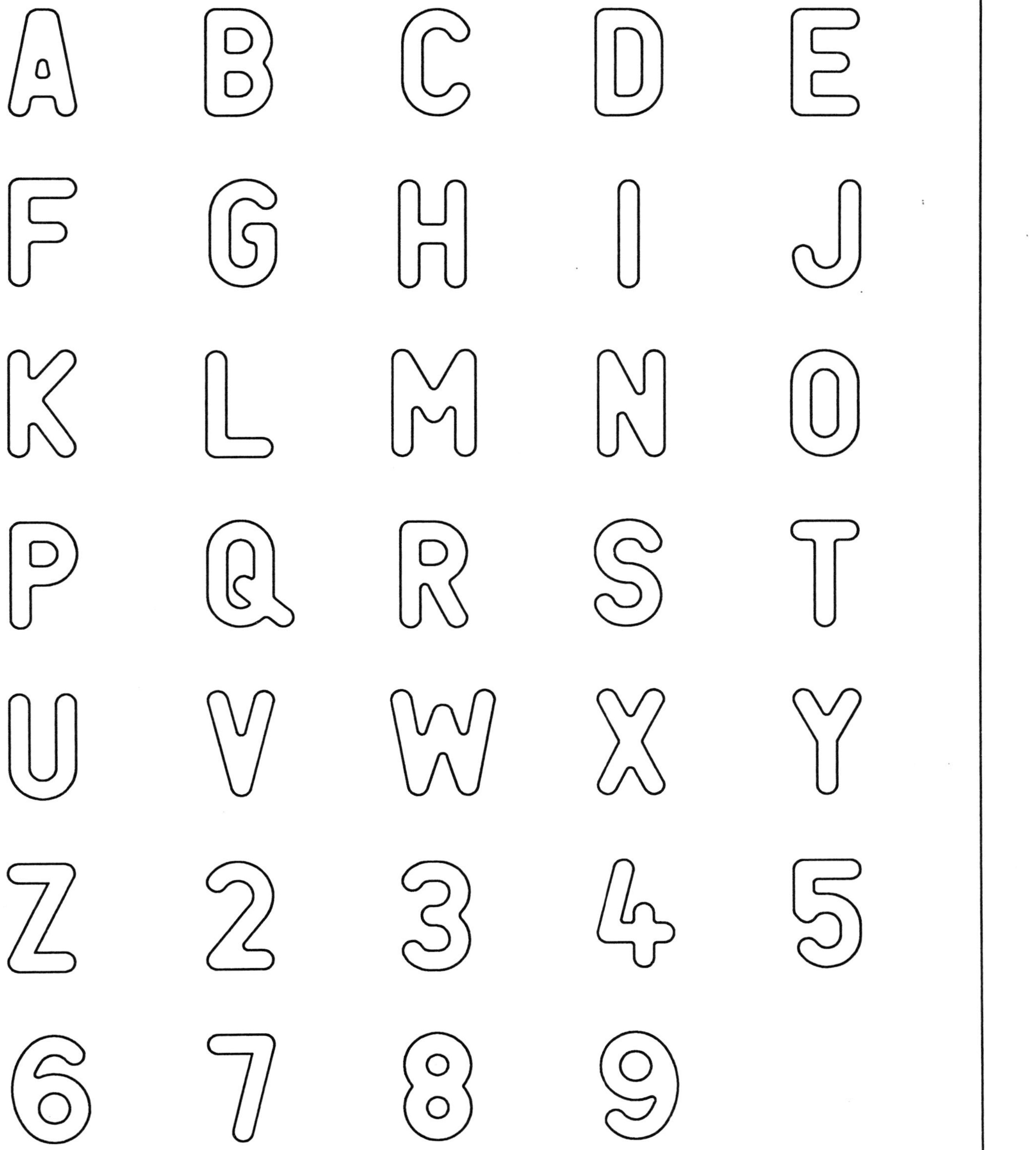

A B C D E
F G H I J
K L M N O
P Q R S T
U V W X Y
Z 2 3 4 5
6 7 8 9

DWG. NO.	TSM—N34

© American Pharmaceutical Association

imprinted consistently across a major axis location (see Illustration 8). Tablet orientation is critical to maintaining a consistent placement of the identification on the tablet and to avoiding side printing, or printing on the tablet band (see Illustration 9).

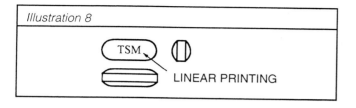

Illustration 8

TSM
LINEAR PRINTING

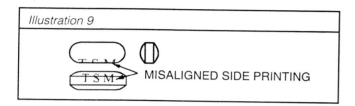

Illustration 9

T S M
MISALIGNED SIDE PRINTING

The two major factors to consider in designing a tablet for linear printing are (1) cup radii and (2) tablet proportions.

Cup Radii

The cup radii, which are the major and minor axis radii, form the tablet's contour, or surface. The cup radii should be as large as possible to reduce rocking of the tablet in the printer's carrier pockets (see Illustration 10). Because the minor axis controls the degree of rocking, the size of the minor axis radius should be emphasized in the tablet design.

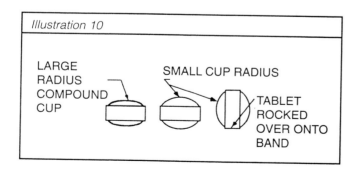

Illustration 10

LARGE RADIUS COMPOUND CUP

SMALL CUP RADIUS

TABLET ROCKED OVER ONTO BAND

The cup radii will also affect the printing window. The size of the printing window determines the maximum character size that can be printed on the tablet's surface. Illustration 11A shows that a large cup radius provides a wide printing window, whereas a medium cup radius provides only a narrow printing window. On tablet drawings, an approximation of the printing window is usually shown on the face view as a phantom line (see Illustration 11B).

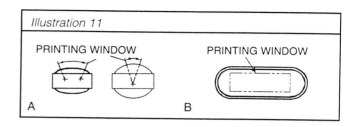

Illustration 11

PRINTING WINDOW   PRINTING WINDOW

A   B

Tablet Proportions

A tablet's proportions can affect the degree to which rocking occurs. To reduce tablet rocking, the difference between the tablet's minor axis, or width, and the tablet thickness should not be less than .060 inch; a difference range of .075–.090 inch is preferable. Cup depth, which can also affect rocking, should be at least 24% of the total tablet thickness (see Illustration 12). Both proportions must be met to prevent tablet rocking. If the stipulated difference between the minor axis and tablet thickness is met, but the cup depth is less than 24% of the tablet thickness, the resultant increase in band thickness may cause the tablet to rock onto its side.

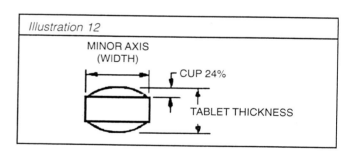

Illustration 12

MINOR AXIS (WIDTH)

CUP 24%

TABLET THICKNESS

Tablet Detail Drawings

Prior to manufacturing of any tooling, a detailed drawing of the proposed tablets must be generated. Whether creating a design for a new product or modifying the design of an existing one, tooling manufacturers can aid in preparing tablet drawings. A tablet detail drawing should contain the following basic information:
- A face view with full dimensions of the tablet periphery

4

© American Pharmaceutical Association

- For round tablets, a single side view
- For shaped tablets, side views of the major and minor axes
- Cup depth, land, and cup radius
- For compound cup tablets, all radii locations

If a tablet identification is present, the following information is needed:

- Height, width, and spacing for each character
- Location of the identification relative to the periphery's latitude and the centerline's longitude
- Details and notes for techniques to prevent picking
- Stroke specifications

Because drawings for most shaped tablets usually require at least three views, a B-size (11- by 17-inch) sheet is suggested. An A-size (8 1/2- by 11-inch) sheet is usually sufficient for the face and side views required on drawings of round tablets. (A detail drawing of each side of the tablet printed on separate sheets is recommended.) If a drawing's size is reduced for facsimile transmission, the text should be checked again for legibility. Tablet drawings created on a B-size sheet usually require a minimum text height of 1/8 inch [3.175 millimeter].

If a tablet drawing lacks the required information and the tooling for the product is purchased later from a different vendor, an inconsistency in the product may occur. The new vendor needs the following information to ensure product consistency:

- Tablet detail drawing for each side of the tablet
- For round tablets, samples of the upper and lower punches
- For shaped tablets, sample punches and a sample die
- Description of any past problems with the tooling, including:
  - Premature fatigue
  - Picking and capping
  - Reduced press speed needed to improve tablet quality
  - Tablet coating problems (e.g., chipping, abrasion, and lack of identification clarity)
  - Printing problems (e.g., inconsistent tablet orientation resulting in side printing and the need to reduce printer conveyor speed)

With this information in hand, the tooling manufacturer may suggest changes in tablet design, tooling material, and punch variables that will improve tooling life and tablet quality.

Tablet Land

The tablet land is the narrow plane perpendicular to the tablet's periphery, which creates a junction between the tablet's periphery and cup (see Figure 35, Illus. A; page 66). The two reasons for incorporating a land into a tablet's design are to (1) reduce nicks on punch tip edges and (2) increase the strength of tip edges. The following discussion of the separate illustrations in Figure 35 explains why adding a land to a tablet design improves the function of tip edges.

Effect of Land on Tip Edges

Illustration B of Figure 35 shows that a punch tip without a land has a sharp punch tip edge. As the cup depth increases, the tip's edge strength decreases. Detail A shows a deformed tip edge, which can occur easily on sharp edges during press setup or when tooling is mishandled. Adding a minimum .002-inch blended land will remove the sharp tip edge and minimize deformities to the edge caused by mishandling; however, a land this small will not effectively improve the tip's edge strength.

Illustration C of Figure 35 shows deflection of the tip edge caused by excessive compression force. When a punch begins compressing powder into a tablet form, the force is initially higher at the tip edge; then the compression force is distributed across the cup's surface. Cup depth, dwell time, and applied tonnage can affect the occurrence of tip edge deflection and the equal distribution of force across the entire cup surface. Choosing the appropriate land width is essential to reducing tip edge deflection. Because the dwell time and tonnage needed to produce a new tablet are usually not known at the tablet design stage, the cup depth category is used to determine the appropriate land width.

FIGURE 35. GUIDELINES FOR PUNCH TIP LAND

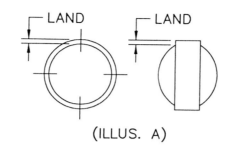

(ILLUS. A)

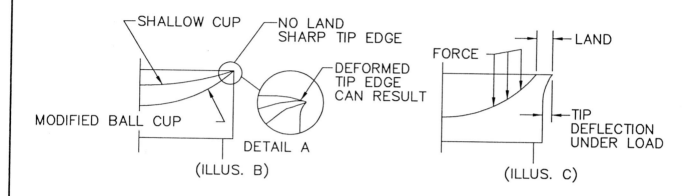

SHALLOW CUP

NO LAND SHARP TIP EDGE

DEFORMED TIP EDGE CAN RESULT

MODIFIED BALL CUP

DETAIL A

(ILLUS. B)

FORCE

LAND

TIP DEFLECTION UNDER LOAD

(ILLUS. C)

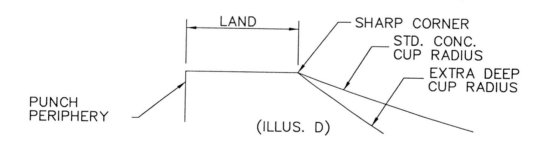

LAND

SHARP CORNER

STD. CONC. CUP RADIUS

EXTRA DEEP CUP RADIUS

PUNCH PERIPHERY

(ILLUS. D)

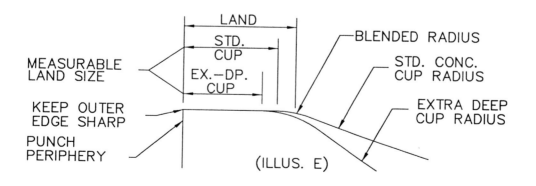

LAND

STD. CUP

EX.-DP. CUP

MEASURABLE LAND SIZE

BLENDED RADIUS

STD. CONC. CUP RADIUS

EXTRA DEEP CUP RADIUS

KEEP OUTER EDGE SHARP

PUNCH PERIPHERY

(ILLUS. E)

DWG. NO.	TSM–N35

© American Pharmaceutical Association

Minimum Land Widths

Land width is the straight line distance starting at the punch's periphery and ending at the junction of the land with the cup's surface. This junction forms a sharp corner (see Figure 35, Illus. D). Where applicable, tablet detail drawings should indicate the land widths before the sharp corners are blended.

Table 9 lists the minimum land widths for round and shaped tablets. The appropriate land width is determined by the tablet's *cup depth category*. For round tablets, the *O.D.* and actual cup depth determine if a tablet's cup depth category is shallow, standard, deep, extra-deep, or modified ball. Matching the tablet's diameter and cup depth with the appropriate punch tip diameter and cup depth, respectively, in Table 10 on page 68 gives the cup depth category.

For shaped tablets, the *minor axis* and actual cup depth determine a tablet's cup depth category. Although the concave punch tip tabulations in Table 10 apply to round tablets, this table can also be used to determine a shaped tablet's cup depth category. Matching the minor axis and cup depth of a shaped tablet with the appropriate punch tip diameter and cup depth, respectively, determines the tablet's cup depth category. The cup depth category is then correlated with the appropriate minimum land width in Table 9.

Measurable Land

Measurable land is the land that remains after a blended radius is applied to the junction of the land with the cup. A blended radius, which is a fillet or curved transition between two mating surfaces, is normally used to remove sharp corners on a contoured surface (see Figure 35, Illus. E).

The actual width of a measurable land is affected by the (1) size of the blended radius and (2) cup radius and depth. Based on the same land requirements, Illustration E shows the measurable land of two cup depth categories. The standard cup depth has a larger measurable land. Difficulty in controlling how much material is removed, or blended, increases as the cup depth increases.

TABLE 9. MINIMUM LAND WIDTHS

CUP DEPTH	LAND WIDTHS	
	SHAPES	ROUNDS
SHALLOW	REMOVE SHARP TIP EDGE	REMOVE SHARP TIP EDGE
STANDARD	.004 [.102]	.003 [.076]
DEEP	.005 [.127]	.004 [.102]
EXTRA-DEEP	.006 [.152]	.005 [.127]
MOD. BALL	.008 [.203]	.007 [.178]
F.F.B.E.	.004 [.102]	.003 [.076]

NOTE: VALUES PERTAIN TO MINIMUM LAND WIDTHS BEFORE BLENDING.

NOTE: The TSM Committee recommends that a land be specified for all tablets or punches with a cup depth of standard or greater.

© American Pharmaceutical Association

TABLE 10. PUNCH TIP TABULATIONS

PUNCH TIP DIA. INCHES [MILLIMETERS]	SHALLOW CUP DEPTH	STANDARD CUP DEPTH	DEEP CUP DEPTH	EXTRA-DEEP CUP DEPTH	MOD. BALL CUP DEPTH	FFBE/FFRE CUP DEPTH
1/8 [3.175]	.005 [.127]	.017 [.432]	.024 [.610]	.030 [.762]	.040 [1.016]	.007 [.178]
5/32 [3.970]	.007 [.178]	.021 [.533]	.030 [.762]	.036 [.914]	.049 [1.245]	.008 [.203]
3/16 [4.763]	.008 [.203]	.026 [.635]	.036 [.914]	.042 [1.067]	.059 [1.499]	.009 [.229]
7/32 [5.555]	.009 [.229]	.029 [.737]	.042 [1.067]	.048 [1.219]	.069 [1.753]	.010 [.254]
1/4 [6.350]	.010 [.254]	.031 [.787]	.045 [1.143]	.050 [1.270]	.079 [2.007]	.011 [.279]
9/32 [7.142]	.012 [.305]	.033 [.838]	.046 [1.168]	.054 [1.372]	.089 [2.261]	.012 [.305]
5/16 [7.938]	.013 [.330]	.034 [.864]	.047 [1.194]	.060 [1.524]	.099 [2.515]	.013 [.330]
11/32 [8.730]	.014 [.356]	.035 [.889]	.049 [1.245]	.066 [1.676]	.109 [2.769]	.014 [.356]
3/8 [9.525]	.016 [.406]	.036 [.914]	.050 [1.270]	.072 [1.829]	.119 [3.023]	.015 [.381]
13/32 [10.318]	.017 [.432]	.038 [.965]	.052 [1.321]	.078 [1.981]	.128 [3.251]	.016 [.406]
7/16 [11.113]	.018 [.457]	.040 [1.016]	.054 [1.372]	.084 [2.134]	.133 [3.378]	.016 [.406]
15/32 [11.905]	.020 [.508]	.041 [1.041]	.056 [1.422]	.090 [2.286]	.148 [3.759]	.016 [.406]
1/2 [12.700]	.021 [.533]	.043 [1.092]	.059 [1.499]	.095 [2.413]	.158 [4.013]	.016 [.406]
17/32 [13.493]	.022 [.559]	.045 [1.143]	.061 [1.549]	.101 [2.565]	.168 [4.267]	.016 [.406]
9/16 [14.288]	.024 [.610]	.046 [1.168]	.063 [1.600]	.107 [2.718]	.178 [4.521]	.016 [.406]
19/32 [15.080]	.025 [.635]	.048 [1.219]	.066 [1.676]	.113 [2.870]	.188 [4.775]	.016 [.406]
5/8 [15.875]	.026 [.660]	.050 [1.270]	.068 [1.727]	.119 [3.023]	.198 [5.029]	.016 [.406]
11/16 [17.463]	.029 [.737]	.054 [1.372]	.073 [1.854]	.131 [3.327]	.217 [5.512]	.020 [.508]
3/4 [19.050]	.031 [.787]	.058 [1.473]	.078 [1.981]	.143 [3.632]	.237 [6.020]	.020 [.508]
13/16 [20.638]	.034 [.864]	.061 [1.549]	.083 [2.108]	.155 [3.937]	.257 [6.528]	.020 [.508]
7/8 [22.225]	.037 [.940]	.065 [1.651]	.089 [2.260]	.167 [4.242]	.277 [7.036]	.020 [.508]
15/16 [23.813]	.039 [.991]	.069 [1.753]	.094 [2.388]	.179 [4.547]	.296 [7.518]	.020 [.508]
1 [25.400]	.042 [1.067]	.073 [1.854]	.099 [2.515]	.191 [4.851]	.316 [8.026]	.025 [.635]

NOTES:

1. DUE TO DEFORMATION FROM THE HOBBING PROCESS, LARGE F.F.B.E. AND F.F.R.E. PUNCH FACES MAY BE SLIGHTLY CONVEX. AS A RESULT, THE WORKING LENGTH DIMENSION MAY VARY ACROSS THE PUNCH FACES; THE VARIATION SHOULD BE CONSISTENT WITHIN A SET OF TOOLING.
2. TIP TABULATIONS FOR SHAPED PUNCHES ARE DETERMINED BY CORRELATING THEIR MINOR AXIS DIMENSION WITH THE APPROPRIATE PUNCH TIP DIAMETER IN THIS TABLE.

© American Pharmaceutical Association

Tool Steels, Compression Forces, and Fatigue Failure

Tool Steels

Toughness, resistance to wear and corrosion, strength, and resistance to distortion and warping during heat treatment are the most important properties of a tool steel. These properties are determined by the steel's chemical composition and the conditions under which it is manufactured. For purposes of comparison, the steels used to manufacture tablet press tooling have been grouped in three categories: general-purpose, wear-resistant, and corrosion-resistant.

General-Purpose Steels

Most tablet press punches are manufactured from S1, S5, S7 or 408 (3% nickel) tool steel. The S series steels provide a good combination of toughness and wear resistance, and have a proven record of performance in tablet production. At one time, 408 or 3% nickel steel was the industry standard because of its superior toughness. However, the S grades, which have only a slight loss in ductility as compared to 408 steel, offer much improved wear characteristics and have all but replaced 408 as the preferred general-purpose steel for punches.

Wear-Resistant Steels

A2, D2, and D3 grades are high-carbon, high-chromium steels used for their excellent wear resistance. Among all the steels commonly used for press tooling, D3 has the highest wear resistance. Its low toughness rating, however, almost exclusively limits its use to dies. D2 rates slightly lower in abrasion resistance than does D3, but its increased toughness makes D2 suitable for manufacturing punches, provided the cup design is not too fragile. A2, which is a compromise between the general-purpose S grades and D2 in toughness and wear, can be used for punches and dies.

Tungsten carbide, while not actually a steel, is extremely wear resistant and is commonly used to line dies.

Although punch tips can be manufactured from tungsten carbide, its use is restricted to applications where tip fracture caused by high compression forces is not likely. Such punches are quite expensive and require special setup and alignment procedures. The tooling supplier should be consulted about these procedures.

Ceramic materials, such as partially stabilized zirconia, can also be used as die liners. Due to their low coefficient of friction, these materials offer longer wear, higher corrosion resistance, and lower required force for tablet ejection than do either steel or tungsten carbide liners.

Corrosion-Resistant Steels

S1, S7, and 408 steels provide some protection against mildly corrosive materials; more severe corrosion problems demand the use of stainless steel (440C) tooling. From the standpoint of wear, 440C falls between the S and D grades of tool steel. Because 440C has a low toughness rating (comparable to that of D3), the punch must have a strong cup design to avoid problems with tip fractures.

Refined Tool Steels

One measure of a tool steel's quality is the rate of inclusions. Inclusions are unwanted impurities or voids that are present to some degree in all steels. After heat treatment, inclusions give rise to localized areas of stress concentration where microscopic cracks can later develop. Remelting the original steel ingots in a vacuum-tight shell allows the impurities, in the form of dissolved gases, to be expelled from the shell. This process of "vacuum remelting" further reduces the level of impurities and improves the steel's quality. The performance of tooling made from this remelted steel is subsequently improved. When punch tip fracture is a problem, tooling suppliers may recommend a remelted or premium grade of a particular steel as a means of eliminating the problem.

© American Pharmaceutical Association

Chemical Composition of Steels

Carbon and alloy steels—the two main categories of steel—contain carbon, manganese, and usually silicon in varying percentages; they can also contain copper and boron as specified additions. To qualify as a *carbon steel*, a steel's maximum concentrations of manganese, silicon, and copper must not exceed 1.65%, .60%, and .60%, respectively. With the exception of boron and deoxidizers, no other alloy element is intentionally added. *Alloy steels* comprise those steel grades that exceed the above limits, as well as any grade to which an element other than those previously mentioned is added to achieve a specific alloy effect.

The effects of the following chemical elements on the properties of hot-rolled carbon and alloy bars are considered individually. In practice, the effect of a particular element often depends on the presence and quantities of other elements in the steel. For example, the total effect of a combination of elements on the hardness of a steel is usually greater than the sum of their individual effects. This interrelation should be considered when a change in a specified analysis is being evaluated. (With the exception of sulfur and phosphorous, Table 11 details the chemical composition of pharmaceutical tool steels.)

Carbon

Carbon is the principal hardening element in steel; each additional increment of carbon increases the hardness and tensile strength of steel in the as-rolled, or normalized, condition. As carbon content exceeds approximately .85%, the resultant increase in strength and hardness is proportionately less for each increment added. Upon quenching, the maximum attainable hardness also increases with increasing carbon; however, the rate of increase is very small for carbon contents above .60%.

Conversely, a steel's ductility and weldability decrease as its carbon content increases. Ductility is the ease with which metal flows during the high pressures of compression. Carbon also has a moderate tendency to segregate within the ingot. Because carbon has a significant effect on steel properties, its segregation is frequently more important than the segregation of other elements in the steel.

Manganese

Manganese, which is present in all commercial steels, contributes significantly—but to a lesser degree than does carbon—to a steel's strength and hardness. The effectiveness of manganese depends largely on and is directly proportional to a steel's carbon content.

Manganese has a greater ability than any of the commonly used alloy elements to decrease the critical cooling rate during hardening, thereby increasing a steel's hardenability. This element is also an active deoxidizer and shows less tendency to segregate within the ingot than do most of the other elements. Manganese also improves a steel's surface quality because it tends to combine with sulfur, thereby minimizing the formation of iron sulfide. Iron sulfide can cause hot-shortness (i.e., the susceptibility of a steel to crack and tear when the ingot is rolled).

Silicon

Silicon is one of the principal deoxidizers used in manufacturing carbon and alloy steels. Depending on the steel type, the amount of silicon can vary up to .35%; greater amounts are used in some steels (e.g., silicomanganese steel). The combined effects of these two elements produce steels with unusually high strength, good ductility, and shock resistance (toughness) in the quenched and tempered conditions. At these larger concentrations, however, silicon has an adverse effect on machineability and increases the steel's susceptibility to decarburization (i.e., removal of carbon) and graphitization (i.e., conversion into graphite).

Chromium

Chromium is used in constructional alloy steels primarily to increase hardenability, provide improved resistance to abrasion, and promote carburization. Chromium is surpassed by only manganese and molybdenum in its effect on hardenability. A chromium content of 3.99% has been established as the maximum limit for constructional alloy steels. Exceeding this limit for chromium content puts a steel in the heat-resisting or stainless steel category.

© American Pharmaceutical Association

Of the common alloy elements, chromium forms the most stable carbide, which gives high-carbon high-chromium steels exceptional wear resistance. Because this carbide is relatively stable at elevated temperatures, chromium is often added to steels used for high-temperature applications.

Vanadium

Vanadium improves the strength and toughness of thermally treated steels, primarily by its ability to inhibit grain growth over a fairly broad quenching range. This element also forms strong, stabile carbides. At contents of .04 to .05%, vanadium increases the hardenability of medium-carbon steels with a minimum effect upon grain size. Above this content, insoluble carbides form, and the hardenability effect per unit added decreases with normal quenching temperature. However, increasing the austenitizing temperatures can increase the hardenability of a steel with these higher contents of vanadium. Austenite is a solid solution of carbon and, sometimes, other solutes that can occur as a constituent of steel under certain conditions.

Tungsten

Tungsten, another stabile carbide former, increases wear resistance and red hardness (i.e., the ability to retain hardness at elevated temperatures). Most tungsten alloys are used for applications that require hardness retention at elevated temperatures.

Molybdenum

With the exception of manganese, molybdenum exhibits a greater effect on hardenability *for each unit added* than do the other common alloy elements. Because it is a nonoxidizing element, molybdenum is highly useful in melting steels when close control of hardenability is desired. Molybdenum is unique in the degree to which it increases the high-temperature tensile and creep strengths of steel. Its use also reduces a steel's susceptibility to temper brittleness.

Nickel

Nickel is one of the fundamental alloy elements. When present in appreciable amounts, it improves toughness, particularly at low temperatures; provides a simplified and more economical thermal treatment; increases hardenability; and improves corrosion resistance. Its presence also reduces distortion of the steel during quenching.

Nickel lowers the critical temperatures of steel, widens the temperature range for effective quenching and tempering, and retards the decomposition of austenite. Further, nickel does not form carbides or other compounds that might be difficult to dissolve during heating for

TABLE 11. CHEMICAL COMPOSITION OF TOOL STEELS

CHEMICAL ELEMENT	PERCENTAGE OF CHEMICAL ELEMENTS								
	408	S1	S5	S7	A2	D2	D3	440C	O1
CARBON	.50	.40–.55	.50–.65	.45–.55	.95–1.05	1.40–1.60	2.00–2.35	.95–1.20	.90
MANGANESE	.50	.10–.40	.60–1.00	.20–.80	.00–1.00	.00–.60	.00–.60	.00–1.00	1.20
SILICON	.25	.15–1.20	1.75–2.25	.20–1.00	.00–.50	.00–.60	.00–.60	.00–1.00	.40
CHROMIUM	.75	1.00–1.80	.00–.35	3.00–3.50	4.75–5.50	11.0–13.0	11.0–13.5	16.0–18.0	.50
VANADIUM		.15–.30	.00–.35	.00–.35	.15–.50	.00–1.10	.00–1.00		.20
TUNGSTEN		1.50–3.00					.00–1.00		.20
MOLYBDENUM		.00–.50	.20–1.35	1.30–1.80	.90–1.40	.70–1.20		.00–.75	
NICKEL	3.00							.00–.50	
COBALT						.00–1.00			

© American Pharmaceutical Association

austenitizing. All of these factors contribute to easier and more successful thermal treatment. Nickel's relative insensitivity to variations in quenching conditions is insurance against costly failures to attain the desired properties, particularly when the furnace is not equipped for precision control.

Cobalt

Cobalt is used primarily to increase the red hardness of steel. D2 is the only tool steel that contains this alloy element.

Sulfur and Phosphorous

Sulfur and phosphorous, which are present in almost all steels, are considered to be impurities. Their concentrations in tool steel should not exceed .03 to .05%; greater concentrations will affect the strength of the steel.

Hardness of Tool Steels

The abrasion resistance of a steel usually increases as its hardness increases; conversely, the steel's ductility and toughness decrease. Tooling that exceeds the recommended hardness range may fracture during use, whereas tooling that is too soft may wear rapidly. Punches that are F.F.B.E. or are deeper than the TSM standard concave may require a different hardness for the fragile punch tip than is required for the head and barrel. Secondary tempering of punch tips made from certain steels reduces the hardness of the tip and helps eliminate tip breakage during compression. In this process, the punch tips are subjected to high temperatures and then cooled slowly. Punches made from S7 and D2 steels do not require a

second tempering to produce durable punch tips, whereas punches made from S5 steel are routinely tempered a second time to reduce tip hardness.

The hardness of punches and dies can be checked with a nondestructive tester such as the Rockwell Tester, which determines hardness by measuring the depth to which its steel or diamond points penetrate the surface of the tool steel. The Rockwell Tester has two scales, A and C, for measuring tool hardness. The A scale, which uses a minor weight load to penetrate the steel surface, leaves a small indentation. This superficial testing should be considered for checking fragile punch tips. The more commonly used C scale penetrates the surface more deeply, thereby giving a more accurate reading of the hardness under the surface. The resultant raised surface around the indentation should be removed by blending or polishing the tool before it is used in a press.

Accurate measurements of the tip hardness for shaped punches are very difficult to obtain due to the critical alignment required between the punch supports and the penetrator. Unless the tip has undergone secondary tempering, only the hardness of the barrel needs to be measured for shaped punches. Dirt, grease, scale, and burrs on a tool surface can also alter the final hardness reading. To achieve positive results, tooling surfaces should be cleaned or smoothed before readings are taken.

Because of the limited surface area contact, the Rockwell hardness measurements for diameters or curved surfaces on tooling are lower than the actual hardness. When checking punches with 3/4- or 1-inch barrel diameters, .5 points should be added to the indicated hardness to obtain the actual hardness. Table 12 lists the typical hardness ranges of pharmaceutical tool steels.

TABLE 12. TYPICAL HARDNESS READINGS FOR TOOL STEELS

ITEM	HARDNESS RANGES (Rc)								
	408	S1	S5	S7	A2	D2	D3	440C	O1
PUNCH	48–56	54–56	50–59	54–58	58–60	58–60	58–60	56–58	55–60
DIE					60–62		62–64	56–58	

© American Pharmaceutical Association

Punch Tip Force Ratings

The question tablet manufacturers ask most frequently of tooling suppliers is, "How much tonnage [force] can I use with this cup design without risking punch tip cracking?" Virtually every user of tablet presses has at one time or another been faced with problems related to punch tip fracture. The consequences of tool breakage go well beyond just the cost of replacing the tools. Additional inspection procedures, rejected batches of tablets, and operator and equipment safety concerns are related issues. Two important steps in good tablet production procedures are (1) knowing the force limits for each set of tooling used in production operations and (2) properly setting and maintaining that limit on the press overload mechanism.

Historically, most press suppliers and tooling manufacturers developed their own charts and graphs for determining the allowable compression force for various punch tip designs. Initially, this information was limited to round concave and F.F.B.E. tooling. As shaped tooling became more prominent, techniques for translating the data for round tooling to other configurations, such as capsules and ovals, were formulated. The resultant punch tip pressure guides were, at best, only a rough approximation of the force capacity for shaped punches. Tooling users found the published figures to be too conservative in many cases and too high in others.

Today, advanced desktop computer hardware and sophisticated stress analysis software, which are capable of modeling complex shapes, have enabled tooling designers to calculate punch tip force ratings for all tablet shapes with a high degree of accuracy. The punch tip force ratings for TSM round tooling listed in Table 13 (see page 74) were derived using a finite element analysis (FEA) to model exact cup designs. From the FEA of hundreds of capsules and ovals, a calculation method for determining the force ratings of shaped tooling was derived. This method can also be used to calculate tip force rating for nonstandard sizes of round tooling. Although the calculations required for capsules and ovals take a little more time than simply looking up the force rating in a table, the greater accuracy of the resultant force rating is well worth the investment.

The maximum recommended compression forces in this manual are based on the fatigue limit for S5 tool steel. These values may be increased by 10% for S1 or S7 steel; however, the values should be reduced by 15% for D2, D3, and 440C steels.

Punch Tip Force Ratings for Oval, Round, and Capsule-Shaped Tooling

Because the cup's minor axis (width), major axis (length), and configuration can vary greatly in capsule- and oval-shaped tooling, the compression force rating for this type of tooling cannot be covered by simple charts. However, extensive analysis has shown that the maximum allowable pressure (i.e., force per unit area) that can be exerted on the punch face for oval and capsule shapes is strongly related to a cup shape factor. This factor is defined as the ratio of the cup depth to the minor axis dimension. The compression force rating is then computed by multiplying the allowable pressure associated with the calculated shape factor by the cross-sectional area of the punch tip. Calculating compression force ratings for shaped tooling comprises four major steps.

Step 1: Calculate the Shape Factor
For rounds, capsules, and ovals with a single cup radius, the shape factor *SF* is found by dividing the cup depth *D* by the width *W* (see Illustrations 1 and 2).

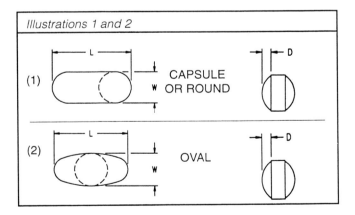

Illustrations 1 and 2

(1) CAPSULE OR ROUND

(2) OVAL

For ovals with a compound cup on the minor axis (see Illustration 3), the minor radius is used to determine the equivalent cup depth *De* and width *We*. (A compound cup is a cup design with two or more radii per axis.) As indicated by the phantom circle on Illustration 3, this

© American Pharmaceutical Association

TABLE 13. PUNCH TIP COMPRESSION FORCES FOR TSM ROUND TOOLING

PUNCH TIP DIA.		COMPRESSION FORCE BY CUP DEPTH (IN KILONEWTONS)						
		SHALLOW CONCAVE	STANDARD CONCAVE	DEEP CONCAVE	EXTRA-DEEP CONCAVE	MODIFIED BALL	F.F.B.E.	F.F.R.E.
1/8	[3.175]	5.0	3.5	2.6	2.0	1.2	3.5	3.5
5/32	[3.970]	7.5	5.0	4.0	3.4	1.9	5.2	5.4
3/16	[4.763]	11.0	7.5	6.0	5.0	2.8	7.2	7.7
7/32	[5.555]	15.5	10.5	7.5	7.0	3.7	9.5	10.5
1/4	[6.350]	20.0	14.0	10.5	10.0	4.8	12.5	13.7
9/32	[7.142]	25.0	18.0	15.0	13.0	6.0	14.5	17.3
5/16	[7.938]	31.0	23.0	19.5	16.0	7.5	17.5	21.0
11/32	[8.730]	38.0	29.0	24.0	19.5	9.0	21.0	26.0
3/8	[9.525]	45.0	36.0	30.0	23.0	11.0	24.0	31.0
13/32	[10.318]	53.0	42.0	36.0	27.0	13.0	27.0	36.0
7/16	[11.113]	61.0	49.0	43.0	32.0	16.5	31.0	42.0
15/32	[11.905]	70.0	58.0	50.0	36.0	17.0	36.0	48.0
1/2	[12.700]	80.0	66.0	57.0	42.0	19.5	41.0	54.0
17/32	[13.493]	91.0	75.0	65.0	47.0	22.0	46.0	61.0
9/16	[14.288]	100.0	85.0	74.0	53.0	25.0	52.0	69.0
19/32	[15.080]	113.0	95.0	83.0	59.0	27.0	58.0	77.0
5/8	[15.875]	125.0	106.0	93.0	65.0	30.0	64.0	85.0
11/16	[17.463]	151.0	129.0	114.0	79.0	37.0	68.0	103.0
3/4	[19.050]	181.0	154.0	137.0	94.0	44.0	81.0	122.0
13/16	[20.638]	211.0	182.0	162.0	110.0	51.0	95.0	144.0
7/8	[22.225]	245.0	212.0	188.0	128.0	59.0	110.0	167.0
15/16	[23.813]	281.0	244.0	218.0	146.0	68.0	127.0	191.0
1	[25.400]	320.0	278.0	249.0	166.0	77.0	144.0	217.0

1. THE GIVEN TIP DIAMETERS AND CUP DEPTHS (SHALLOW, STANDARD, ETC.) CORRESPOND TO THE TSM CONFIGURATIONS IN TABLE 10 (SEE PAGE 68). FOR OTHER CUP DEPTHS AND TIP DIAMETERS, THE CALCULATION METHOD FOR ROUNDS, OVALS, AND CAPSULES SHOULD BE USED.

2. THESE FIGURES SHOULD BE USED ONLY AS A GUIDE.

3. TO CONVERT THE KILONEWTON RATINGS TO U.S. TONS (2,000 LB), DIVIDE BY 8.896.

4. TO CONVERT THE ABOVE RATINGS TO LONG TONS (2,240 LB), DIVIDE BY 10.

5. EMBOSSING CAN GIVE RISE TO AREAS OF SIGNIFICANT STRESS CONCENTRATION ON A PUNCH FACE. IT IS SUGGESTED THAT THE COMPRESSION FORCES BE REDUCED BY 20% (MULTIPLIED BY .80) FOR TOOLING WITH EMBOSSING.

© American Pharmaceutical Association

procedure can also be used to determine De and We for rounds with a compound cup. These dimensions can be determined graphically by extending the minor radius until it intersects the plane of the land, as shown, and then using a scale to measure De and We.

If the location of the center of the minor radius is known, De and We can also be calculated directly as follows:

$De = R - Y$,

where R equals the cup radius, and Y equals the distance from the center of the minor radius to the land.

$We = 2X$,

where X equals the distance from the center of the minor radius to the outside edge of the tablet.

Dividing De by We gives the SF for this configuration.

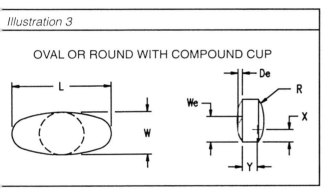

Illustration 3

OVAL OR ROUND WITH COMPOUND CUP

Step 2: Determine the Maximum Allowable Pressure

Table 14 (see pages 76 and 77) lists the allowable cup face pressures for various shape factors. The maximum allowable pressure P is obtained by correlating the SF value with the appropriate value for allowable pressure in Table 14. For cross-sectional areas given in inches, P is expressed as units of pounds per square inch (lb/in²). Accordingly, for cross-sectional areas given in millimeters, P is expressed as units of kilonewtons per square millimeter (kN/mm²).

> NOTE: This procedure can also be used to calculate compression force ratings for round tooling not covered in Table 13.

Step 3: Calculate the Punch Tip Cross-Sectional Area

Cross-sectional area A can be calculated using the formulas listed below. Width W and length L dimensions should be given in inches or millimeters.

For round tooling:
$A = .785\,(W^2)$

For capsule-shaped tooling:
$A = .785\,(W^2) + W\,(L - W)$

For oval-shaped tooling:
$A = .785\,WL$

This formula yields exact values for round and capsule shapes. The values calculated for ovals are an approximation and are usually within 5% of the true cross-sectional area; any errors are on the conservative side (i.e., calculated value is less than actual area). Exact values for ovals can be obtained from tooling suppliers.

Step 4: Calculate the Compression Force Rating

The compression force rating F for the punch tip is now determined by multiplying the maximum allowable pressure P by the cross-sectional area A.

$F\,(\text{lb}) = P\,(\text{lb/in}^2) \times A\,(\text{in}^2)$, or

$F\,(\text{kn}) = P\,(\text{kN/mm}^2) \times A\,(\text{mm}^2)$

> NOTE: The calculated force ratings apply to S5 steels. These values should be *increased* by 10% for S1 or S7 steel and *decreased* by 15% for D2, D3, and 440C steels. Further, embossing can give rise to areas of significant stress concentration on the punch face. For engraved tooling, the calculated force ratings should be reduced by 20% (multiplied by .80).

Sample Calculations of Compression Force Ratings

The Compression Force for a Capsule-Shaped Cup (see Illustration 4) is calculated as follows.

TABLE 14. PUNCH TIP PRESSURE RATINGS VERSUS SHAPE FACTORS
(FOR ROUND, CAPSULE, OVAL, AND COMPOUND-CUP OVAL TOOLING)

SHAPE FACTOR (SF)	ALLOWABLE PRESSURE (LB/IN²)	ALLOWABLE PRESSURE (kN/MM²)
.000	110,000	.758
.005	108,000	.745
.010	105,500	.727
.015	103,000	.710
.020	101,000	.696
.025	98,500	.679
.030	96,500	.665
.035	94,500	.652
.040	92,500	.638
.045	90,500	.624
.050	88,500	.610
.055	86,500	.596
.060	84,500	.583
.065	82,600	.569
.070	80,800	.557
.075	79,100	.545
.080	77,400	.534
.085	75,800	.523
.090	74,200	.512
.095	72,650	.501
.100	71,100	.490
.105	69,550	.480
.110	68,000	.469
.115	66,500	.458
.120	65,000	.448
.125	63,600	.438
.130	62,300	.430
.135	61,000	.421
.140	59,700	.412
.145	58,400	.403
.150	57,100	.394
.155	55,900	.385
.160	54,700	.377
.165	53,600	.370
.170	52,500	.362

NOTE: THESE FIGURES SHOULD BE USED ONLY AS A GUIDE.

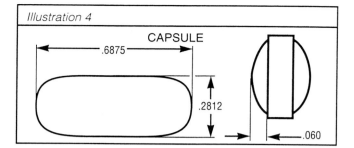

Illustration 4

1. Calculate shape factor:
$SF = D/W$
$SF = .060/.2812 = .213$

2. Determine maximum allowable pressure:
Correlate the SF of .213 with its corresponding maximum allowable pressure in Table 14; in this example, P equals 43,000 lb/in² (value is interpolated).

3. Calculate punch tip cross-sectional area:
$A = .785(W^2) + W(L - W)$
$A = .785(.2812)^2 + (.2812)(.6875 - .2812)$
$A = .176$ in²

4. Calculate compression force rating:
$F = P \times A$
$F = (43,000 \text{ lb/in}^2)(.176) = 7,568$ lb [34 kN]

The Compression Force for a Compound Cup (see Illustration 5) is calculated as follows.

1. Calculate shape factor:
$SF = De/We$
$SF = .063/.188 = .335$

For this cup configuration, We and De are determined graphically by extending the minor radius R until it intersects the plane of the land; De and We are then measured. If the location of the center of the minor cup radius relative to the outside edge of the tablet is known, the De and We can be calculated as follows:

$De = R - Y = .093 - .030 = .063$
$We = 2X = 2(.094) = .188$
$SF = De/We = .063/.188 = .335$

2. Determine maximum allowable pressure:
Correlate the SF of .335 with its corresponding maximum allowable pressure in Table 14; in this example, P equals 18,500 lb/in².

© American Pharmaceutical Association

. Calculate punch tip cross-sectional area:
$A = .785 (WL)$
$A = (.785) (.312) (.625) = .153$ in²

. Calculate compression force rating:
$F = P \times A$
$F = (18,500$ lb/in²$) (.153$ in²$) = 2,830$ lb [13 kN]

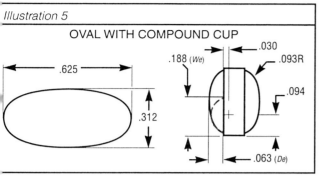

Illustration 5

OVAL WITH COMPOUND CUP

'atigue Failure of Punch Tips

ne failure of machine components subjected to repeat-
l loading cycles is known as fatigue failure. At stress
vels close to the ultimate stress limit of a material,
tigue failure may occur after only a few hundred load-
g cycles. Conversely, stress levels below approxi-
ately 50% of the ultimate stress limit will usually
low an infinite number of loading events to take place
ithout failure occurring. The stress level that provides
rtually indefinite life is known as the endurance, or
tigue, limit of the material.

gure 36 on page 79 shows a generalized stress versus
cle-life curve for a high-strength tool steel. Close
amination of the characteristic fatigue curves for fer-
us materials, such as tool steels, reveals several
portant points about fatigue failure. First, the
durance limit corresponds to a cycle life in the neigh-
rhood of one to four million loading cycles. Unless
e operating stress level is known in advance for a par-
ular component, at least one million loading events
e needed to assess whether the design is adequate for
e working environment. In the case of tablet tooling,
e quantity of tablets made during the research and
velopment stages is rarely sufficient to meet this cri-
rion. As a result, problems associated with punch tip

TABLE 14. (CONTINUED)

SHAPE FACTOR (SF)	ALLOWABLE PRESSURE (LB/IN²)	ALLOWABLE PRESSURE (kN/MM²)
.175	51,400	.354
.180	50,300	.347
.185	49,200	.339
.190	47,750	.329
.195	46,650	.322
.200	45,550	.314
.209	44,450	.306
.210	43,500	.300
.215	42,500	.293
.220	41,500	.286
.225	40,500	.279
.230	39,500	.272
.235	38,500	.265
.240	37,500	.259
.245	36,500	.252
.250	35,500	.245
.255	34,500	.238
.260	33,500	.231
.265	32,500	.224
.270	31,500	.217
.275	30,500	.210
.280	29,500	.203
.285	28,500	.196
.290	27,500	.190
.295	26,500	.183
.300	25,500	.176
.305	24,500	.169
.310	23,500	.162
.315	22,500	.155
.320	21,500	.148
.325	20,500	.141
.330	19,500	.134
.335	18,500	.128
.340	17,500	.121
.345	16,500	.114
.350	15,500	.107

NOTE: THESE FIGURES SHOULD BE USED ONLY AS A GUIDE.

breakage usually do not become apparent until long after a product enters the manufacturing stage.

Another point to consider from an analysis of fatigue curves is the logarithmic relationship between stress and cycle life. A 25% reduction in stress, for instance, results in a tenfold increase in tooling life. Punch breakage is usually the result of stress levels that exceed the maximum allowable limit for infinite life by less than 20%. For this reason, only relatively minor design changes to the punch cup are needed to eliminate fatigue failure.

Finally, fatigue damage is cumulative. When a part is over-stressed, the microscopic damage inflicted reduces the useful life of that part by a percentage approximately equal to the number of cycles accumulated at that stress level divided by the predicted cycle life from the fatigue curve. Intermittent periods of excessive stress followed by long periods of stress levels below the fatigue limit can extend the time to failure well beyond the range of one to four million cycles. This explains why some tooling sets produce hundreds of millions of tablets before the tools crack.

© American Pharmaceutical Association

FIGURE 36. STRESS VERSUS CYCLE LIFE FOR TOOL STEEL

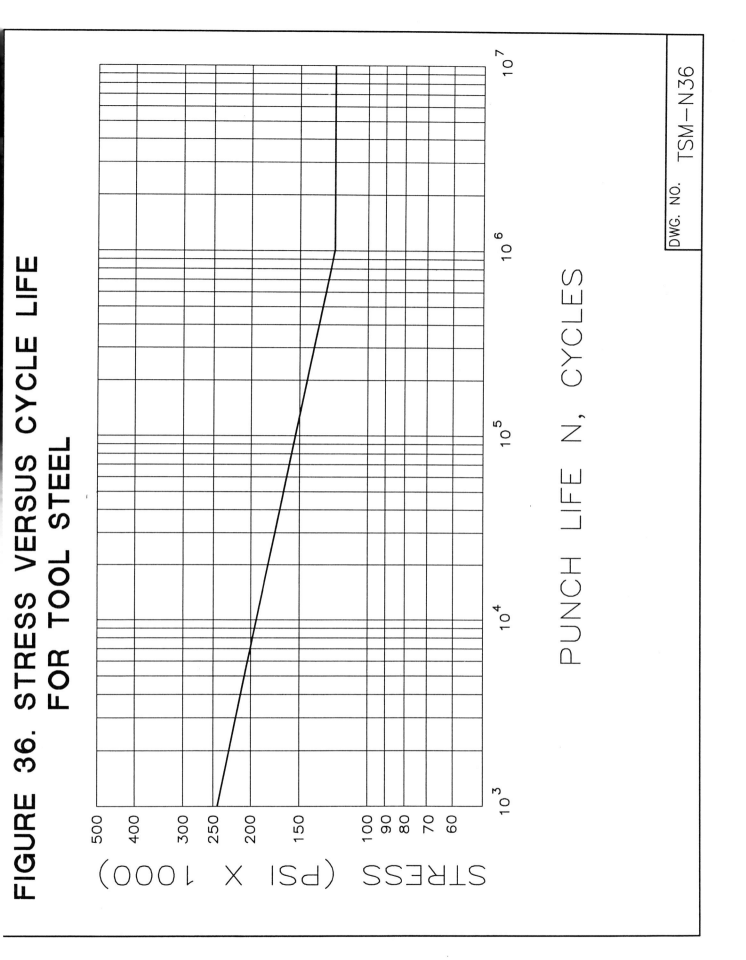

DWG. NO. TSM—N36

© American Pharmaceutical Association

Notes:

© American Pharmaceutical Association

Tooling Procurement, Inspection, and Maintenance

o processes are more important to producing the esired quantity and quality of tablets than the proper rocurement, inspection, and maintenance of tablet oling. Every tablet manufacturing division should tablish standard operating procedures (SOP) for these ocesses.

Standard Operating Procedures

he TSM Committee offers the following procedures as guide in setting up a SOP program and does not imply at any such program should consist of or be limited to e information presented here. These guidelines can be ilored to meet the needs of individual manufacturing visions.

Tablet and Tooling Directory

tablet and tooling directory should be developed, aintained, and made available to all personnel volved in decisions or procedures that affect tablet anufacturing. Such a directory provides documenta- on control, serves as a communication aid, and is a ocurement reference. Specifically, the directory is a st of tablet products and the punches used to produce em. The directory should include:

- Name of product
- Product embossed code
- Product number
- Tablet size (not thickness) and shape
- Punch position (upper or lower)
- Punch embossing
- Tablet drawing number
- Tablet drawing revision number
- Tooling supplier drawing number
- Directory revision date

The information for the upper and lower punches should be placed on separate lines because the upper and lower faces of a tablet often carry different emboss- ing. If the punch is not a B-type, this should also be noted in the directory. The directory is a ready source of information for the "Sample Tablet Tooling Approval Form" (see Figure 37, page 82).

Control of Tooling Drawings

A single group or department should be responsible for maintaining master files and issuing copies of all tablet and tooling drawings. This group participates in the process of approving tooling drawings. Specific steps in the process include the following:

- Establish a suggested procedure for approving drawings that includes, at a minimum, review and approval of all drawings by the production and quality assurance departments, as well as the appropriate engineering, marketing, and regulatory affairs departments.
- Establish a master file that consists of the original tablet, tooling, and/or hob drawings with the appro- priate approval signatures.
- Keep a listing of all copies of approved drawings in satellite files. If the drawings are modified or elimi- nated, copies of earlier drawings should be collect- ed and destroyed.

Procurement of Tooling

Use of the "Quote/Order Form" (see Figure 38, page 83) for tooling will ensure that the essential items have been specified on each purchase order. The purchase order should include, but not be limited to:

- Respective tablet/tooling drawing number(s) or hob number(s)
- Identification number(s) to be engraved/imprinted on each tool (These numbers provide a method of maintaining records.)

FIGURE 37.   SAMPLE TABLET TOOLING APPROVAL FORM

TO: MANUFACTURING AND/OR TECHNICAL SERVICE MANAGER(S)

FROM: COMPANY OR INDIVIDUAL PRODUCT AND/OR TOOLING COORDINATOR

SUBJECT: TABLET TOOLING APPROVAL FOR PRODUCT(S)

APPROVAL OF: DRAWING(S) [   ]   HOB(S) [   ]

TOOLING SUPPLIER: _____   PURCHASE ORDER: _____

The following new tooling drawing(s) and hob(s) are approved:

PRODUCT STRENGTH, SIZE & SHAPE	PUNCH EMBOSSING POSITION	USER DRAWING NO.	SUPPLIER DRAWING NO.
XXXXX, 50 MG. 5/16 DIA.	UPPER: ZZZ 102	B-NNNNN-R	P-ABCW-EX
XXXXX, 50 MG. 5/16 DIA.	LOWER: XXXXX	B-NNNNN-R	P-ABCX-EX
YYYYY, .5 GM. .281 x .718 CAPSULE	UPPER: ZZZ 501(S)	B-NNNNN-R	P-ABCY-EX
YYYYY, .5 GM. .281 x .718 CAPSULE	LOWER: YYYYY	B-NNNNN-R	P-ABCZ-EX

Name _____

Title _____

Phone No./FAX No. _____

cc: Manufacturing Manager, Technical Service or Engineering Manager (if not listed above), Purchasing, Tooling Procurement Initiator (if not listed above), Tooling Supplier

1. (S) means the tablet is scored.
2. The information in the table should be included in any notice of tooling approvals sent to the supplier.

© American Pharmaceutical Association

FIGURE 38. QUOTE/ORDER FORM

_____ DATE _____ P.O. NO. _____

Company _____

Address _____

_____

User Contact _____

Phone No. _____ Fax No. _____

Previous Order Ref. No. _____

Required Date _____   Shipping ☐ Standard ☐ Overnight

Press Model No. _____ No. of Stations _____

Tooling Size ☐ B Size ☐ D Size ☐ Other _____

Punch Mat. ☐ Stand. ☐ Prem. ☐ Other _____

Die Mat. ☐ Prem. ☐ Lined W/C ☐ Other _____

Availability Of Samples ☐ Tools ☐ Dwgs. ☐ Tablets

Upper Tablet Face Dwg. No. _____

Upper Punch (quantity) _____ Price _____

Tooling Replacement ☐   New ☐

Embossed ☐
Plain ☐
Bisect Line ☐

Description

Lower Tablet Face Dwg. No. _____

Lower Punch (quantity) _____ Price _____

Tooling Replacement ☐   New ☐

Embossed ☐
Plain ☐
Bisect Line ☐

Description

Tablet Shape/Size (circle one)

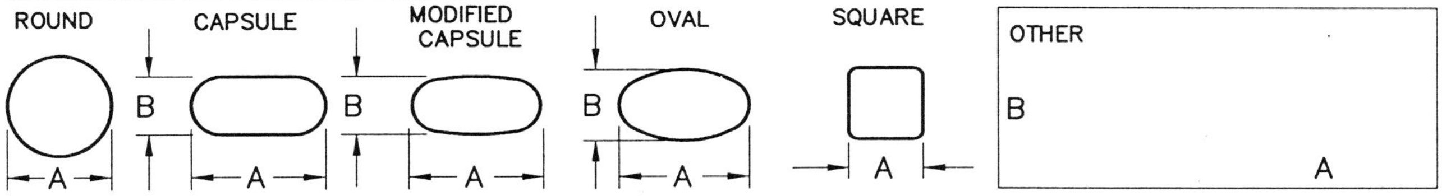

ROUND CAPSULE MODIFIED CAPSULE OVAL SQUARE OTHER

DIM.A _____ DIM.B _____

Tablet Profile (circle one)

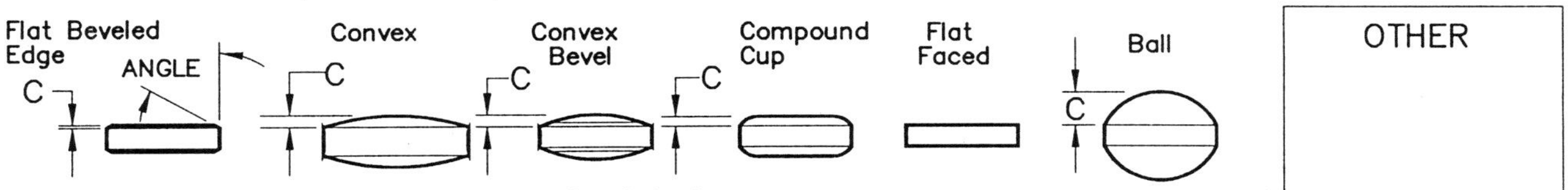

Flat Beveled Edge ANGLE Convex Convex Bevel Compound Cup Flat Faced Ball OTHER

Cup Depth C= _____ Land= _____ Bevel Angle= _____

Product Name _____

Existing ☐   New ☐
Film—Coated ☐   Sticky ☐
Abrasive ☐   Corrosive ☐

Tool Marking Requirements

Punches _____
Dies _____
_____

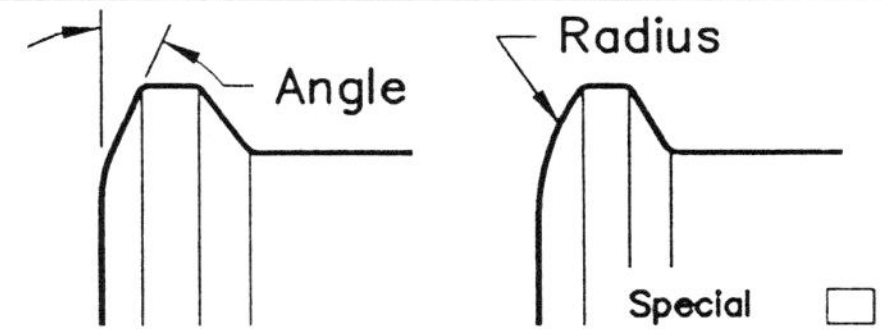

Angle   Radius

T.S.M. Head ☐   T.S.M. Semi—Domed ☐   Special ☐

DIE INFO.	EXTRA OPTIONS	KEYS	KEY ORIENTATION

Die Quantity _____

Die Size
.945 ☐
1.1875 ☐
1.500 ☐

DIE GROOVE PROTECTION
RADIUS ☐   SHOULDER ☐

Polished Heads ☐   Chrome Tips ☐
Tip Relief on Lower ☐   Chrome Other ☐
Bakelite Relief on Lower ☐   _____
Tapered Dies_ (+.003 on Dia.3/16 Deep)
1 End_ ☐   2 Ends_ ☐

Woodruff ☐
Hi—Pro ☐
Parallel ☐
Screw—in Key ☐
Secondary Key Slot ☐

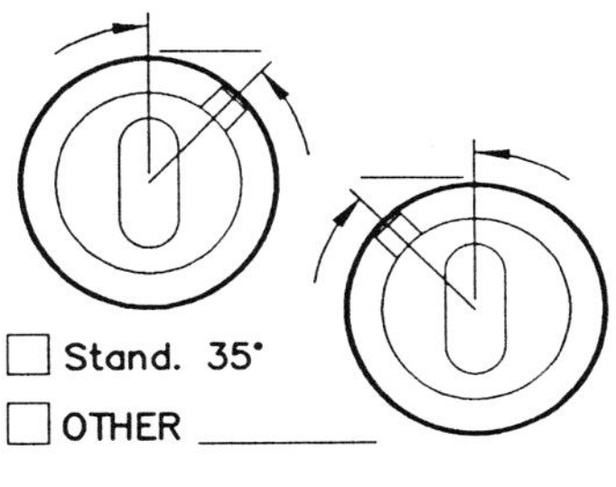

☐ Stand. 35°
☐ OTHER _____

(THIS FORM MAY BE COPIED)

© American Pharmaceutical Association

- Logo description and punch orientation, if applicable
- Punch and die size
- Type of tooling design: TSM, European, etc.
- Steel type for punches and dies
- Make and model of tablet press
- Number of tooling stations on the tablet press (It is recommended that the quantity on each order include 10% or more extra punches and 5–10% extra dies.)
- Punch and die materials
- Type of punch key, if applicable
- Tooling options (i.e., chrome punch tips, tapered dies, etc.)

> **NOTE:** Interchanging shaped punches and dies made by different manufacturers is not a good practice. If a punch is ordered for use with another manufacturer's die, the punch supplier will request a sample of the die to check the fit of the tools.

Initial Inspection of Tooling

Upon receipt of a set of tablet tooling, the following inspection could be considered for all or a portion of the tools received. The dimensions should be documented on a preprinted form, such as Figure 39. As part of the routine maintenance of tooling, this inspection should be repeated periodically and documented accordingly.

- Inspect the logo for accuracy, size, and, if applicable, position.
- Measure tooling according to the instructions in the discussions of "Measuring Punches" and "Die Measurements" on pages 88–91 and 98–99, respectively.
- Perform a hardness test on a percentage of the punches and dies to ensure that the specified hardness has been achieved. (See Table 12 and the discussion of "Hardness of Tool Steels" on page 72.)

Storage of Tooling

Each set of tooling should be identified and stored separately in an environment that is controlled to prevent oxidation and subsequent rusting. See the discussion of "Storage of Tooling," presented on the last page of this section.

Disbursement and Usage of Tooling

When disbursing a set of tooling, the following procedures should be considered and documented accordingly on a preprinted form, such as the sample form in Figure 40 on page 86.

- Visually inspect the appropriate set of tooling to ensure that the tooling is not damaged and that a sufficient number of tools are available for the press in which they are to be used.
- Examine the tools to ensure a proper fit between the upper and lower punches and the respective die.
- Document the product name, strength, and code number of the material to be compressed.
- Document the identification number of the press on which the tools are to be used.
- Document the identification number(s) of the individual batches that are compressed with the tooling.
- Calculate and document the current status of the standard that is used to determine the periodical inspection of the tooling (i.e., number of batches, number of tablets produced, etc.).

Maintenance of Tooling

The following is a general list of the steps taken to maintain tooling. The discussion of "Punch and Die Maintenance" on the following pages gives step-by-step instructions for these important procedures.

- Clean per approved procedures, and inspect for wear or damage those tooling sets used in press runs.
- Refurbish worn or damaged tools per approved procedures.
- Discard and document accordingly tools that are worn or damaged beyond repair. Deface identifiable markings on any discarded tool.
- Measure a tool selected to replace a discarded one to ensure a proper fit with the remaining tools in that set. All tooling should meet TSM specifications.
- Periodically inspect tooling and document the results as specified earlier in the discussion of "Initial Inspection of Tooling."

4

© American Pharmaceutical Association

FIGURE 39. PUNCH AND DIE INSPECTION SHEET

PRODUCT NUMBER	PRODUCT NAME		CODE

	UPPER PUNCH		LOWER PUNCH	
DWG. No.	EMBOSSING/BISECT	DWG. No.	EMBOSSING/BISECT	

TYPE OF TOOLING	☐ ROUND ☐ ODDSHAPED ☐ FLAT FACE BEVELED EDGE ☐ FLAT FACE ☐ CONCAVE ☐ OTHER _____

TOOLING SUPPLIER	P.O. No.	MACHINE TYPE USED ON	TOOLING TYPE ☐ NEW ☐ REPLACEMENT

HOB APPROVAL (NEW) PUNCH TIP & IMAGE SLUG VS DRAWING OR OVERLAY	UPPER ☐ ACCEPT ☐ REJECT	LOWER ☐ ACCEPT ☐ REJECT	APPROVALS/DATE	
			TECH. SERVICE	MFTG

	UPPER		LOWER		DIE		COMMENTS
	ACC.	REJ.	ACC.	REJ.	ACC.	REJ.	
HARDNESS Barrel 10%							
EMBOSSING vs DRAWING OR OVERLAY 100%							
FACE & SURFACE DEFECTS Nicks, pits, cracks 100%							
WORKING LENGTH Indicator 100%							
OVERALL LENGTH Indicator 100%							
KEY FIT/KEY TO HEAD Go/No Go 100%							
TIP CONCENTRICITY Indicator 100%							
HEAD Go/No Go 100%							
PUNCH BARREL O.D. Go/No Go 100%							
PUNCH TIP SIZE Micrometer 100%							
TIP TO BARREL Over all vs MAX. w/or w/o Chamfer 100%							

DIES	DIE		COMMENTS	DIES	DIE		COMMENTS
	ACC.	REJ.			ACC.	REJ.	
O.D. Micrometer 100%				3/16" RADIUS AND EDGE PROTECTION			
I.D. Punch Tip or Bore Gage 100%				DIE CONCENTRICITY O.D.			
CHAMFER I.D. Hand Comparator 100%				DIE SQUARENESS			
HEIGHT Micrometer 100%				INSPECTOR		DATE	

TOOLING APPROVALS		
MANUFACTURING	QUALITY CONTROL (NEW)	TECH. SERVICE (NEW)

© American Pharmaceutical Association   (THIS FORM MAY BE COPIED)   85

FIGURE 40. TABLET TOOLING USAGE AND REPAIR CARD

PRODUCT/STRENGTH	
PRODUCT No.	
DATE RECEIVED	
VENDOR NAME	
DRAWING No.	TOP
	BOTTOM

DIE SIZE		QUANTITY
UPPER (UP)		QUANTITY
LOWER (LP)		QUANTITY
SHAPE		TABLETS/BATCH

LOCATION	
SET No.	
CARD No.	

ISSUES

DATE	BATCH	MACHINE No.	UP-LP-DIE	ISSUED TO

RETURNS

DATE	UP-LP-DIE	RETURN BY	AUTH. BY

DESTRUCTION

DATE	No./TYPE	DESTROY BY	VERIFY BY	REASON	COMMENTS

(THIS FORM MAY BE COPIED)

© American Pharmaceutical Association

Punch and Die Maintenance

Proper maintenance is the most important factor in maximizing the life of punches and dies. Maintaining tooling also minimizes many compression problems such as variations in tablet weight and thickness, and picking, sticking, or capping of tablets. The cost of maintenance equipment and the time spent in maintaining tooling will be amply recovered by the savings realized in prolonged tooling life and reduced incidence of problems during tablet production.

The person responsible for tooling maintenance must be conscientious, adaptable, and, most importantly, fully trained in the techniques of handling and polishing tooling. A person with basic mechanical knowledge is ideal for the job; however, previous engineering knowledge is not essential.

The following instructions for maintaining punches and dies cover the most common polishing techniques; the supporting illustrations apply mainly to B- and D-type tooling. These techniques along with the appropriate modifications to equipment, if required, can be applied to other tooling types.

A record of the polishing of tooling and inspection of tooling dimensions is an excellent aid in determining when to purchase backup sets of tooling, thereby reducing the risk of downtime in tablet production. (See Figure 39, "Punch and Die Inspection Sheet.")

> Although the techniques for punch and die maintenance described in this manual have been used successfully, the TSM Committee has no control over their application and, therefore, cannot accept liability arising from their use.

Cleaning Tooling

Punches and dies removed from the press should be cleaned and inspected before any maintenance is performed. An ultrasonic bath is ideal for cleaning tooling. If another system is used, the liquid cleaner should be nontoxic and should not cause rust. After cleaning, tooling must be handled carefully to prevent moisture from the operator's fingers remaining on the tooling and causing rust.

This section describes all aspects of punch and die maintenance; however, only the operations that bring tooling to an acceptable running condition should be performed. Because the operations are abrasive in nature, excessive or unnecessary maintenance will reduce tooling life. After all repair work is done, tooling should be cleaned again by the described method.

Safety Procedures

Before proceeding with the actual maintenance of tooling, the following safety procedures should be noted.

- DO wear safety glasses at all times.
- DO maintenance procedures in good lighting.
- DO the work according to the maintenance manual and training that have been provided.
- DO protect yourself from sharp punch edges and keyway slots.
- DO use all provided safety guards.
- DO secure loose clothing, hair, and jewelry.
- DO ensure that tools are securely and squarely clamped before turning on a machine.
- DO use cotton wool to clean rotating punches.
- DO NOT leave chuck keys in a motorized chuck.
- DO NOT apply excessive pressure to polishing bobs; slipping may occur.
- DO NOT use cloths to wipe punches clean while punches are rotating.
- DO NOT use a chuck without the guard in place.
- DO NOT wear gloves when operating moving components.

Typical Maintenance Equipment

The following equipment is used for general cleaning and polishing of tooling and for tooling repairs, such as removing burrs, chips, and bruises.

A motorized polishing chuck with a magnetic brake is used for general cleaning and polishing of plain concave punches and for cleaning of die bores (see Illustration 1). The motor is fitted with a backplate and a 5-inch, standard three-jaw chuck, which is gear scrolled and self-centering.

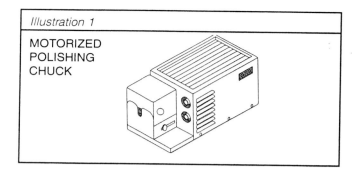

Illustration 1

MOTORIZED POLISHING CHUCK

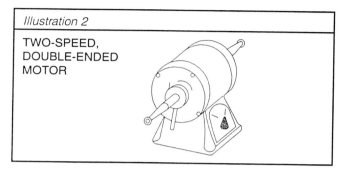

Illustration 2

TWO-SPEED, DOUBLE-ENDED MOTOR

Collet-type lathes are also very effective for cleaning and polishing tooling.

A two-speed, double-ended motor is used to polish and debur F.F.B.E., shaped, and embossed punch tips, including the breaklines (see Illustration 2). The motor can be supplied with two standard adapters for nylon brushes and an adapter for a brass-wheel type brush.

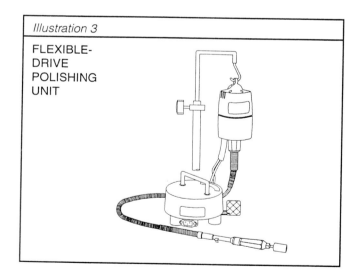

Illustration 3

FLEXIBLE-DRIVE POLISHING UNIT

A flexible-drive polishing unit is used with a motorized polishing chuck to polish plain concave punches, large F.F.B.E. punches, and die bores (see Illustration 3). The flexible-drive unit has a motor, handpiece, and stand from which the unit is suspended.

An air-driven hand-held polisher is an alternative to the flexible-drive polishing unit. The hand-help polisher requires an air supply of 80 psi/6 bar.

Maintenance Materials

The following materials are commonly used in maintaining and handling punches and dies. Variations of listed materials may also be considered.

Materials used with motorized polishing chucks and flexible-drive polishing units include:

- Radius gauges (inch and/or metric sizes)
- Felt bobs (various sizes)
- Nylon brushes
- Diamond-polishing compound (grades from 0–2 microns to 8–12 microns)

Materials used with double-ended polishing motors include:

- Nylon brushes (wheel-type or pencil-type)
- 2-inch brass brushes (wheel-type)
- Polishing paste or compounds

Additional materials used in the maintenance and handling of punches and dies include:

- Lapping sticks (various sizes)
- Cotton wool
- Self-adhesive, fine emery sheet (600-grit)
- Self-adhesive, fine emery sheet (320-grit)
- Medium emery cloth strip (180-grit)
- Coarse emery cloth strip (80-grit)
- Scotchbrite sheet
- Arkansas stone
- Magnifying glass
- V blocks
- Corrugated PVC strips
- Length gauge

Handling Punches

The most important factor in tooling maintenance is appreciating the delicate nature of punch tips. Although a punch tip is designed to withstand several tons of pressure in a press, it is very easily damaged by the slightest contact with a hard surface. Therefore, a punch tip should never come in contact with (1) any part of

© American Pharmaceutical Association

other punch, whether in the press, on a bench, or in storage; (2) any part of the press; (3) any metal tools or equipment such as a vice, polishing unit, etc.; and (4) any part of a metal storage container.

Many punches and dies are damaged beyond repair each year by mechanical damage (e.g., bruising and chipping) while they are out of the press. This unnecessarily high cost could be reduced, or even eliminated, if the maintenance operator imagines the punch tips to be made of glass and treats them accordingly. Using strips of corrugated PVC sheets, of the type used for roofing materials, to segregate punches during handling and maintenance prevents them from rolling into each other or off the bench (see Illustration 4). The PVC strips are 5.06 inches [130 millimeters] wide and have a 1.19-inch [30-millimeter] profile. Using racks or storage boxes can also reduce damage.

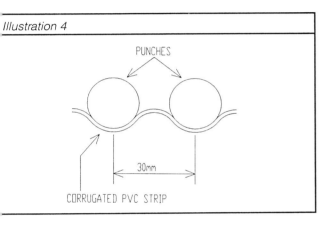

Illustration 4

Maintenance personnel should be discouraged from wiping punch tip faces with their fingers. Fingerprints on clean punches often cause corrosion, which is very difficult to remove.

Measuring Punches

Maintaining working lengths of punches within a specified range is critical to avoiding problems in tablet production. Excessive deviations from TSM standards for tip-to-barrel concentricity, tip sizes, and tip radii can result in damaged tooling and poor-quality tablets.

Checking tooling dimensions is recommended as part of routine maintenance procedures. The following

equipment used to check these dimensions is shown in Illustrations 5 and 6:

• Comparator
• Pointed brass anvil
• Ball anvil
• Length gauge
• Appropriate punch holder (B- or D-type)
• Vertically held V block, used in place of a punch holder (see Illustration 8)
• Micrometer (see Illustration 9)
• "Go-No Go" Gauge (see Illustration 10)

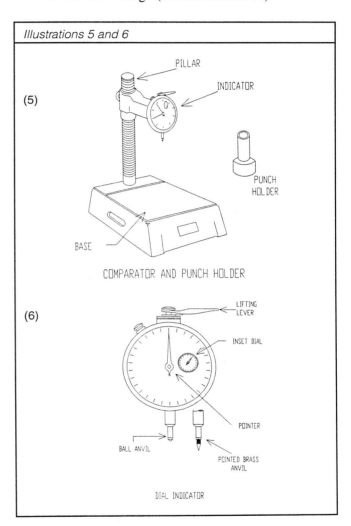

Illustrations 5 and 6

Setting Up the Comparator

The comparator is used to measure overall length, working length, and tip-to-barrel concentricity of a punch. An optical comparator with overlays can also be used to check head profiles, tip profiles, and overall length. The described steps for setting up the comparator should be followed carefully.

1. Fit appropriate anvil into dial indicator on the comparator.

   NOTE: The pointed brass anvil is used for punches with embossing or bisect lines and for punches with small tips and deep concavities. The ball anvil is used for flat and plain concave punches (see Illustration 6).

2. Place the length gauge on the comparator base under the dial indicator anvil, while depressing the lifting lever.
3. Move the dial indicator unit on the pillar until it makes contact with the length gauge.
4. Continue to move the indicator until the pointer has made a sufficient revolution of the dial to measure the appropriate depth of the punch concavity or bevel; then set the indicator to zero.

   NOTE: The number of revolutions of the pointer will be shown on the small inset dial (see Illustration 6).

5. Remove length gauge.

Measuring Overall Length

1. Place punch in holder with tip in recessed end and head pointing up.
2. Place holder on base of comparator; depress lifting lever to raise anvil; and slide punch and holder under the anvil.
3. Lower the anvil carefully onto the head flat and record the indicator reading.

The overall length is not critical because wear of the tip edges only marginally affects variations in tablet weight. Also, embossing and breaklines, which protrude above the tip surface, can affect the measurement of overall length.

Measuring Working Length

1. Place punch in holder with head in recessed end and tip pointing up (see Illustration 7).
2. Place holder on base of comparator; depress lifting lever to raise anvil; and slide punch and holder under the anvil.
3. Lower the anvil carefully onto the punch face and find the deepest point by moving the punch and holder around until the dial indicator shows the minimum reading.

4. Subtract this minimum reading from the measured overall length and compare the difference to the theoretical or calculated cup depth. If the punch meets TSM standards, the difference in lengths should closely approximate the cup depth.

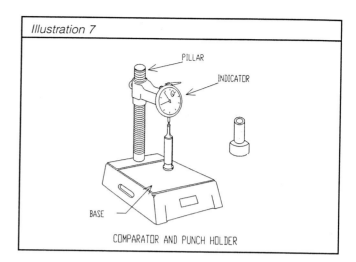

Illustration 7

PILLAR
INDICATOR
BASE
COMPARATOR AND PUNCH HOLDER

The working length is the *most critical* punch dimension because it controls tablet weight and thickness. The working lengths of all punches in a set must be within ±.001 inch [±.025 millimeter] of each other. If the punches do not meet this standard due to wear, reworking, etc., the working lengths should be adjusted according to the instructions given in "Maintaining Accurate Punch Lengths" on page 94.

Measuring Cup Depths

1. Obtain the theoretical depth of the cup from the tooling drawing, or calculate the depth using the formula for cup depths.
2. To find the actual cup depth, subtract the measured working length from the measured overall length.

   NOTE: Again, the cup depth is not a critical dimension with regard to controlling tablet weight.

Measuring Tip-to-Barrel Concentricity

1. Set up the comparator with a ball anvil and V block.
2. Place V block on comparator base; place punch in V block with the outside edge of the punch tip or tip straight under the indicator anvil to ensure sufficient register on the dial (see Illustration 8).

© American Pharmaceutical Association

3. Carefully rotate the punch and note pointer deflection, which should not exceed .001 inch [.025 millimeter] T.I.R.

NOTE: T.I.R., or total indicator reading, is the difference between the highest and lowest readings taken during one rotation of the punch. Eccentricity, or deviation from T.I.R, that exceeds .001 inch [.025 millimeter] is excessive and could be caused by poorly manufactured tools, mishandling of tools, or excessive compression force applied to tools in the press.

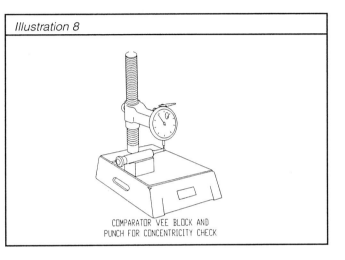

Illustration 8

COMPARATOR VEE BLOCK AND
PUNCH FOR CONCENTRICITY CHECK

Measuring Punch Barrel Diameters

1. Measure barrel diameter with a micrometer.
2. Check the tolerances shown on tooling drawings or relevant tolerance charts (see Figures 8–11, pages 22–25) to determine if the diameters meet specifications.

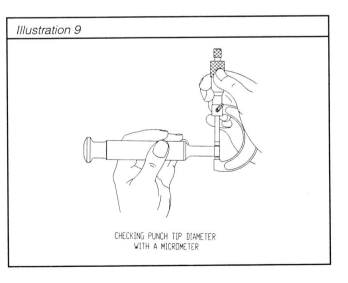

Illustration 9

CHECKING PUNCH TIP DIAMETER
WITH A MICROMETER

Measuring Punch Tip Diameters

1. Measure tip diameters with a micrometer (see Illustration 9).
2. Check the tolerances shown on tooling drawings or relevant tolerance charts (see Figures 8–11, pages 22–25) to determine if the diameters meet specifications.

Checking Radii of Concave Punches

• Using radius gauges that are thin steel templates and contain a range of internal and external radii, check the radius of punch faces. When the gauge is compared to the punch face, there should be a good match of radii.

Checking Punch Head and Neck Profile

1. Using a "go–no go" gauge (see Illustration 10), check the punch head first by passing it through the "go" end; then check that the head does not pass through the "no go" end.

NOTE: An alternative method is to use an optical comparator.

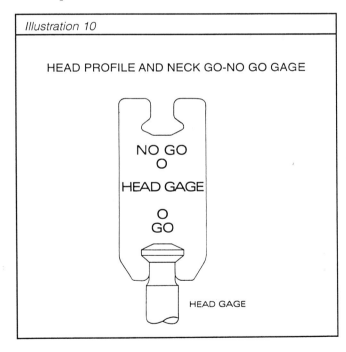

Illustration 10

HEAD PROFILE AND NECK GO-NO GO GAGE

NO GO
O
HEAD GAGE
O
GO

HEAD GAGE

2. Reject any punch that cannot pass through the "go" end or that passes through the "no go" end.

NOTE: The same gauge can be used for punch heads that have the same specifications, but are used in different presses.

© American Pharmaceutical Association

Inspecting Punches

After tools have been removed from the press and cleaned to remove all granulation and oil, they should be inspected to determine their condition before any maintenance is considered.

Inspecting Punch Tips

1. Use a magnifying glass to inspect the outside of tip edges for bruising (see Illustration 11). A toolmaker's microscope can also be used.

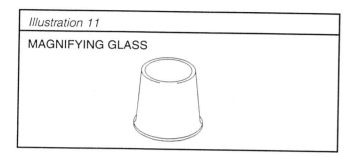

Illustration 11

MAGNIFYING GLASS

2. Check tip edges for raised burrs by visually inspecting the tip edge and/or by drawing a finger nail across the tip edge (see Illustration 12). Be careful not to leave finger prints on the punch.

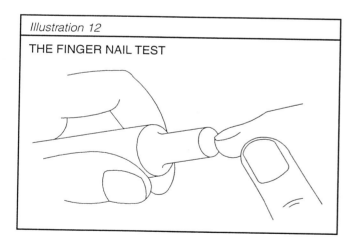

Illustration 12

THE FINGER NAIL TEST

3. Visually inspect tip straights for scoring.

Inspecting Punch Faces

1. Use a magnifying glass to inspect punch faces for abrasion.
2. Visually inspect punch faces for corrosion.

Inspecting Punch Bodies

1. Use a magnifying glass to check for scoring or binding on punch barrels or stems.
2. Visually inspect punch bodies for corrosion.

Inspecting Punch Heads

1. Use a magnifying glass or toolmaker's microscope to inspect punch heads for any signs of damage (see Illustration 13).

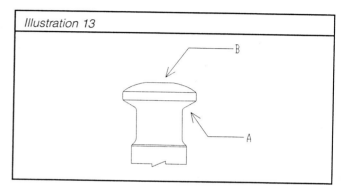

Illustration 13

2. Check under the head for irregular or excessive wear of the inside head angle (see Illustration 13A).
3. Check the top of the head, head flat, and outside head radius or angle for irregular or excessive wear (see Illustration 13B).

These are the most common forms of head damage. If either type of damage is present, problems with the press are indicated.

Inspecting Presses

Performing the following press checks should determine the cause of damage to punches.

1. Pay close attention to the press's lubrication, cleanliness (particularly punch guides), and applied pressure; head wear is usually caused by one or a combination of these factors. In some cases, head wear is caused by excessive tablet ejection pressure.

NOTE: If lubricant becomes contaminated with the granulation or powder, its lubricating properties are destroyed and excessive wear will result.

2. If punches are not free to move under their own weight in the punch guides with the antiturning

© American Pharmaceutical Association

device loosened, remove punches and then clean guides thoroughly with a stiff turret brush. Return punches to cleaned guides.

3. If head wear is severe, steel has been removed from the punches and probably deposited in the press, in cam tracks, or on the pressure rollers. Check press cams and pressure rollers before the press is used again. If the steel particles are rolled under pressure into the punch heads, further damage is inevitable.

NOTE: Tools are subjected to very high pressures: a load of several tons in point contact with the punch head is normal during tablet compression.

Punch Repairs

Common maintenance procedures for punches include repairing damaged heads, repairing chipped or bruised tip edges, removing burrs from inside punch tips, and polishing punches. Only trained personnel should perform the following procedures.

Repairing Punch Heads

1. Set up equipment: motorized polishing chuck, 80- and 180-grit emery cloth, and cotton wool.
2. Set punch in polishing chuck with the head protruding. Take care to prevent damage to punch tip.
3. Turn on polishing chuck.
4. Holding an 80-grit emery cloth in the fingers, wipe over the damaged portions of the punch head. Apply firm pressure until all marks are removed. Or if the head is severely damaged, apply pressure until the marks are smooth to the touch.
5. Polish punch head with an 180-grit emery cloth.
6. Clean punch head with cotton wool.
7. Be sure to clean the equipment to prevent coarse emery grit from interfering with the fine polishing of the punches.

Repairing Chipped or Bruised Tip Edges

1. Measure the tip diameter with a micrometer.
2. Set up equipment: motorized polishing chuck; cotton wool; and a 600-grit, self-adhesive emery sheet applied to a hard flat surface, such as a 12-millimeter wide, hardwood lapping stick (see Illustration 14).

3. Set the punch in the polishing chuck with the tip protruding.

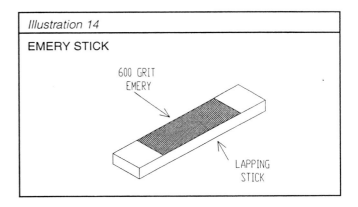

Illustration 14

EMERY STICK

600 GRIT EMERY

LAPPING STICK

4. Turn on motor.
5. Very carefully apply the emery sheet to the outside diameter of the punch tip, making sure the surface of the emery sheet is parallel to the side of the tip. Move the emery stick back and forth (see Illustration 15A).
6. Do not allow more than one-fourth of the emery stick to protrude beyond the end of the tip (see Illustration 15B), or rounding of the tip will occur.

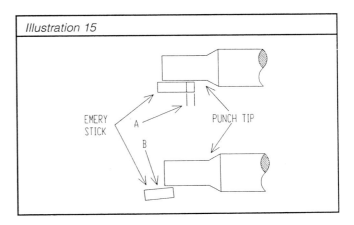

Illustration 15

EMERY STICK   A   PUNCH TIP
B

7. Do not remove any more metal than is absolutely necessary to eliminate the damage. Only burrs or metal raised above the level of the surrounding surface can be removed; any dents or chips can only be disguised.
8. Clean the tip edge by wiping with cotton wool.
9. Check the amount of metal removed by again measuring the tip diameter with the micrometer.

NOTE: A technique of applying the emery stick alternately with an Arkansas stone is often effective in repairing tip edges.

© American Pharmaceutical Association

Removing Burrs Inside Tip Edges

1. Set up equipment: motorized polishing chuck, Arkansas stone, and cotton wool.
2. If a burr is raised inside the punch tip (see Illustration 16A) remove it with an Arkansas stone held against the rotating tip (see Illustration 16B and C).

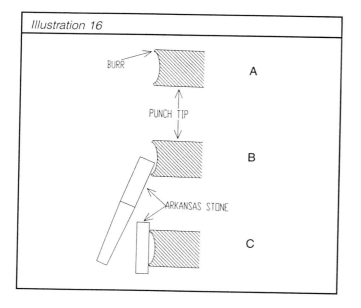

3. If the tip has a breakline or other embossing that prevents this operation from being carried out with the punch rotating, carefully move the stone by hand around the tip edge of a stationary punch.
4. Ensure that the stone does not touch any part of the punch face other than the extreme edge. Take particular care with embossed punches.
5. Clean tip edge with cotton wool.

Maintaining Accurate Punch Lengths

1. From a set of punches that need reworking of head flats, select the punch that has the shortest working length.
2. Using this length as a standard, remove sufficient material with a surface grinder from the head flats of the remaining punches to bring the working lengths of all the punches to within ±.001 inch [±.025 millimeter] of the TSM specification.

NOTE: Using a surface grinder is a skilled operation and should be done by an experienced operator who is aware of the delicate nature of tablet punches. Consult your tooling supplier about the maximum reduction in punch head thickness.

3. Mark reworked punches as such and store them separately from other sets of punches.
4. If only one or two punches in a set are badly worn, replace them with the spare punches. Measure and, if necessary, standardize the replacement punches.
5. If many of the punches are worn, rework the head flats of all the worn punches.
6. Check the diameter of head flats on punches that underwent surface grinding. The head flat diameters must be smaller than the neck diameter or breakage under pressure is likely (see Illustration 17).
7. If the punches do not meet the minimum length, replace them.
8. Polish the reworked punch heads.

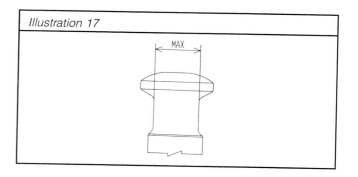

Polishing of Punches

Punch tips can be completely spoiled by excessive or improper polishing that can remove the knife edge of punch tips in seconds. Each punch tip is machined to a very high degree of accuracy and can tolerate only very slight wear before causing excessive "flash" or "collaring" of tablets. This excessive material left on the edges of tablets results from rounding of the tip edge, which creates a space between the tip and the die.

Because all polishing operations abrade the surface, polishing must be kept to a minimum. The four most common errors in polishing punches are:

- Rounding of the outside diameter of the tip (see Illustration 18A)
- Rounding of the edge of the tip face (see Illustration 18B)
- Distortion of the tip face (see Illustration 18C)
- Distortion of embossing (see Illustration 18D)

© American Pharmaceutical Association

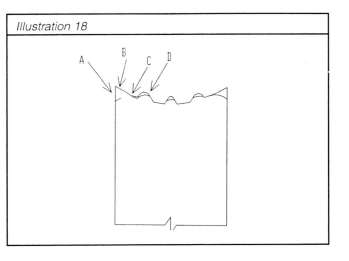

Illustration 18

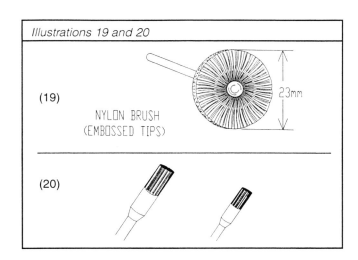

Illustrations 19 and 20

(19) NYLON BRUSH (EMBOSSED TIPS) 23mm

(20)

Polishing Compounds

Various grades of diamond paste or milder abrasive compounds are used to polish punch tips (see Table 15). These compounds are very abrasive, particularly the coarser diamond pastes. Unless used very sparingly, excessive removal of metal will occur with subsequent reduction of punch life.

Polishing Tools

One of the most important points of polishing punch tips is ensuring that the polishing tools (brushes or bobs) are of a size and form appropriate to the tip being polished.

Polishing Brushes are used for all small F.F.B.E., shaped, and embossed punch tips, including the breakline. A nylon wheel brush, similar to the type used in dental work, is recommended; the brush diameter should not exceed .91 inch [23 millimeters] (see Illustration 19). Alternatively, a pencil brush can be used in a handpiece (see Illustration 20). A pencil brush is recommended when a mirror surface finish is needed to prevent granulation from sticking inside the embossing of a punch face.

Felt Bobs are used for plain concave and large F.F.B.E. punch tips. For plain concave tips, the end of the bob should be spherical and have the same radius as the tip concave (see Illustration 21A). The diameter of the bob end should be smaller than the punch tip diameter (see Illustration 21B).

For large F.F.B.E. tips, the bob's radius should be slightly smaller than that of the punch tip (see Illustration 21C); the bob's diameter should be approximately two-thirds the diameter of the punch face (see Illustration 21D).

Table 15. Polishing Compounds and Tools

Use	Tool	Compound
Cleaning and polishing embossed, shaped, and small F.F.B.E. tips with good surface finish	Nylon brush	Mild abrasive compound
Polishing embossed, shaped, and small F.F.B.E. tips with deteriorating surface finish	Nylon brush	Diamond paste (0–2 microns)
Final polishing of plain round (concave or convex) and large F.F.B.E. tips with good surface finish	Felt bob	Diamond paste (0–2 microns)

1. Separate felt bobs and nylon brushes should be kept for each grade of polishing compound.

2. When punch tips are severely deteriorated, it may be necessary to use a 14-micron diamond paste with either a felt bob or nylon brush. To give the final required high polish, a final polishing with a 3-micron diamond paste is recommended.

3. Coarse emery grit should not be allowed to contaminate the felt bob or polishing compounds.

© American Pharmaceutical Association

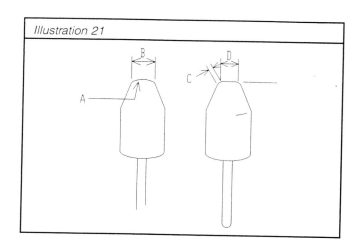

Illustration 21

Felt bobs should be shaped with a file as the bob is rotated in the polishing handpiece. The bob and punch tip radii must match exactly, or the punch tip will be distorted. A radius gauge should be used to obtain the exact radius.

Using Polishing Equipment

Polishing equipment for tablet tooling includes a (1) polishing unit with motor and handpiece, (2) motorized polishing chuck, and (3) two-speed double-ended motor.

Polishing of Punch Barrels is usually done with a motorized chuck to remove corrosion or discoloration from punch bodies and to polish punch tips and heads.

1. Set the punch in the chuck with the tip and half of the barrel protruding. If the tool is a shaped punch, remove the key.
2. Turn on the motor to rotate the punch.
3. Lightly polish the punch barrel with a Scotchbrite sheet. If the punch is severely corroded, use a 600-grit emery sheet.
4. Polish only to the point of removing the corrosion or discoloration. Further polishing could reduce the barrel diameter.
5. To polish tip diameter, hold a 600-grit, emery lapping stick parallel to the punch tip and apply pressure carefully. Move the emery stick back and forth across the tip to avoid rounding of the tip edge.
6. Turn off motor; remove punch; and push a wad of clean cotton wool into the chuck to protect the punch tip from being damaged by the contact with the backplate. Reverse the position of the punch so that the head is protruding from the chuck.

7. Using a Scotchbrite sheet, lightly polish the remainder of the punch barrel.
8. To polish punch heads, use a 180-grit emery sheet. Avoid excessive polishing of the dwell flat, which could reduce the punch length.

Polishing of Plain Tip Faces is done with a motorized polishing chuck and a flexible-drive polishing unit, or with an air-driven hand-held polisher.

1. Be sure any bruises or chips in the tip edge have been dealt with before polishing the tool.
2. Be sure safety guard is in place.
3. Set the punch in the polishing unit with the tip protruding.
4. Fit a bob into the handpiece.
5. Apply a small quantity of polishing compound to the bob.
6. Turn on the unit to begin rotation of the punch.
7. Turn on the handpiece.
8. During the operation, keep elbows and forearms firmly on the bench top or some other rigid support to maintain control of the polishing tool. Always use the protective fences to prevent injury to hands.
9. Apply the end of a rotating bob to the punch face, making sure the punch is rotating in the opposite direction of the bob. Move the handpiece from side to side, pivoting away from the punch face (see Illustration 22).

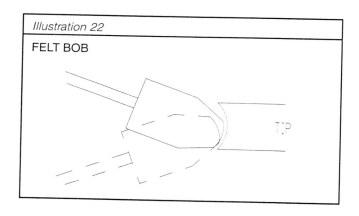

Illustration 22

FELT BOB

TIP

10. Wipe the punch face and inspect it. If the desired finish has not been achieved, repeat the operation.
11. After polishing is completed, check the working length of the punches. If the punch lengths do not fall within ±.001 inch [.025 millimeter] of the length of the reference punch, rectify the problem (see "Maintaining Accurate Punch Lengths").

© American Pharmaceutical Association

Illustration 23 shows the operator's view of this polishing method; the arrows indicate the pivoting of the polishing tool from side to side. An alternative method is to mount the bob on a fixed-drive chuck while holding the punch in the hand.

Illustration 23

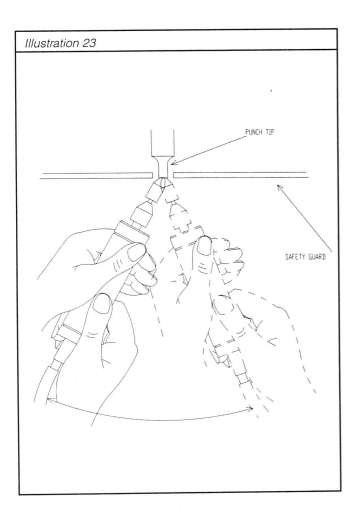

The bob radius must fit the radius of the concave punch tip (see Illustration 24A). An oversized bob with an incorrect radius (see Illustration 24B) can cause severe wear of the punch tip edge (see Illustration 24C). Conversely, if the bob is undersized, it will not polish around the tip edge and might distort the face (see Illustration 24D).

An internal radius gauge can be used to check the bob radius. If the bob radius is too small, it should be increased by removing material from the center of the convex. If the radius is too large, it should be reduced by removing material from the outer edge of the convex.

© American Pharmaceutical Association

Illustration 24

FELT BOBS

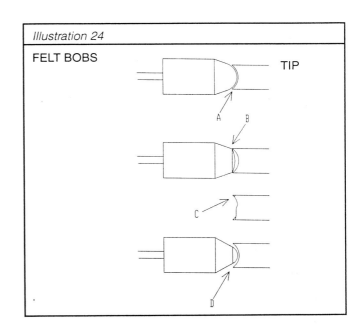

TIP

Polishing of Plain F.F.B.E. Tip Faces is a similar operation to that for plain concave tips, with the exception that the bob should be dressed flat with a chamfer (see Illustration 25).

Illustration 25

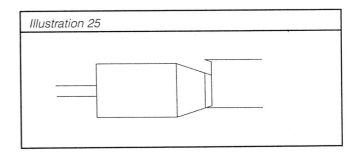

1. Follow steps 1–8 for polishing plain concave tips.
2. Apply the end of the felt bob to the tip face, keeping the flat end of the bob parallel with the flat surface of the punch face. Move the bob from side to side across the punch face (see Illustration 26).

Illustration 26

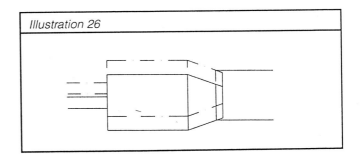

NOTE: The bevel on the edge of the bob should be smaller than the bevel on the punch face; otherwise, wear of the tip edge will occur.

Polishing of Embossed Punches requires different equipment and polishing tools.

1. Be sure any bruises or chips in the tip edge have been dealt with before polishing the tool.
2. Set up equipment: double-ended polishing motor, nylon brushes, polishing compound, and polishing fluid.
3. Turn on motor.
4. Apply a small quantity of polishing compound to the punch tip face.
5. Hold the punch in the hand as shown in Illustration 27, supporting the punch in the left hand and rotating the punch against the brush with the right hand.

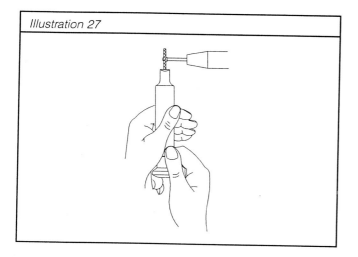

Illustration 27

6. Carefully rotate the tip, applying very light pressure (i.e., do not flatten nylon brushes against the tip).
7. Avoid polishing the outside edges of the punch tips, especially when the tips have a blended land (see Illustration 28A); otherwise, problems with tablet production will occur.
8. Make sure the bristles of the brush move from inside the cup to the outside edge (see Illustration 28B), never from the outside edge into the cup (see Illustration 28C).
9. If the polishing compound becomes dry and sticks to the tip face, moisten the compound with polishing fluid.
10. Clean the tip face.
11. Inspect the finish. If acceptable, go on to the next punch; if not, repeat the operation.

NOTE: Experience will aid in determining the time required to polish a tool; an experienced operator can polish a complete set of tools in a very short time.

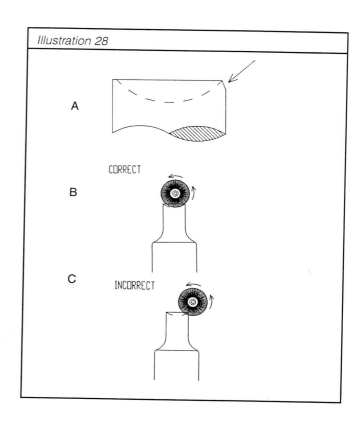

Illustration 28

A

CORRECT

B

C

INCORRECT

Die Maintenance

The following measurements and inspections of dies should be performed upon initial receipt of a set of tooling, and as part of the routine maintenance of dies.

Die Measurements

Die Height is measured with a micrometer (see Illustration 29). An alternative method is to use a comparator with a ball anvil on the dial indicator.

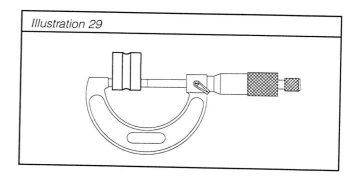

Illustration 29

Die O.D. is measured with a micrometer (see Illustration 30).

Round Die Bores are measured by passing the bore through the "go end" of the appropriate "go-no go" plug gauge (see Illustration 31). If the bore is the cor-

© American Pharmaceutical Association

ect size, the "go" end will pass through the bore, whereas the "no go" end will not. A micrometer can also be used to measure round die bores.

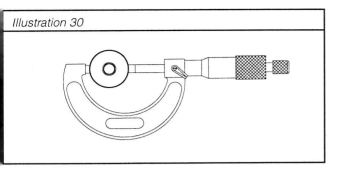
Illustration 30

NOTE: More sophisticated methods, such as air gauging or a spring-loaded probe attached to a measuring scale, are available for measuring round die bores.

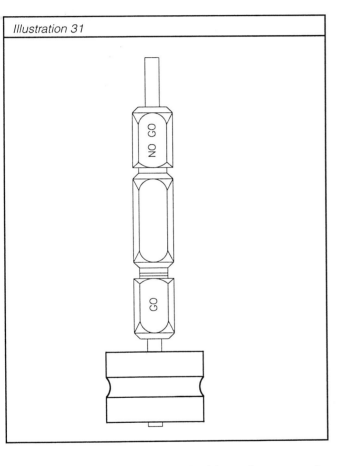
Illustration 31

Shaped Die Bores are measured with a micrometer; the major and minor axes are measured with this gauge. An optical comparator with accurately drawn overlays is then used to check the configuration of the bore.

NOTE: An alternative method to checking shaped die bores is to insert the punch tip into the bore.

Concentricity of Round Die Bores is measured with a comparator. The die is placed in a V block and the ball anvil of the dial indicator is lowered into the die bore (see Illustration 32). The die is then rotated by hand until the total deflection of the dial indicator is observed. The deflection, or T.I.R., should not exceed .001 inch [.025 millimeter].

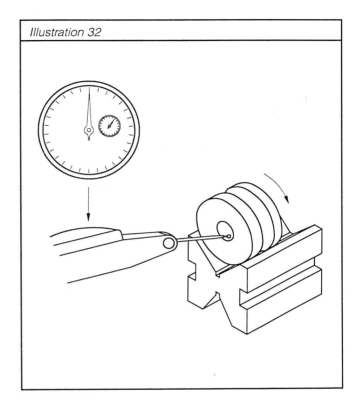
Illustration 32

Die Inspection

Before any repairs are made, the dies should be inspected for (1) compression rings in the bores, (2) wear or binding in the bores, (3) corrosion, and (4) burrs or bruising on the O.D.

Die Repairs

Repairs to dies should be kept to a minimum because any polishing of the die bore will result in an increased clearance between a punch tip and the die bore. Distortion of the die bore can also occur. Under normal working conditions, wiping the die bore and the O.D. with a clean cloth should be sufficient.

Under extreme conditions, and only as a last resort, die bores may be polished. If polishing is warranted, the following method is recommended.

© American Pharmaceutical Association

1. Set up equipment: motorized polishing chuck, flexible polishing unit with handpiece, felt bobs, diamond paste, and polishing fluid.
2. Make sure the felt bob is slightly smaller than the die bore. If necessary, abrade the bob with a clean emery cloth to a size slightly less than the punch tip diameter. The bob's O.D. should be slightly smaller than the die's inner diameter.
3. Put felt bob into polishing handpiece
4. Position die in the polishing chuck so that the chuck grips the die O.D. and the die rotates true.
5. Smear diamond paste on felt bob and moisten the compound slightly with polishing fluid.
6. Turn on both units.
7. Insert rotating felt bob into die bore; using light pressure, move the bob back and forth.
8. Do not allow the bob to protrude more than a quarter of its length from the end of the die bore; otherwise, the bore size will increase rapidly at each end of the die. Also, do not polish the center of the bore excessively; this could cause barrel-shaped bores and lead to problems with tablet ejection.
9. Remove the die from the chuck, and clean the bore with cotton wool.
10. Inspect the finish. If unsatisfactory, repeat the operation.

Storage of Tooling

Tooling must be stored carefully to prevent corrosion. Of the several storage methods, one method is to store tooling in a cabinet; another is to store tooling in specially designed plastic storage boxes. These storage containers allow transport of the tooling with minimum handling. Further, operators should wear cotton gloves to handle tools. Applying a light coating of a thin, non-toxic lubricant will protect tooling from rust. If punches and dies have been stored for long periods between use, they should be inspected periodically to ensure corrosion is not occurring.

Useful Hints

- Use spare punches frequently to maintain punch length compatibility.
- Do not polish chrome-plated tooling because the chromium will be removed.
- Design a safe and practical storage system that will extend tooling life.
- Design a compact and user-friendly layout for the punch and die room.
- Use a custom-designed cart, rack, or tray (with separations that prevent punches from moving) to carry tooling from storage to the press.
- To avoid shortages, keep an inventory record of consumables such as diamond paste, polishing bobs and brushes, etc.

The procedures described in this section for cleaning, repairing, and polishing punches and dies are part of a general maintenance program. Following these procedures will help to prolong tooling life and avoid production problems. If such problems do occur, the troubleshooting tables in Section 6 list corrective actions for the most common tablet and tooling problems.

© American Pharmaceutical Association

Troubleshooting Tablet Production Problems

Problems encountered during tablet production may be caused by deficiencies in the granulation, the tablet press, or the compaction tooling. Many times, a deficiency in one component leads to improper functioning of and/or damage to the other components. A third of all production problems are caused or made worse by ignoring three basic rules:

- Keep compression pressure as low as possible.
- Clean and lubricate the machine properly.
- Keep punches and dies in good condition.

Adhering to the third rule requires paying attention to the factors that can affect the service life of punches:

- Product corrosion
- Excessive compression force (overloading)
- Cam wear on punch heads
- Damage caused by improper handling or accidentally running punches together in the press
- Insufficient land size
- Internal punch defects
- Excessive hardness of punch tips
- Excessively deep cup depth
- Worn compression rollers
- Worn cam tracks
- No lubrication of compression rollers
- Poorly lubricated granulation
- A malfunction of the automatic system that oils punches

Advantages of Quality Tooling

Careful consideration and implementation of the many factors involved in a good, workable tooling program will reap benefits in many ways. A well thought-out design is necessary to produce the highest quality product at the lowest overall cost. The designer must consid-

er the practicality of manufacturing tooling to exact specifications, as well as the needs of production, packaging, and marketing personnel.

Quality of tooling is far more important than the price. Failed tooling can result in hundreds to thousands of dollars lost by a product not being available for the market, the labor expended in the remanufacturing of an unmarketable product, and/or the labor expended in reworking of poor-quality tablets.

The number of tablets that the tools will produce during their useful life and the resultant tooling costs per tablet will be a function of the tooling design, the tool steel and hardness selected, and the quality of the tooling maintenance program. The time required to implement the tooling for a new tablet design will be a function of the correctness and completeness of the information supplied to the tooling supplier.

Tooling suppliers have gained a wealth of experience in dealing with many compressing problems. Tooling users should not hesitate to contact their supplier if the need arises. The suppliers will be pleased to help whenever they can in the solution of any tablet compressing problem.

Of the two troubleshooting guides that follow, Table 16 describes common production problems with tablet quality; Table 17 deals with the most common tooling problems that occur during tablet production.

Tablet Problems

The impact of distributing tablets of poor quality is not limited merely to a diminished corporate image. If a poor-quality tablet provides an improper dosage amount, the well-being of those who purchase the product can be affected. The importance of producing a

© American Pharmaceutical Association

high-quality product cannot be overemphasized: the tablet manufacturer's livelihood depends on the company's commitment to using high-quality tooling and presses to manufacture high-quality tablets. The following troubleshooting guide to tablet problems is an excellent resource for determining the source of and correcting the most common problems related to tablet quality.

TABLE 16. PRODUCTION PROBLEMS WITH TABLET QUALITY

TABLET PROBLEM	POSSIBLE CAUSE(S)/CORRECTIVE ACTION(S)

A. Nonuniform tablet weight 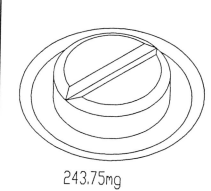 250.00mg 243.75mg	1. Erratic punch flight
	CHECK FOR/ACTION
	  a. Free movement of punch barrels in guides (Guides must be clean and well lubricated.)
	  b. Excessive press vibration
	  c. Worn or loose weight-adjustment ramp
	  d. Proper operation of lower-punch control devices
	  e. Limit cam on weight-adjustment head missing, worn, or incorrectly fitted
	  f. Check dust seals
	  g. Check that antiturning device is set correctly
	  h. Reduce press speed
	
	2. Granulation lost or gained after proper filling of die
	CHECK FOR/ACTION
	  a. Tail over die missing or not lying flat on die table
	  b. Recirculation band leaking
	  c. Excessive vacuum pressure, or nozzle improperly located
	
	3. Feeders starved or choked
	CHECK FOR/ACTION
	  a. Incorrect setting of hopper spout adjustment
	  b. Granulation bridging in hopper
	  c. Wrong fill cam in use
	  d. Excessive recirculation of granulation
	
	4. Dies not filling
	CHECK FOR/ACTION
	  a. Excessive press speed
	  b. See A3 and A5
	  c. Check speed or shape of feeder paddle
	
	5. Lower punch pulled down before die is filled
	CHECK FOR/ACTION
	  a. Inadequate recirculation of granulation
	  b. Recirculation scraper missing or bent
	
	6. Poor scrape-off of granulation
	CHECK FOR/ACTION
	  a. Scraper blade bent, worn, or not lying flat; bad spring action
	
	7. Nonuniform punch length
	CHECK FOR/ACTION
	  a. Check that working length is within ±.001 inch of TSM specification
	
	8. Projection of die(s) above die table
	CHECK FOR/ACTION
	  a. Clean die pocket or check die dimension

© American Pharmaceutical Association

TABLE 16. PRODUCTION PROBLEMS WITH TABLET QUALITY (CONT.)

TABLET PROBLEM	POSSIBLE CAUSE(S)/CORRECTIVE ACTION(S)
A. Nonuniform tablet weight (continued)	9. Automatic weight-control system not working correctly **CHECK FOR/ACTION** a. Check that system's settings and operation are correct; see manufacturer's handbook 10. Wide variation in thickness of lower punch heads **CHECK FOR/ACTION** a. Check that head thickness of lower punches is within ±.010 inch of TSM specification
B. Nonuniform tablet thickness (Not pictured)	1. Nonuniform tablet weight **CHECK FOR/ACTION** a. See A 2. Bouncing of pressure rollers **CHECK FOR/ACTION** a. Improper setting for overload release b. Press operating near maximum density point of granulation; increase thickness and/or reduce weight within allowable tablet tolerances c. Pressure rollers not moving freely; punch faces in poor condition d. Air trapped in hydraulic overload system e. Worn pivot pins on roller carriers 3. Nonuniform punch lengths **CHECK FOR/ACTION** a. Check that working length is within ±.001 inch of TSM specification
C. Nonuniform tablet density (friability) 	1. Nonuniform tablet weight and thickness **CHECK FOR/ACTION** a. See A and B b. See capping in G 2. Unequal distribution of granulation in die bores **CHECK FOR/ACTION** a. Stratification or separation of granulation in hopper b. Excessive recirculation (This causes classification of granulation because only finer mesh material escapes the rotary feeders.) 3. Particle segregation or stratification in hopper **CHECK FOR/ACTION** a. Reduce variations in particle size; reduce machine vibration; reduce machine speed 4. Low moisture content **CHECK FOR/ACTION** a. Add moisture to aid bonding
D. Excessive vibration of press (Not pictured)	1. Worn drive belt **CHECK FOR/ACTION** a. Inspect drive belt 2. Mismatched punch lengths **CHECK FOR/ACTION** a. See A-7

© American Pharmaceutical Association

TABLE 16. PRODUCTION PROBLEMS WITH TABLET QUALITY (CONT.)

TABLET PROBLEM	POSSIBLE CAUSE(S)/CORRECTIVE ACTION(S)
D. Excessive vibration of press (continued) (Not pictured)	3. Press operating near maximum density point of granulation **CHECK FOR/ACTION** a. Increase tablet thickness and/or reduce its weight within allowable tablet tolerances 4. High ejection pressure **CHECK FOR/ACTION** a. Worn ejection cam b. Add more lubrication to granulation, or taper dies c. Barrel-shaped die bores 5. Improper pressure-release setting **CHECK FOR/ACTION** a. Increase pressure to the tooling's limit
E. Dirt in product (black specks) (Not pictured)	1. Dust, dirt, or press lubrication in the granulation **CHECK FOR/ACTION** a. Clean press more frequently b. Excessive or wrong press lubrication c. Use proper punch dust cups and keyway fillers d. Rubbing of feeder components e. Punch-to-die binding
F. Excessive loss of granulation (Not pictured)	1. Incorrect fit of feeder to die table **CHECK FOR/ACTION** a. Feeder base set incorrectly (i.e, too high or not level) b. Bottom of feeder pans worn due to previous incorrect settings; relap pans, if necessary 2. Incorrect action of recirculation band **CHECK FOR/ACTION** a. Gaps between band's bottom edge and die table b. Binding in mounting screw c. Inadequate pressure on hold-down spring 3. Insufficient scraping of die table **CHECK FOR/ACTION** a. Worn or binding scraper blade b. Outboard scraper edge allowing granulation to escape 4. Granulation lost from die prior to upper punch entry **CHECK FOR/ACTION** a. Tail over die not lying flat on table 5. Granulation lost at compression point **CHECK FOR/ACTION** a. Compression occurring too high in the die b. Excessive suction or misdirected exhaust nozzle 6. Excessive sifting **CHECK FOR/ACTION** a. Excessive clearance between lower punch tip and die bore b. Excessive fine particles in the granulation c. Tapered dies installed upside down

© American Pharmaceutical Association

TABLE 16. PRODUCTION PROBLEMS WITH TABLET QUALITY (CONT.)

TABLET PROBLEM	POSSIBLE CAUSE(S)/CORRECTIVE ACTION(S)

G. Capping and lamination

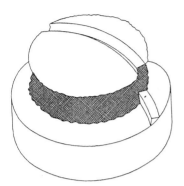

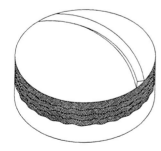

1. Air entrapment
   CHECK FOR/ACTION
   a. Compress granulation higher in the die
   b. Reduce press speed
   c. Precompress granulation
   d. Reduce quantity of fine particles in the granulation
   e. Reduce cup depth on punches
   f. Taper dies
   g. Ensure that punch-to-die clearance is correct

2. Excessive pressure
   CHECK FOR/ACTION
   a. Reduce tablet weight and/or increase its thickness within allowable tolerances
   b. Adjust pressure

3. Ringed or barrel-shaped die bore
   CHECK FOR/ACTION
   a. Reverse dies
   b. Hone or lap bores
   c. Compress granulation higher in the die

4. Too rapid expansion of tablet upon ejection
   CHECK FOR/ACTION
   a. Taper dies

5. Weak granulation
   CHECK FOR/ACTION
   a. Increase quantity of binder; use stronger binder

6. Excessively dry granulation
   CHECK FOR/ACTION
   a. Increase level of lubricant

7. Excessive lubrication of granulation
   CHECK FOR/ACTION
   a. Decrease level of lubricant; blend all ingredients fully before adding lubricant

8. Punch cavity too deep
   CHECK FOR/ACTION
   a. Use punches with less concave depth

9. Punch tips worn or burred
   CHECK FOR/ACTION
   a. Refurbish or replace punches

10. Lower punch set too low at tablet take-off (Reworking or refurbishing punches can cause this.)
    CHECK FOR/ACTION
    a. Set lower punch tip flush with top of die

11. Tablet take-off bar set too high
    CHECK FOR/ACTION
    a. Adjust take-off bar

© American Pharmaceutical Association

TABLE 16. PRODUCTION PROBLEMS WITH TABLET QUALITY (CONT.)

TABLET PROBLEM	POSSIBLE CAUSE(S)/CORRECTIVE ACTION(S)

H. Picking and sticking

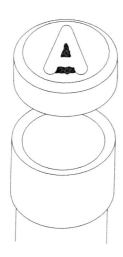

1. Excessive moisture
   CHECK FOR/ACTION
   a. Check moisture content of granulation
   b. Check room humidity

2. Punch face condition
   CHECK FOR/ACTION
   a. Pits on punch faces and/or improper draft on embossing; try repolishing punch faces
   b. Try chrome-plating punch faces

3. Insufficient compaction force
   CHECK FOR/ACTION
   a. Increase tablet weight and/or reduce its thickness within allowable tolerances

4. Inadequate lubrication of granulation
   CHECK FOR/ACTION
   a. Check and/or adjust level of lubricant used

5. Poor embossing design
   CHECK FOR/ACTION
   a. Redesign embossing per TSM guidelines, or consult tooling supplier

I. Mottled or marked tablets

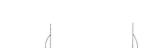
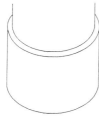
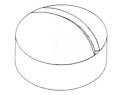

1. Contamination of granulation, usually by grease or oil
   CHECK FOR/ACTION
   a. Check oil seals on upper punch guides
   b. Reduce lubrication of upper punches to an acceptable level
   c. Fit oil/dust cups to upper punches

2. Contamination of granulation from chutes, feed hoppers, take-off bar, or rubbing together of feed paddles
   CHECK FOR/ACTION
   a. Clean and reset components correctly

3. High moisture content of granulation
   CHECK FOR/ACTION
   a. Re-dry granulation

4. Oversized granulation particles
   CHECK FOR/ACTION
   a. Reduce particle size

J. Indistinct breakline or embossing

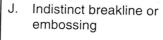
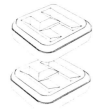

1. Incorrect embossing design
   CHECK FOR/ACTION
   a. Redesign embossing per TSM guidelines, or consult tooling supplier

2. Worn punch tips
   CHECK FOR/ACTION
   a. Replace punches

3. Excessively coarse granulation
   CHECK FOR/ACTION
   a. Reduce particle size

© American Pharmaceutical Association

TABLE 16. PRODUCTION PROBLEMS WITH TABLET QUALITY (CONT.)

TABLET PROBLEM	POSSIBLE CAUSE(S)/CORRECTIVE ACTION(S)

TABLET PROBLEM

POSSIBLE CAUSE(S)/CORRECTIVE ACTION(S)

J. Indistinct breakline or embossing (continued)

4. Inadequate binder
   CHECK FOR/ACTION
   a. Increase binder strength

5. Picking
   CHECK FOR/ACTION
   a. Compress granulation at a lower pressure

K. Double impression of embossing

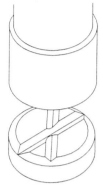

1. Rotation of punches
   CHECK FOR/ACTION
   a. Adjust antiturning device
   b. Use keyed punches

L. Chipping or splitting

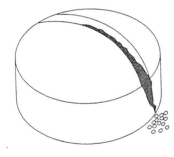

1. Poor surface finish on punch tips; worn punches and dies
   CHECK FOR/ACTION
   a. Polish punch tips; replace punches and dies

2. Poor tooling design (e.g., sharp embossing or bisect lines)
   CHECK FOR/ACTION
   a. Polish punch tips; replace punches and dies

M. Splitting of layered tablet

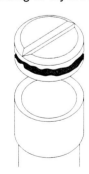

1. Excessive pressure
   CHECK FOR/ACTION
   a. Decrease pressure

2. Excessive lubrication of granulation
   CHECK FOR/ACTION
   a. Reduce amount of lubricant

NOTE: Table reprinted with permission from *Pharmaceutical Dosage Forms*, Vol. 2, 2nd. ed. New York: Marcel Dekker, Inc.; 1989: 603–607.

Tooling Problems

Most tablet manufacturers face the expensive problem of damaged tooling during some stage of tablet production. Often, the problem could easily be avoided by using the press correctly. If left unchecked, the damage could result in the cost of a new set of tools or even major repairs to the press.

Table 17 is a troubleshooting guide to the tooling problems most commonly encountered during tablet production. Each problem is described, details of the problable causes given, and, when possible, corrective actions suggested. If the problem cannot be rectified, suggestions to prevent recurrence of the problem are given.

To help readers isolate the problem, illustrations showing the likely damage accompany the description of all but two problems. However, to aid clarity, the damage shown is exaggerated; the actual damage will be far less pronounced.

TABLE 17. PRODUCTION PROBLEMS WITH TOOLING

	TOOLING PROBLEM	CAUSE(S)	CORRECTIVE ACTION(S)	COMMENTS
	(1) The tip has cracked across the face of the concave and then broken away.	1. Excessive hardness for application. Excessive pressure.	None: discard tool; consult tooling manufacturer.	Tools should always be run at the minimum pressure required to achieve a satisfactory tablet.
	(2) The tip has cracked and broken away along the angle between the bevel and tip face.	2. See cause for 1.	See action for 1.	A crack will always follow the line of least resistance, which may be the sharp angle between the punch face and the embossing.
	(3) The tip has cracked and broken away along the angle between a breakline and a concave tip face.	3. Excessive hardness. Areas of concentrated stress near breakline or on embossing (i.e., abrupt change of surface contour). Excessive pressure.	See action for 1.	See comments for 2.
	(4) The tip has cracked and broken away along the embossed lettering.	4. See cause for 3.	See action for 1.	See comments for 2.

© American Pharmaceutical Association

TABLE 17. PRODUCTION PROBLEMS WITH TOOLING (CONT.)

	TOOLING PROBLEM	CAUSE(S)	CORRECTIVE ACTION(S)	COMMENTS
	(5) *This die shows a typical wear pattern in the bore.*	5. Normal die wear caused by continuous pressure at the compression area in the bore.	Examine dies with magnifying glass and monitor tablet ejection. When possible, compress tablets in different areas of the die to spread wear, and reverse the die when one end is worn. Check that correct steel was chosen. If wear is a serious problem, consult tooling manufacturer.	If allowed to go too far, the die wear can lead to ejection problems and other problems associated with punch tightness. If a known abrasive granulation is to be compressed, the tooling manufacturer can possibly offer a more wear-resistant material for tooling.
	(6) *The edge of the tip has been damaged outside the press.*	6. Mishandling of punch (punch has collided with or been dropped onto a hard surface). Accidental damage occurred during fitting of punches to the press.	Carefully remove damage by blending and polishing. Exercise extreme care when handling tools; the tips are very fragile. Train personnel to handle tools properly.	Careful examination of this type of damage will reveal clues to its cause. (a) If the damage has caused the tip to spread beyond its diameter, the damage most likely occurred out of the press. (b) The texture of the surface causing the damage will be transferred to the damaged part.
	(7) *The punches have met in the press; damage occurred where the opposing punch has a breakline.*	7. Contact between upper and lower punches in the press.	Carefully remove dents by blending and polishing. Do not run the press without granulation at setup; manually turn over the dies until all are filled with granulation.	In some presses, if tools are run or even turned without granulation, the punches can meet, causing damage.
	(8) *Again, the punches have met in the press, but the opposing punch has no breakline.*	8. See cause for 7.	See action for 7.	See comments for 7.
	(9) *Pressure has started to spread the punch tip; working length may not yet be affected. The spreading will probably occur on both upper and lower punches.*	9. Excessive pressure (first stage for upper and lower punch).	In the early stages before working length is affected, punch damage can be removed by blending or polishing. Check all punch lengths before reusing the set; other punches may have been damaged.	This type of damage can be checked by measuring the tip diameter at the extreme edge and at the lower end. If these dimensions vary, damage has occurred.

TABLE 17. PRODUCTION PROBLEMS WITH TOOLING (CONT.)

	TOOLING PROBLEM	CAUSE(S)	CORRECTIVE ACTION(S)	COMMENTS
	(10) Lower punch is over-pressured to the point where the stem is distorted and the working length is reduced.	10. Excessive pressure (final stage for lower punch).	None: the final stage of over-pressure cannot be rectified; the punch is permanently distorted.	Rolling the punch barrel on a flat surface is a simple way to check for this type of damage: the punch tip will be seen to rotate out of true.
	(11) Excessive pressure will have the same effect on the upper punch as on the lower; see (10).	11. Excessive pressure (final stage for upper punch).	See action for 10.	See comments for 10.
	(12) The head flat has worn to the point where fragments of metal are being removed from the punch head.	12. Excessive pressure and damaged or worn pressure roller. Foreign matter between pressure roller and punch head.	Reduce pressure; replace lubricant; repair pressure roller. Spalling of the head deposits metal particles in the press: clean press throughout. Consult tooling manufacturer.	If not tackled early, this type of damage can lead to serious wear and damage to the tools and the press.
	(13) Scoring of the punch barrel is caused by a lack of lubrication and/or the presence of foreign matter in the punch guides.	13. Tightness of the punch barrel in the turret leading to possible scoring and pick up of metal, which leads to increased tightness. Poor lubrication.	If possible, polish punch to restore original condition. Check that guides are clear of granulation and metal particles. Pay particular attention to the punch sockets in the turret. Check working length before reworking punch. Ensure that the lubrication system is clean, correct, and operative.	Many tooling problems are caused by tightness; marking of the barrel is a definite indication of trouble. If the lubrication becomes contaminated with the granulation, its lubricating properties are destroyed and excessive wear occurs.
	(14) The punch is not rotating, and the pressure roller may be running tight, causing wearing of the head in only one spot. (Shaped punches do not rotate.)	14. Excessive pressure. Lack of lubrication. Tight punches or pressure rollers.	Check that head flat is not too small to achieve satisfactory dwell time during compression. Check underside of head for damage. If warranted, polish head. Resolve pressure problem; ensure that punch and pressure roller can move freely; ensure adequate lubrication.	Press damage is possible.

10

© American Pharmaceutical Association

TABLE 17. PRODUCTION PROBLEMS WITH TOOLING (CONT.)

	TOOLING PROBLEM	CAUSE(S)	CORRECTIVE ACTION(S)	COMMENTS
	(15) The ejection cam is causing wear on the lower punch head.	15. A rotating punch is running very tight on ejection, causing a radial pattern of wear. Insufficient head flat. Excessive pressure. Damaged, bruised, or scored compression roller.	Polish head or increase size of head flat. Ensure that punches can operate freely at all times. Resolve ejection problem; to ease ejection loads, taper dies. Always use minimum pressure needed to compress tablets. Ensure that surface of compression roller is clean and free of burrs or bruising. Check cam for excessive wear; clean and remove any metallic particles from the cam track and pressure rollers.	If the head flat is too small, the compression force is concentrated on a small area and ultimately will cause the center of the head to fail. Tooling is subjected to continuous high pressure and eventually the structure of the steel will break down. If punches are tight, unnecessary pressure is applied to tooling, cams, and compression rollers. If not corrected, damage to punch heads or compression rollers will transfer rapidly to all the punches in the press.
	(16) Tight punches have caused excessive wear to the inside head angle. (Damage to press cams is likely.)	16. Punch has become tight in the die or press turret due to lack of lubrication. Incorrect cam angle on punch heads. Bruised or scored press cams.	None: discard the punch. Determine cause and ensure that replacement punch moves freely (i.e., punch should fall freely under its own weight when antiturning device is loosened). Clean the press to remove metal particles. Ensure that punch guides are clean and correct lubrication is applied. Check that cam angle is compatible with the press cams. Inspect cams for bruises and scores; if needed, repolish or replace cams.	The top of the punch head may also be damaged. This kind of damage leaves metal particles in the press.
	(17) This damage is similar to (16), but the punch was not allowed to rotate, resulting in part of the head breaking off.	17. This problem is similar to 16, but the punch is not rotating due to the use of a keyed punch or tightening in the turret.	None: discard the punch. Determine cause of problem, and ensure that replacement punch is loose (i.e., punch should fall freely under its own weight when the antiturning device is loosened). Clean the press to remove metal particles.	See comments for 16.

© American Pharmaceutical Association

TABLE 17. PRODUCTION PROBLEMS WITH TOOLING (CONT.)

	TOOLING PROBLEM	CAUSE(S)	CORRECTIVE ACTION(S)	COMMENTS
	(18) *The punch barrel has snapped in the press.*	18. Upper punch is possibly being prevented from entering the die due to tip breakage (see 1, 2, 3 or 4); the head then strikes part of the punch guide system and breaks the barrel. Excessive tightness.	Discard tool; monitor condition of tooling at all times to avoid tightness and excessive pressure.	With unenclosed presses, the broken part may be ejected from the press with considerable force, endangering personnel and equipment.
	(19) *The punch snapped in the press, but this time the head has broken off.*	19. Due to wear and refurbishing, head flat has become larger than the neck diameter. When compression force is applied, the punch is unsupported at the neck and breakage results.	None: discard tool and monitor the condition of tools in use, especially after refurbishing. Ensure that all metal fragments are removed from the press.	Severe damage to the press is almost certain.
	(20) *Burrs are present inside the punch tip (clawing).* (Not pictured)	20. Misalignment of punch tips in die bore. Worn punch guides or die sockets. Eccentricity of punch tips to punch body. Extrusion of product between punch tips and die bores. Excessive feather edge on punch tips, especially deep concave cups.	Ensure that internal chamfer of die bores is sufficient. Check for wear and rectify; check concentricity of punch tips. Ensure that tip-to-die bore clearance is correct. Increase land or flat on tip edge; ensure that land is blended.	
	(21) *The surface finish of the punch face is deteriorated (i.e., pitted or discolored).* (Not pictured)	21. Compression of an abrasive or corrosive granulation.	Ensure that the correct steel has been chosen. Check for sufficient lubrication of the granulation.	

NOTE: Reprinted with permission from *Tooling Problems*, Holland Educational Series, No. 4. Nottingham, England: I Holland Limited; 1988.

© American Pharmaceutical Association

urret Guideway Wear

rret guideways for upper punches are sized suffi-
ntly larger than the punch barrels to allow free
vement of the punches and provide adequate room
lubrication. The resultant clearance also gives rise to
angular end play, which causes the punch tip to be
ghtly off center relative to the die bore as the punch
ers the die. Figure 41 depicts this phenomenon.

1en using punches that meet TSM tolerances in new
rets, tip deflection can be as much as ±.003 inch,
pending upon the press make. Die bore chamfers
sure that the punch tips are guided into the die with-
causing damage to the tooling. As the turret guide-
ys wear, tip deflection increases and the punches

impact the chamfer harder. Excessive deflections and
high impact forces can ultimately lead to dents in the
land or a curling in of punch tips. Serious damage to
inside head angles can also occur as the smooth movement of punches through lifting and lowering cams
becomes increasingly difficult.

Wear in turret guideways is not uniform throughout the
length of the guideway. Loads from the cams and compression rollers force the punch barrels to the backside
of the guideway at the head end and toward the leading
side at the tip end. The net effect is an egg-shaped wear
pattern at the tops and bottoms of the guideways with
very little wear occurring in between. Because of the
wear pattern, establishing a specification as to when a
turret is worn cannot be based on measurements of
guideway bore diameters.

Punch tip deflection, however, is a good indicator of
guideway wear. The procedure for measuring tip deflections is as follows:

1. Cover the die pocket in the station that is to be measured with a thin strip of metal. A blank die can also
   be used.
2. Insert a punch and let it rest on the metal strip or
   blank die.
3. Set up a surface gauge indicator so that circumfer-
   ential tip movement can be measured.
4. Tilt the punch back and forth at the head end and
   measure the T.I.R. at the tip.

Maximum recommended tip deflections may vary
according to the press manufacturer, type of tooling
(i.e., round or shaped), and press speed. As a general
guideline, a maximum range of .012 to .014 inch can be
used. Noticeable punch tip damage and inside head
angle wear should also be considered as indications to
replace a turret.

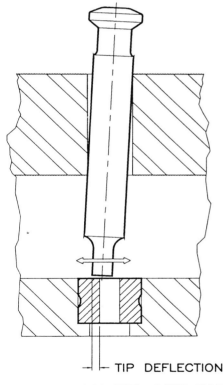

FIGURE 41. PUNCH TIP DEFLECTION

TIP DEFLECTION

USING PUNCH TIP DEFLECTION
AS AN INDICATOR OF WEAR
IN TURRET GUIDEWAYS

DWG. NO.	TSM—N41

The Tableting Specifications Steering Committee
expresses its deepest appreciation to I. Holland
Limited and Thomas Engineering Inc. for sharing
with the Committee and users of this *Manual* the
valuable information contained in the troubleshooting tables. This generous contribution of time and
materials will help users of tableting tools to
increase the service life of their tools and avoid
costly work stoppages.

Tablet Press and Tooling Manufacturers and Distributors

Press Manufacturers and Distributors

Cadmach Machinery Co. Pvt. Ltd.
Ahmedabad, India
Represented by:
Key International, Inc.
480 Route 9
Englishtown, NJ 07726

Courtoy, N.V.
Halle, Belgium
Represented by:
A.C. Compacting Presses, Inc.
1577 Livingston Avenue
North Brunswick, NJ 08902-0366

Wilhelm Fette - GmbH
Schwarzenbek, Germany
U.S. Office:
Fette America
300 Roundhill Drive
Rockaway, NJ 07866

Elizabeth-Hata International, Inc.
Banco Industrial Park
North Huntington, PA 15642

Horn + Noack Pharmatechnik GmbH
Worms, Germany
U.S. Office:
Romaco, Inc.
American Enterprise Park
104 American Road
Morris Plains, NJ 07950

Mutual Corporation (Kikisui Press)
Osaka, Japan
Represented by:
United Chemical Machinery
Supply Inc.
1520 Route 37 West, Suite 2
Toms River, NJ 08756-4142

Kilian & Co., GmbH Maschinenfabrik
Koln, Germany
U.S. Office:
Kilian & Co., Inc.
415 Sargon Way, Unit 1
Horsham, PA 19044

KORSCH Pressen GmbH
Berlin (Borsigwalde), Germany
U.S. Office:
KORSCH America, Inc.
200 Middlesex/Essex Turnpike
Iselin, NJ 08830

BWI Manesty
Liverpool, England
Represented by:
Thomas Engineering, Inc.
575 West Central Road
Hoffman Estates, IL 60195

Riva S.A.
Buenos Aires, Argentina
Represented by:
Supermatic Package Machinery Inc.
7 Speilman Road
Fairfield, NJ 07004

Stokes Merrill, Inc.
2 Pearl Buck Court
Bristol, PA 19007

Tooling Manufacturers and Distributors

Advance Engineering and Manufacturing Company
1 Vance Drive
O'Fallon, MO 63366

Elizabeth Carbide Die Co., Inc.
601 Linden Street
McKeesport, PA 15132

Wilhelm Fette - GmbH
Schwarzenbek, Germany
U.S. Office:
Fette America
300 Roundhill Drive
Rockaway, NJ 07866

I. Holland Limited
Nottingham, England
Represented by:
Holland McGinley Co.
Box 57
Malvern, PA 19355

Key International, Inc.
480 Route 9
Englishtown, NJ 07726

Natoli Engineering Company, Inc.
28 Research Park Circle
St. Charles, MO 63004

Stokes-Merrill, Inc.
2 Pearl Buck Court
Bristol, PA 19007

Thomas Engineering, Inc.
575 West Central Road
Hoffman Estates, IL 60195

Vector Corporation
675 44th Street
Marion, IA 52302

© American Pharmaceutical Association

CW00951557

Self-Intelligence

A Handbook for Developing Confidence, Self-Esteem and Interpersonal Skills

Stephen Bowkett

Published by Network Educational Press Ltd.
PO Box 635
Stafford
ST16 1BF

First Published 1999
© Stephen Bowkett 1999

ISBN 1 85539 055 8

Stephen Bowkett asserts the moral right to be identified as the author of this work.

All rights reserved. No part of this publication may be reproduced, stored in a retrieval system or reproduced or transmitted in any form or by any other means, electronic, mechanical, photocopying (with the exception of the following pages: 29, 30, 31, 37, 46, 48, 49, 50, 87, 88, 89, 90, 101,102, 119, 128, 160, 161, 167, 170, 171, 172, 201, 202, 203, 204, 205), recording or otherwise without the prior written permission of the Publisher. This book may not be lent, resold, hired out or otherwise disposed of by way of trade in any form of binding or cover other than that in which it is published, without the prior consent of the Publisher.

Quotations on p. 9, 10, 21 from Neil Postman & Charles Weingartner, *Teaching as a Subversive Activity* (Penguin Education Specials 1972; originally published by Pitman Publishing), are reproduced by courtesy of Pearson Education.

Quotations on p. 23 from *All Our Futures: Creativity, Culture and Education*, the report by the National Advisory Committee on Creative and Cultural Education (DfEE Publications, © Crown Copyright, 1999), are reproduced by permission of the Controller of Her Majesty's Stationery Office.

Edited by Anne Gibbens
Design/Graphics and Layout by
n.hawkins@appleonline.net

Printed in Great Britain by
Redwood Books, Trowbridge, Wilts.

CONTENTS

Preface

Self-intelligence is about equipping children with an emotional toolkit, and giving them the skills to pick the right tool for the job. Although we might not all be teachers of English, we all can and should play our part in developing the emotional capabilities of our pupils. This we can do through the medium of our subject. This book, intended as a companion volume to *Imagine That...*, is designed to develop emotional resourcefulness in yourself and the children you teach.

Emotional resourcefulness – or 'self-intelligence', as I call it – is the capacity to know and understand yourself and make best use of that understanding. This involves:

- noticing your own emotional responses
- recognising the range of your own talents and potentials
- becoming aware of blocks and limiting beliefs preventing the development of those potentials
- taking responsibility for your current states and then taking direct positive action to modify those states
- making interventions to respond more flexibly to circumstances, incidents, events and situations
- becoming more sensitive to other people's emotions and perceptions (their subjective realities and their responses to those realities), and recognising how these can affect your own state
- developing the capacity to respond more capably to other people's emotions.

> Reason must have an adequate emotional base for education to perform its function.
>
> *Plato*

Structure of the book

It is my intention that every idea and activity in this book should play a part in developing children's emotional resourcefulness. The activities have many spin-off applications in different areas of the curriculum, therefore any overly prescriptive structure would probably be counter-productive. It's likely you will dip into *Self-Intelligence* and try out what takes your fancy, integrating ideas that work for you into your regular classroom practice; they can be used independently, but I anticipate you'll find many useful ways of cross-fertilising techniques when you read them in combination.

Developing self-intelligence breaks down naturally into four key areas, and the layout of the book reflects these:

developing sensory acuity

utilising relaxation and break states

enhancing emotional literacy

encouraging a creative attitude

These four main components, you'll find, overlap and complement one another. The ideas are broadly arranged within sections according to their level of sophistication. Simpler and more straightforward activities tend to be found early on in the sections, while more complex or demanding techniques come later, on the assumption that by then you'll have some specific experience of self-intelligence work. The explanations are often accompanied by photocopiable worksheets (or playsheets, as I prefer to call them).

In the index ideas for ongoing techniques, those which you might use continually as part of your classroom practice, appear in *italics*, and specific activities in **bold**.

As in my previous book, *Imagine That...*, you'll find very little jargon in *Self-Intelligence*. Maybe not surprisingly, I have never needed to know about subordinate noun clauses to get books published, nor about instinctual fusion to practise hypnotherapy and run creative thinking workshops for the past nine years. As Albert Einstein sensibly pointed out, 'Everything should be made as simple as possible, but no simpler.'

Acknowledgements

Every effort has been made to trace and acknowledge ownership of copyright. If any required credits have been omitted or any rights overlooked, it is completely unintentional. The publishers will be glad to make suitable arrangements with any copyright holder whom it has not been possible to contact, and wish to make acknowledgements for material quoted from the following:

Nikos Kazantsakis, *Zorba the Greek* (1961), reproduced on pp. 11 and 78 by permission of Faber & Faber Ltd.; Daniel Brown, *Principles of Art Therapy* (1997), reproduced on p. 13 by permission of HarperCollins Publishers Ltd.; Susan Greenfield, *The Human Brain: A Guided Tour* (Phoenix 1997), reproduced on p. 14 by permission of Weidenfeld & Nicolson; Arne Naess, *Thinking Like a Mountain* (Heretic Books 1988) reproduced on p. 14 by permission of GMP Publishers Ltd.; Joseph O'Connor and John Seymour, *Introducing Neuro-Linguistic Programming* (1993), reproduced on p. 15, and Malcolm Boyd, *Rich with Years* (1994), reproduced on p. 16, both by courtesy of HarperCollins Publishers Ltd.; M. C. Richards, *Crossing Point*, reproduced on p. 181 by permission of University of New England Press

Thanks to A & C Black Ltd for permission to use the three illustrations on pp. 170-2 by David Burroughs, from *Roy Kane TV Detective* by Stephen Bowkett (1998).

Author's acknowledgements

With thanks to Stella Hender for her wonderfully atmospheric drawings (p. 29-31) and to three young artists, Fabian Oppenheimer (p. 70), Julian Oppenheimer (p. 112) and James Murphy (p. 82 and p. 159) for theirs – and, as always, with love to Wendy for her patience and support.

Introduction

A note on marking

Among my earliest memories of mathematics is an occasion when I was about seven or eight years old, and a pupil at Edmund Street Junior School in the Rhondda Valleys, South Wales. We had been set a pageful of problems by our teacher 'Bomber' Evans. Bomber was not in a good mood that day, and so there would be no stories that afternoon about his wartime escapades. Instead, we'd be given more work, or a session of the horrendous 'Music and Movement' in the hall. But the morning followed its regular pattern, despite Bomber's temper; Maths B.M. (Before Milk) and English A.M., with no playtime if we misbehaved. Bomber ran through his explanation of what we had to do, wrote some textbook page numbers on the board, and told us to get on with it – in absolute silence, of course.

I took one look at the first pageful of 'sums' and despaired. I couldn't do this stuff. Bomber's previous explanations meant nothing; they simply didn't connect. I was in alien territory without a guide, and I felt panicky and frightened. A kind of dread came upon me as I glanced across at my mate, Kevin Howells, simply whizzing through the examples. I wasn't able to ask him for help, of course, on pain of punishment. I couldn't ask Bomber, because he'd already made things clear, hadn't he? So all I could do was get on with it, in absolute silence, with that horrible feeling of failure and imminent humiliation welling up inside me.

Because I had no clue about what I was doing, I finished quickly. The rule was that when you were done you had your work marked at the teacher's table. I pretended I hadn't finished for quite some time, hoping one of my classmates would summon up the bravery to be The First. But they were playing the same game, naturally, and anyway my fate was decided for me when Bomber noticed me looking around and called me out to the front.

With a loose-bowelled sense of fatalism I went and stood in trepidation at the Big Table. Bomber pushed his pile of marking aside and concentrated on my work. I got the first example wrong, and as Bomber put the red X by my answer, his other hand came up and slapped me open-palmed across the back of the skull. My embarrassment and shame were complete, I thought, as the other kids stared at me with glee or wide-eyed horror, or in desperation at realising they were up for the same.

I had completed about two dozen sums, and got every one wrong. That meant twenty-four slaps on the skull, twenty-four re-confirmations that I was pretty damned useless at maths. By the time Bomber had marked my book, he'd marked me too, very thoroughly...

That was all a long time ago. I'm grown up now, of course, and can put these things behind me. I can laugh about it and rationalise it away and say, well, it was character-forming. Right? No, not really. And not at all strange to me that I've never forgotten the episode, and that maths is still a strange and frightening land to me, because the ghost of Bomber Evans still haunts the shadows.

> Knowledge is a quest not a commodity.
>
> *Neil Postman &*
> *Charles Weingartner*

> The person who can't make a mistake can't make anything.
>
> *Abraham Lincoln*

> People almost always become what others think they are – becoming is almost always the product of expectation.
>
> *Neil Postman &*
> *Charles Weingartner*

This is an example of what has been called 'state-bound' or 'state-dependent' learning, memory and behaviour. My nervous state regarding maths was anchored within me because of this (and probably other) negative experiences. In that sense I was bound into a response state by what happened. It still echoes now when I meet similar situations, although it no longer has its past power to frighten. My nervousness-over-maths behaviour was a block to me and limited my potential for emotional resourcefulness because it was the only response I had at my disposal.

The techniques in *Self-Intelligence* aim to address this matter by creating a greater repertoire of emotional responses that can be used deliberately and systematically. Change through choice is the name of the game.

But perhaps you think I'm being melodramatic over the Bomber incident, blowing up out of all proportion one event among the millions of things I've seen and done in my life? After all, there must be many occasions I can remember when teachers were kind and supportive and effective in helping me learn. Yes, of course. But we are each the outcome (the ongoing outcome, if I can put it like that) of all the moments through which we've lived. And those moments are woven together deep in our minds to form what I like to call our 'map of reality'. This amounts to our individual, sum-total understanding of what we perceive the world to be, and the part we each play within it. So our opinions, attitudes, beliefs, the extent to which our potentials are fulfilled or inhibited, are profoundly wired-in to the minutiae of the inner map we carry in our heads. And my experience has been that these details are connected, not chronologically, but by significance – so that something which happened to me many years ago may react powerfully with an incident I experience today. Furthermore, although I might recall that earlier incident consciously, its influence could well be entirely nonconscious (subconscious), so that the behaviour which results may seem irrational and inexplicable, and apparently beyond my power to modify.

One of the things that constantly intrigues me about these ideas and the areas they allow me to explore is that each of us embodies a complex weave of themes, sub-themes, motifs and repeating narratives: we retell the story of our own life in whatever we interpret, believe, do and say. I am also astonished anew, day by day, to realise that our behaviours are accessible and modifiable by many different means. If there's something about the way we think, feel or behave that we don't want, then we can change it. Everything is negotiable. Everything is possible.

My spin on the words 'self' and 'intelligence' will become clearer as the book unfolds. Basically, however, I'm talking about the capacity for any individual to know him/herself better. With that knowledge comes understanding, and following understanding, greater control. Another way of expressing this process of self-discovery might be to say that in order to find out about ourselves, we need to look in.

In today's culture especially, we are immersed in notions of targets, goals, outcomes, tables of comparison, standards and competitiveness. The pressure is on for us to ACHIEVE. Being clever is not enough, perhaps. My opinion is that intellectual ability, however much it is developed and expressed, is but one aspect of our cumulative resourcefulness; our self-wealth, which Howard Gardner calls the intelligences or talents – that inner field of potentials which any effective educational system will draw out and allow to be expressed.

Standards for learning are not the same as standards for grading.

Neil Postman &
Charles Weingartner

The subject is me.

Neil Postman &
Charles Weingartner

Regarded in this way, it's clear that our talents operate synergistically if they are each cultivated and nourished according to our individual needs and requirements. And it is my view that emotional resourcefulness underpins all other abilities: literacy, numeracy and the whole spectrum of skills we are required to 'bring on' in children within the context of formal education. Since the mark of an educated person is the ability to manipulate ideas creatively, and since creativity flourishes when a person is confident, unstressed-but-challenged, possessed of high self-assurance and self-esteem, and able to use emotions elegantly, then it follows that offering children the means to enhance their emotional resourcefulness amounts to giving them a sound platform from which to develop the range of their other abilities.

Like Newton, we stand on the shoulders of giants. In presenting my work to you I am indebted to the sparkling insights of people like Howard Gardner, Daniel Goleman, Ernest Rossi and many others (see Bibliography). Ultimately, however, I have found my own way here: this stuff works for me, because I accept that the truest learning comes from one's own direct experience. So, as a previous tutor of mine would have it, I am responsible for what I say, but not for what you hear. Whatever interests you in this book, take it and make it your own. Doing that will give you the deepest understandings of what self-intelligence means.

The self-writing book

I once read a short story called *The Self-Assembling Curry*. I remember it partly because I wished I'd thought of the title, and also because it was a lovely metaphor for something that flew in the face of accepted common sense. What a wonderfully resourceful and self-determining curry it was!

In pale imitation of the title that inspired me, I offer the self-writing book. It is an image I frequently use to explain, to myself and others, the way the mind works – at least to a level of understanding that enables me to do what I do. It also embodies the notion of self-determination, which is part of the ethos underpinning the activities that follow.

If you are constantly or largely stuck with a feeling of frustration, anger, anxiety, fearfulness, failure, apathy, or whatever; or if, more broadly, you feel that things can't change for the better, and indeed may even get worse, then the sense of helplessness can eventually become overwhelming. On the other hand, if you were to entertain the notion that even the deepest and most rooted feelings can be modified by *direct positive action*, then the concept of the self-writing book will make more sense.

There are two underlying principles to this idea:

1. The mind and body are completely interconnected, so that thoughts, feelings and actions interweave in the process of being alive.

2. Each of us has a conscious aspect and a nonconscious aspect to our lives.

Thus, we can speak of conscious thoughts, feelings and actions, and nonconscious thoughts, feelings and actions. To a large extent these divisions are artificial since, as in a lake, who can say where the shallows end and the deeps begin? Yet it is true that many people are out of touch with themselves and fail to pick up or interpret the signals and messages streaming out from the deeper, non-conscious levels. At the same time, often, as we attempt to solve problems through sheer intellectual effort and will-power (determination to act), we may

What a strange machine man is! You fill him with bread, wine, fish and radishes, and out of him come sighs, laughter and dreams.

Nikos Kazantzakis

actually spend much of our time engaged in negative self-talk and what I call 'undeliberate' thought – consciously constructed thoughts which continue to run in our heads, but which we fail to attend to subsequently. (This is a bit like a pop song that goes round and round in our minds: it's there, but we don't notice it after a while, so it carries on by default.) The point is that our undeliberate thoughts contain meanings which may intensify if we allow them to drip-feed into the nonconscious part of the mind. We come to 'buy in' to the scenario they describe, without really having chosen to. And we all know that what we buy, we own. But what we own can also come to own us.

In other words, there is constant two-way communication between the conscious and subconscious parts of ourselves (see Fig. 1). However, we may not consciously attend to our inner wisdoms (inner-tuitions), nor act clearly and decisively to optimise the way we think, feel and act

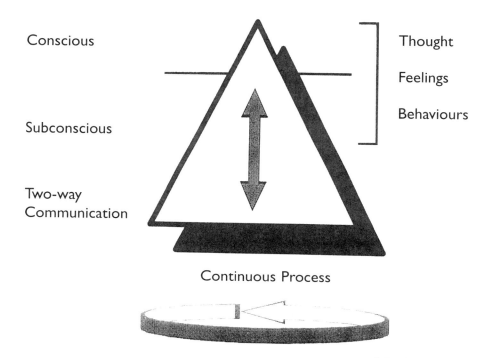

Conscious

Subconscious

Two-way
Communication

Thought

Feelings

Behaviours

Continuous Process

A basic model of the mind

Patterns of behaviour

The process just described frequently creates patterns of behaviour (some 'good', some 'bad') in our lives. It's convenient for us to run on automatic to a large extent, because then we don't need to reflect and make decisions about all the tiny elements of our existence. But if unhelpful patterns start up, through undeliberate thought and/or due to incidents which we may not consciously remember, such patterns may feel as though they're built in to the way we are, beyond our ability to change.

It is widely recognised that action follows thought, habit of action follows habit of thought, and compulsion of action follows compulsion of thought. This is the foundation of affirmations and self-empowerment – and also of catastrophism, the tendency to visualise worst-case scenarios and then worry over them as though they were inevitable. To take the attitude, 'Oh well, that's the reality of the situation. Whatever will be, will be', simply allows catastrophic thinking to continue unchecked. 'Che sara sara' is the antithesis of what self-intelligence is about.

Nonconscious learning

To return to the self-writing book: your conscious point-of-attention as it focuses on this page at this moment is like the nib of a pen as it writes down the latest meaning in your life. Now visualise the rest of that book. Everything that's ever happened to you – or rather, everything as you perceived it to happen, consciously and nonconsciously – is recorded back and back through those pages right to the very earliest entries. That life story corresponds to the 'map of reality' I referred to earlier.

But this is a subtle book and a complex one. To imagine it as I've suggested reflects our conscious perception: that the information is contained chronologically, with the first entries on page one. From this perspective what's most recent is clearest, while what's written in the past fades the further back it goes until, apart perhaps from a few vividly remembered episodes, the earliest part of life is largely forgotten.

Consider it another way, from the nonconscious angle. The book now more closely resembles an organiser. It is wonderfully cross-referenced so that, practically speaking, every piece of information is linked to every other piece. Moreover, information which gives rise to our wealth of beliefs is gathered together into 'chapters', regardless of when those incidents or ideas occurred to us. And every chapter is constantly being updated in light of our current experience, and in light of our ongoing beliefs.

In other words, we learn anyway: meanings are written in at a deep level and are assigned significance based upon previous experiences. Likewise our nonconscious interpretation of those previous experiences may become modified in light of incoming information. This whole seething process of 'meaning-making' produces a multitude of responses which may be either generalised and operative in all areas of our life, or highly specific to certain circumstances. Furthermore, these responses can be pleasant or unpleasant, as far as we are consciously concerned – although experience shows that behind even negative behaviours (phobias, anxieties or whatever) lie *positive intentions* (usually at a subconscious level and unrecognised consciously), since at all levels most of us have a vested interest in surviving and flourishing in the world.

So, if you hold a belief that you can't achieve something, for example, or that a particular emotional state is natural or inbuilt ('I'm a born pessimist', say), then your perception of the world will tend to reconfirm this belief again and again, and through selective awareness that's how the world will appear to treat you. In other words, the world is what our thoughts make it: 'Perception is projection' is the phrase that sums this up – the point being that in most cases we would not be conscious that all of this was going on, and would therefore fail to understand where our pessimistic outlook came from – much less that we could intervene to change it!

> If we view ourselves in a positive way, the world around us becomes empowering.
>
> *Daniel Brown*

Pit Stop 1:

- Each of us is a mind/body system.
- Thoughts, feelings and actions are linked.
- We possess both a conscious and a nonconscious aspect to our lives.
- Everything we've experienced is remembered at a nonconscious level.
- All of that information contributes to the way we think, feel and act now.
- We can learn to live more deliberately and with greater self-determination through direct positive action, using a wide range of interventions for ourselves, or with the aid of a trained professional.
- Greater emotional resourcefulness is one consequence of this process.

We underestimate
ourselves. I
emphasise self.
We tend to confuse it
with the narrow ego.

Arne Naess

Emotional resourcefulness, in the sense that I'm using the phrase, means the ability to recognise and understand emotions in ourselves (and consequently in other people) and to utilise and modify emotions more deliberately. This implies the ability to access emotions directly, so that unhelpful ones can be modified or eliminated, while positive and empowering ones can be 'switched on' as appropriate, and amplified at will. And if you think this is impossible, then I suggest you withhold judgement until after you've finished the book, and verified what I say through trying the activities I offer against a background of further reading from the references listed in the Bibliography.

Brainscapes, mindscapes and wordscapes

In the educational world in recent years there has been a groundswell of interest in 'brain-based' learning strategies based on discoveries in neuroscience about how the human brain functions. Much of the essential information is well summarised in Alistair Smith's book *Accelerated Learning in Practice*, published by Network Educational Press.

Undoubtedly a knowledge of brain function informs the design of more effective learning strategies. However, my interest, and the underpinning of *Self-Intelligence*, lies not so much in how the machinery works as in the principles governing how we behave (think – feel – act), with emphasis on the emotions.

For my purposes, as someone who wants a practical toolkit of techniques to use now – or at least in time for my PSE session with 9H tomorrow morning – it's sufficient to know that the information which reaches my brain results in physical modifications to the way my brain cells (neurones) are wired up. The network of connections between the neurones evolves in light of what I experience. This is to say, my neural landscape – my brainscape – grows and changes through life as I learn.

I have already mentioned the 'map of reality' - all the information that exists in my mind, together with its interconnections and assigned significance. This territory may also be called the 'mindscape', and it is a direct analogue of the brainscape. One implication of this idea is that when patterns of behaviour are modified, by default or through intervention, *new neural connections are made* to accommodate the change. Read Guy Claxton's book *Hare Brain Tortoise Mind* for much more fascinating detail about this subject and the world of the subconscious. Susan Greenfield in *The Human Brain* also offers a more technical confirmation that 'experience is a key factor in shaping the micro-circuitry of the brain'.

What we think and how we feel are expressed constantly in the language we use. The flow of our words has been described as the surface structure reflecting the deep structure of the mindscape. There is a direct link between how we use language (with all its rich tapestry of conscious and nonconscious associations) and our deepest interpretations of reality. And so we can consider the 'landscape of language', our individual wordscapes, as having great importance in our undertaking to enhance the emotional resourcefulness of ourselves and others.

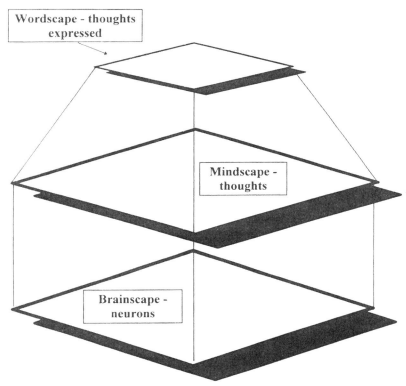

Brainscape, mindscape, wordscape

Jean Paul Sartre compared words with loaded pistols. They carry great energy and power. The meanings we make to survive in the world are embodied in words. We are all 'natural languagers' - we learn language simply as a result of existing among other language users. So part of our exploration of self-intelligence involves unfolding the layers of our language, so as to be able to base many of our interventions for change on what we say and how we say it. Indeed, the basic approach of Neuro Linguistic Programming (NLP) - 'a methodology that leaves behind it a trail of techniques' - seeks personal excellence through the medium of words.

Exploring the context

Let's say a scientist discovers a new kind of parrot in the Amazon rainforest. One way of learning more about the parrot would be to take it back to the lab, notice how it behaved and, perhaps, dissect it eventually to see how the bits were put together.

Another approach – the ecological approach – would be to observe the parrot in its natural surroundings, to see how it interacted with the environment in which it lived. It might also be helpful to know something about how that parrot evolved, adapting itself to current conditions.

How marvellous it would be, surely, if an investigative procedure existed that could achieve the best of both worlds, combining the understandings of the reductionist in the laboratory with the ecological/holistic approaches.

Exploring the ecology, or the context in which an emotion occurs, can lead to profound insights, enabling one to use that emotion more powerfully as a resource. To be able to do it for oneself is a high-level skill, although many naturally intuitive people take such an ability for granted – and here let me explain that I use the word 'intuition' in a particular way, to mean 'inner tuition'. Like most abilities it can be developed, since it lies more or less latent in all of us. To some extent the activities in *Self-Intelligence* amount to a programme of systematic intuition. And in case you're wondering, that programme does combine the laboratory and the ecological processes of discovery.

Our lives cry out for intrinsic meaning.

Malcolm Boyd

The creative edge

My previous book, *Imagine That...*, subtitled 'a handbook of creative learning activities for the classroom', advocates the view that creative thinking allows children to manipulate ideas in their heads, rather than simply accumulate dead knowledge and react to it subsequently – i.e., think reactively or 'guess the right answer'.

Reactive thinking is exemplified by the question, 'What is the capital of France?' This is a closed question targeting a specific piece of information based on a single link between 'capital' and 'France'. The meaning embedded in that link has come from an outside authority, and it is value-laden and judgmental. Which is to say that whether or not I get the answer right, a judgement is made, however implicitly, about my ability to understand, learn and remember. Because I might get the answer wrong, my risk-taking behaviour in trying out possible answers is inhibited. I shut up rather than speak out – and we're right back to the way I felt all those years ago in Bomber Evans' classroom.

The approach of creative thinking, on the other hand, is to explore possible answers, based on the premises that answers are best regarded not as right or wrong, but as more or less useful to our purposes, and that the process of invention is more important than the product invented. From this platform, the elements of the creative approach can be summarised as follows:

- uses and encourages open questioning where varied manipulation of ideas is the primary purpose
- implies many possible answers (which are more or less useful)
- relies upon individual learners' current resources of knowledge and understanding, and encourages access to outside authority as appropriate
- is non-judgmental, co-operative, cumulative
- supports 'risk-taking' answers and celebrates diversity
- seeks to draw out individuals' world pictures – the network of meanings they've already made
- aims to create resourceful learning states by incorporating positive feedback during the thinking process, leading to multiple strategies for achieving goal-oriented outcomes

And so, if we return to the idea of 'capital' and 'France' and process those ideas through a creative thinking approach, we come up with questions like:

- Why do you think Paris is the capital of France?
- How do you find out why it is?
- When do you know you have enough information to reach a conclusion?
- How can you test your conclusion?
- What does it mean for a place to be a capital?
- What conditions does a place need to fulfil to be a capital?
- Investigate other capitals – are some places better suited to be capitals than others?
- Why is this? How do you know?
- Can a town or village be a capital?
- Who decides which place becomes a capital?
- Are there other ways of deciding which place becomes a capital? (Find three, choose the way you think works best, and explain why.)
- Do you think your town / village could be a capital? Why is that?
- Would you like it to be a capital? Why?
- What other meanings for the word 'capital' can you think of / find out? Are they linked? If so, how? (How do you find out?) etc...

The creative thinking process and the quest for self-intelligence

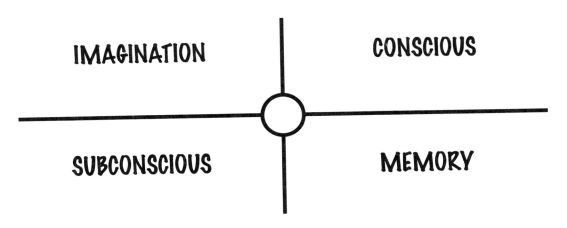

- Thinking-feeling-acting is an elegant dance of energy between these aspects of mind.
- We see with the mind's eye, hear with the mind's ear, touch with the mind's hands, feel with the mind's heart.
- What we conceive and admit, we believe. What we believe, we act upon.
- Experiences are 'anchored' in our lives, both past and future; strung like beads on a necklace.
- Language is a powerful and transforming meaning-making process.

The creative approach can and must also be applied to the quest for greater self-intelligence. In a positive learning loop, it requires playfulness, curiosity and perseverance, and leads to greater self-confidence, insight and independence. This book is intended as a companion volume to *Imagine That....* They can be used independently, but I anticipate you'll find many useful ways of cross-fertilising techniques when you read them in combination.

> I want to be what I was when I wanted to be what I am now.
>
> *Anonymous*

Mix and Match

Accessing emotions, removing blocks to learning, and using memory and imagination to modify systems of belief does not amount to a mysterious process: it requires no special talent to employ the techniques I offer, nor are you in any way 'meddling' with other people's minds or feelings. If you accept that being more emotionally resourceful provides a sound platform for developing other skills across the curriculum, then why not explore ways of achieving this? By the time you've sifted through the activities you will have realised all sorts of applications for my self-intelligence games, simulations and exercises.

Another point I'd like to make is that self-intelligence is a capacity that we can all develop further in ourselves. Perhaps the most effective means of allowing children to grow in this way is for us to use the techniques for ourselves first of all, and become adept with them. You may prefer to work alone, or with a partner. The advantage of this is that you have someone there to help you understand the techniques and find your way through them, and maybe subsequently discuss ways of adapting the activities to fit more closely with your needs and circumstances.

Neil Postman and Charles Weingartner have argued that success at school is best measured by behavioural changes in the students. Which is to say that what lies at the heart of education also lies at the heart of individuals...

... So Explore!

1) List your dominant emotions, ones which you experience often and more strongly than others.
2) Give each one a number on a scale of 1-6 for intensity, where 1 means you feel the emotion faintly and 6 means you feel it powerfully.
3) If any of the emotions you listed in (1) are negative or unpleasant, consider that these emotions might serve a positive purpose in your life, and speculate as to what that purpose might be.
4) Take the most positive emotion in your list and give it a colour, a shape, a size, a texture, a temperature, a weight and, if you wish, a sound and an aroma. (You needn't drop into stereotypical thinking and, for instance, make anger red and sharp, as Mars from the Planets Suite plays in the background...) Let your ideas come along without any special effort: let them just pop into your head.
5) Go through the same process for any negative emotion in your list.
6) Compare each of these emotions to an aspect of the weather, an animal, a machine, a kind of person.
7) Re the emotions compared to an aspect of the weather – in each case suggest some positive aspect of those weather conditions.
8) Re the emotions compared to an animal – suggest some positive quality of the animal in each case.
9) Re the emotions compared to a machine, suggest a useful function for the machine in each case.
10) Re the emotions compared with kinds of person, think of five questions you'd like to ask each person about any aspect of his or her life.

11) Draw a large circle on a blank sheet of paper. Pretend that circle represents you. Prepare to draw other, subsidiary circles which represent positive or negative issues in your life. The rules are:

- The larger the subsidiary circle, the more significant the issue to you.
- Subsidiary circles which overlap are somehow connected (in ways perhaps that you do not completely understand or have not fully explored).
- Circles drawn inside the main circle represent issues which are more or less internal. i.e., other people cannot pick up clues about this issue in your appearance, speech or behaviour.
- Circles overlapping the edge of the main circle represent issues which you are expressing to a greater or lesser degree, i.e., other people can pick up clues about this issue in your appearance, speech or behaviour.
- Subsidiary circles drawn outside the main circle represent external issues, which may be a person, an event, a place, or a combination of these (see p.131-2 for further clarification).

Example of Circle Diagram

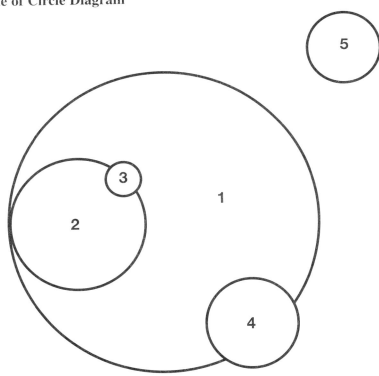

1. Main circle – represents yourself
2. Represents a significant issue that's entirely inside.
3. Represents a smaller issue linked to 2.
4. Represents a fairly significant issue that's in the process of being expressed.
5. Represents some external matter that has not yet affected you (moving towards you), or one that you've experienced and which is now 'moving away'.

Once you have drawn the circle diagram – which is to say, begun to map out your emotional landscape – you can develop the technique in various ways:

a) Put the diagram in an envelope and open it after three months. Note how things have changed in the meantime.
b) Ask yourself 'what if?' questions. What if particular subsidiary circles were larger or smaller? What if inner issues were more obviously expressed? What if current issues were replaced by others of my own

choosing? What if I could arrange for this to happen – what would I need to do? What if negative issues were looked at in a positive light? And so on.

c) **Future Base**: Draw a circle diagram of how you'd like to be at some point in the future. Think about what would need to change for this to become a reality.

d) Take a closer look at the 'ingredients' of subsidiary circles. What emotions are attached? What are the positive and negative ingredients of the circle? How would a change in the circle (pick a change) affect the other circles on the map? How would that change feel to me?

e) **Mind-read**: Draw somebody else's circle diagram. (What you express about them is telling you something about yourself.) Think about why you have reached these conclusions. How can your insights make you more effective in dealing with this person? If they don't, what would you need to do to achieve greater effectiveness?

f) **Scrapbook and Journal**: If certain emotions have a dominating influence in your life, learn more about those emotions. Collect extracts from fiction, poems, items from newspapers and autobiographies that define and describe your chosen emotions. Take time to write about your emotions; what triggers them, how it feels while they're happening, what effects they cause, what things lessen or intensify them. Personify the emotion and write a 'day in the life' of the emotion in the first person, referring to yourself in the third person.

g) **Back to Basics**: Explain important emotions as though to someone who has never experienced them. Use any descriptive technique available to clarify as far as you can what these emotions are like.

h) **Fantasy Scenario**: Pretend a chosen emotion simply didn't exist anywhere in the world or in the human psyche. What differences would result?

12) Try this – it's called *The Necklace Technique*:

- Pick an issue, emotion, potential.
- Pretend it's a thread reaching back through your life.
- Pretend that 'contributory incidents' are beads on that thread. Acknowledge that the size, colour, spacing, texture, etc., of the beads have significance, but that you don't have to know at this stage what it is.
- Take time to sit quietly and gather up an impression of the thread in the most appropriate way for you – which could be as visual images, impressions of sounds, impressions of textures, physical feelings...
- Without making any special effort, imagine you are drifting back along the thread, encountering the beads as you go. At this stage, simply notice the beads are there. You may be aware that some beads are very significant, and you may want to know more about them – i.e., to understand what they represent in your life. If this is the case, read the activity called *Control Panel* on p.108 before you proceed.
- However far you progress with the Necklace Technique, acknowledge to yourself that you have done good work to further your self-understanding, and by implication the emotional resourcefulness of the students in your care.

13) Try three other activities from this book before you use any activities with children.

Any plan is bad which is not susceptible to change.

Italian proverb

Direct positive action

Emotions exist for reasons we can uncover. Dealing with the emotional landscapes of our lives does not mean ignoring feelings or suppressing them, nor does it often mean confronting them. Rather, we act positively and decisively, mindfully and elegantly to explore them. This process results in an increased awareness, which results in greater self-understanding. And from that firm basis of understanding, we inherit control.

We all have a vested interest in emotional resourcefulness, becoming more self-intelligent. So that, for example, because we understand anger more thoroughly we can modulate it, instead of automatically responding angrily to some anger-provoking situation. And if we choose not to express anger at all, then we have at our disposal other emotions that could serve our purposes more beneficially and powerfully... And consider those times when you've done something which filled you with pleasure, joy and a sense of achievement. What if you could have those same feelings just whenever you wanted them – either as an underpinning for a particular task, or just as a treat? And how would it empower you, how will you feel, when you can face the future with more than just hope – with a positive and directed anticipation of success and potentials fulfilled?

Self-Intelligence invites you to range across the world of the emotions so that you gain more experience of them, deliberate and systematic experience. And in that experience lies ownership, authority, and then mastery. Once you have come to realise that for yourself, you are ready to hand over the same power and control to your students. Be assured, you are not meddling with dangerous forces or things you can't understand. Our emotions are us, and we have a right to use them for our own benefit. You are not being asked to do the job of a psychologist, counsellor or therapist, you are not being asked to reveal any private and personal information to anyone, nor are you requiring your students to do so. Nor, can I add, should you feel disconcerted that there is no National Curriculum documentation telling you what to do and how to do it in this area! Thankfully, in my view, no SAT test exists to measure the parameters you're working with – because we are dealing here with the lifeblood of a school, which runs deeper than any political agenda. You will notice the results of your work, and students will certainly feel the difference in themselves. As these changes permeate through the school, the whole institution will change. And this will be the platform on which other future benefits are built.

> I hear and I forget,
> I see and I remember,
> I do and I understand.
>
> *Chinese proverb*

> Success is measured in terms of behavioural changes in students.
>
> *Neil Postman &*
> *Charles Weingartner*

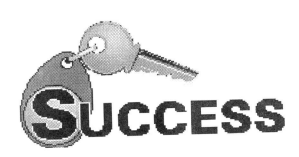

Pit Stop 2

Thinking habits (technically called 'cognitive distortions') which can limit our capacity for self-intelligence include:

- **All-or-nothing**: You see things in terms of black and white. If something isn't perfect, then it's a complete failure.
- **Over-generalisation**: Seeing a single negative event as an ongoing, and often escalating, crisis. This can lead quickly to habit and then compulsion of thought.
- **Labelling**: Putting a label on to yourself, an event or someone else. This essentially turns a verb into a noun, emphasising an object rather than a process. Combined with other cognitive distortions, it can have seriously detrimental results: for example, something doesn't turn out quite right for you so, 'I'm a loser.' Another person behaves, let's say, in a thoughtless way, so 'He's a total moron.' Such a thinking habit helps stoke up negative emotions and provide an instant trigger point for their expression.
- **Negative filtering**: Selecting only the negative aspects of what happens in your life so that pre-existing beliefs are reconfirmed, and filtering out positive experiences as unimportant: you deny or suppress them, usually nonconsciously. The result is that a single negative experience is magnified and outweighs many positive experiences, which are trivialised. (Positive filtering also exists, of course. It's called looking at the world through rose-tinted glasses, and is often a protective device.)
- **Mind-reading**: Guessing or anticipating what someone will think, say or do, and jumping to negative conclusions. This is linked to Fortune-telling, where you behave as though an unpleasant consequence has already occurred ('I'm bound to do badly in this OFSTED inspection!').
- **Emotionally-weighted Reasoning**: Assuming your negative perceptions reflect things as they really are. If you are angry, then you live in an angry world.
- **'Should' limiters**: 'Should' prevents expansion. If you 'should' do something, then you automatically imply that a 'but' follows. This leads to inertia and often a sense of guilt that you 'should, but haven't' taken action. 'Should' projected on to someone else can lead to anger, resentment and frustration when they 'should, but didn't' take action.
- **Personalisation**: Taking on yourself the blame for some external event, when the blame lies elsewhere, or is not even a factor.
- Want to change some of these? Read on.

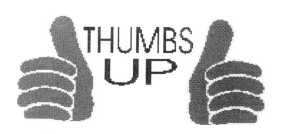

A Note on All our Futures

The National Advisory Committee on Creative and Cultural Education (NACCCE) was established in February 1998 by the Secretary of State for Education and Employment, the Rt. Hon. David Blunkett MP, and the Secretary of State for Culture, Media and Sport, the Rt. Hon. Chris Smith MP, under the chairmanship of Professor Ken Robinson of Warwick University.

NACCCE's terms of reference were 'to make recommendations to the Secretaries of State on the creative and cultural development of young people through formal and informal education: to take stock of current provision and to make proposals for principles, policies and practice'.

My own input to the Committee's work was to form part of an advisory group under Professor Robinson's auspices to discuss the nature of 'creativity' and to translate basic definitions and principles into practical activities that teachers could use with pupils immediately, and which would fit easily into the framework of the solidly-in-place but seemingly ever-changing National Curriculum.

I was at pains to point out that the emotional component of any educational experience is fundamental to the quality of the learning experience. In short, children (and adults, too, actually) learn best when they are interested, motivated, involved, unstressed, and when they can see the personal relevance of what it is they are being required to learn.

In recent years I have given much thought to putting this preaching into practice. Among the most substantial results have been my books *Imagine That...* and the present *Self-Intelligence*. It is highly refreshing to see that the final report by the NACCCE – *All Our Futures: Creativity, Culture and Education* – opens with a foreword by David Blunkett which begins, 'Creative and cultural education can help raise educational standards by boosting a child's self-confidence and self-esteem.' It is my sincere wish that the educational world will take note, and in the process realise also that boosting a child's self-confidence and self-esteem can raise standards in all areas, not least in the fields of creative and cultural education.

What one does, one becomes

Spanish proverb

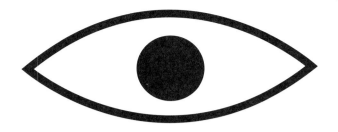

Section One

DEVELOPING SENSORY ACUITY

*T*his, more straightforwardly, means developing the ability to notice things. I can remember as a fourteen-year-old being complimented by the teacher in an art class because I had noticed a mole on the chin of the girl our group was sketching. The art teacher looked at my work and nodded. 'Very well observed,' he said. ' Well done.' It took me twenty minutes to work out what he'd been referring to.

As a writer, I know that often the difference between a readable piece of fiction and one that sparkles is to be found in the inclusion of small details. Those details have to be noticed before they can be used. And as a hypnotherapist, I have been trained to observe subtle nuances in what people say and in how they look and react. Those of you familiar with the field of Neuro-Linguistic Programming (NLP) will know that 'noticing the nonverbals' is a key component of that 'technology'.

In terms of self-intelligence, being emotionally capable involves being sensitive to the way other people feel. We are bundles of contradictions, often saying one thing when our voice tonality, facial expression or body posture imply something else. Similarly, in order to change ourselves we need first to be aware of ourselves (and self-awareness, it goes without saying, is a world apart from self-consciousness).

In today's busy outwardly looking culture, where we have a run-up to Christmas instead of a gentle stroll, many people have lost the knack of being attentive and sensitive to themselves. This section aims to address the issue and redress the balance, developing 'acuities' which have use far beyond the immediate purposes of this book.

Active Noticing

The pupil asked, 'Sir, what is the best way to learn?'
The teacher replied, 'If you have finished your rice, then wash your bowl.'

from a traditional Chinese parable.

Our subconscious minds contain everything we know. Our conscious minds contain all that we are aware of at this moment. Although this is undoubtedly a simplification, it will serve our purposes well; for as Einstein said, 'Always make things as simple as possible, but no simpler.' Our conscious point-of-attention, like a narrowly focused spotlight, illuminates and brings into awareness things that are outside of ourselves and within us, to constitute what we call an experience – not that we notice very much, because both outside and inside things are going on that we cannot or do not attend to, for whatever reason. To some extent, then, we are the passive recipients of experience, noticing only certain aspects of whatever is happening.

Active Noticing is a technique that will be called upon time after time throughout this book. In a way it is no more than 'paying attention', although not exactly the same as our perennial wish for children to listen to what we are saying and look at what we've written on the board. It amounts to a raising of awareness, moment by moment, of how we feel as we move through our day. It helps create a sense of 'living deliberately' as Robin Williams put it so elegantly in the film *Dead Poets' Society*. Active noticing ideally becomes a habit that allows us to make our experiences more meaningful, highlighting the minutes that make up our lives. John Lennon said that life is something that happens while we're busy making other plans. As we notice what we're doing and how we feel, we don't lose the capacity to make plans, but we do become mindful of the moment, with all its richness and texture.

- **Noticing the breath**
  Now, and for the next minute, be aware of your breathing. There's no need to change your breathing in any way, just notice it.

- **Noticing your body**
  Become aware of the position of your body in the chair; notice the weight, the physical presence of your body. Be aware of any areas of tension (forehead? neck and shoulders? jaw?). Notice how you are holding this book. Suddenly feel the weight of the book, the texture of the paper. Turn a page and be aware of the sound that makes.

- **Noticing your feelings**
  Become aware of your emotions now. However faint or subtle, you're feeling something. Now perhaps isn't the time to try to track those emotions back to their roots: simply take some quiet time to notice them, and make notes afterwards.

- **Noticing your environment**
  Let your awareness expand a little and notice what's around you: colours, sounds, positions of things. Play with this awareness. Notice smaller and smaller things, then relax and have a sense of 'the whole picture'.

Pennywork

This is a basic activity which allows children to notice details and understand that differences exist between apparently similar objects. It's a simple little exercise that you might use only once or twice, but it offers a lead in to *noticing* as a useful skill, which can then be more widely applied in many other contexts.

Basic activity

- Hand out pairs of pennies to the groups and ask children to spot differences between the coins and note them down.

- Be prepared initially to hear that there are no differences, and suggest that the children look more closely. Mention if you like that as of writing the record for differences stands at 31! Allow any mark, blemish, scratch, etc., to count as a difference, since this is an exercise in noticing. Groups will very quickly pick up different dates, the one penny/new penny distinction, subtle differences in the Queen's profile, and others.

- Gather feedback to compile a 'definitive list' of differences, where any nick in a coin counts as a single difference (rather than every nick in each coin being one).

Extension activities/variations

- Ask children to speculate about the design details of certain coins. Why do they have different sizes and designs? What do the words on coins refer to? What could the abbreviations mean? Look at paper money and discuss the subtleties of the design. Why is it so complicated, etc.?

- Have children design their own coinage and paper money, emphasising the point that every aspect of the design should serve a purpose, whether that be decorative, symbolic or practical.

- Open out discussion about the difference between cost and value. Where appropriate, explore children's feelings about money, wealth, charity, and so on. Once these feelings have begun to be defined and described, comb through other self-intelligence activities to allow children to use those feelings more effectively.

Literacy Link

Scatterwords – Prepare a sheet containing a number of similarly spelt words and ask the children to notice the differences. Extend the exercise by matching the visual word with the way it's said, again keeping children primed to notice subtle distinctions.

GROUPING	Pairs or small groups, then larger groups or whole class for feedback
TIME	10 minutes for activity plus time afterwards for feedback
EQUIPMENT	Bag of coins
SKILLS DEVELOPED	Observation, visual acuity, discussion
AGE	Across the range

Best Guess

GROUPING	Whole class initially, then smaller groups can work independently
TIME	20-30 minutes per session
EQUIPMENT	Black-and-white pictures
SKILLS DEVELOPED	Observation, deduction, speculation, discussion
AGE	Across the range

Basic activity

● Using a picture such as Illustration 1, ask the children to mention things they can *actually see*. Even the most obvious things count as good observations - 'It's a black and white picture, Miss!'

● It may be necessary early on to point out the difference between a pure observation, a deduction and a personal opinion or value judgement. Point out the differences between statements such as

● ' A firework has gone off above the rooftops.'
' The firework has frightened the cat.'
' I think there are some kids up the road and they scared the cat.'
' Fireworks are dangerous and should be banned.'

- in other words, keep the activity tight by focusing first on observable details.

● Proceed by inviting deductions – because the rocket has gone off, it may have frightened the cat. Because there are few or no leaves on the trees, and fireworks are being let off, it's probably Bonfire Night. Because there are puddles on the pavement, it was probably raining earlier.

● Extend the activity by invoking other senses. If the picture were in colour, what colours would there be, do you think? If we could turn up the volume in the picture, what sounds would we hear? (Deductions and speculations based on personal opinion are acceptable here.)

● Continue by saying to the children, 'OK, let's pretend we can actually step into that picture now. After the count of three, let's do it...' Ask what other impressions come to mind, and encourage kinaesthetic/gustatory responses. Feel the different types of bricks in the wall and describe the differences. What can you smell as you stand there on that street corner? Pick up a leaf and scrunch it up. How does that feel? What sounds does the leaf make?

● Exercise the imagination by telling the children that now they're in the picture, they can notice lots of other things going on around them, outside the scope of the visible picture. Collect ideas and acknowledge everyone's contribution, so that no child dominates the imagined scenario.

● Move on to emotions. How does the cat feel at that moment? Describe the feeling in detail. How do the children feel at Bonfire Night? (Not so much how they feel about it: we're exploring emotions now, rather than gathering opinions.) If 'excitement' is one response, ask if Bonfire Night excitement is different from birthday excitement, holiday excitement, etc. Urge children to be as detailed and specific as possible in making distinctions like these.

● Conclude the activity by having the children 'step back out' of the frame - 'let's pretend' exercises like these are powerful and absorbing, so it's always advisable to reorient the children in the here-and-now. You might then invite ideas as to what might happen to the cat now, or have children talk about their own memories of Bonfire Night, etc.

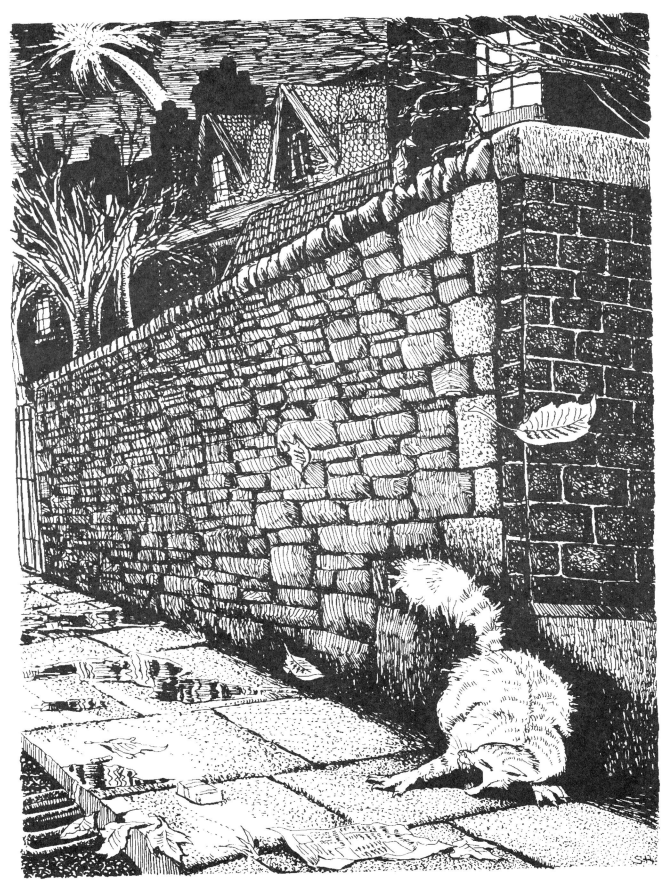

Illustration 1

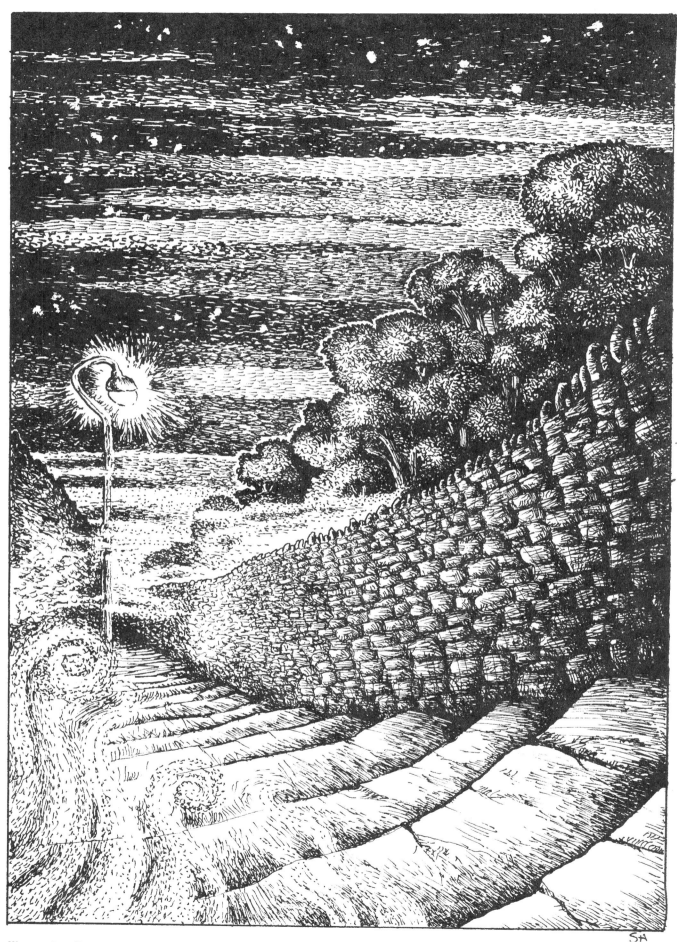

Illustration 2

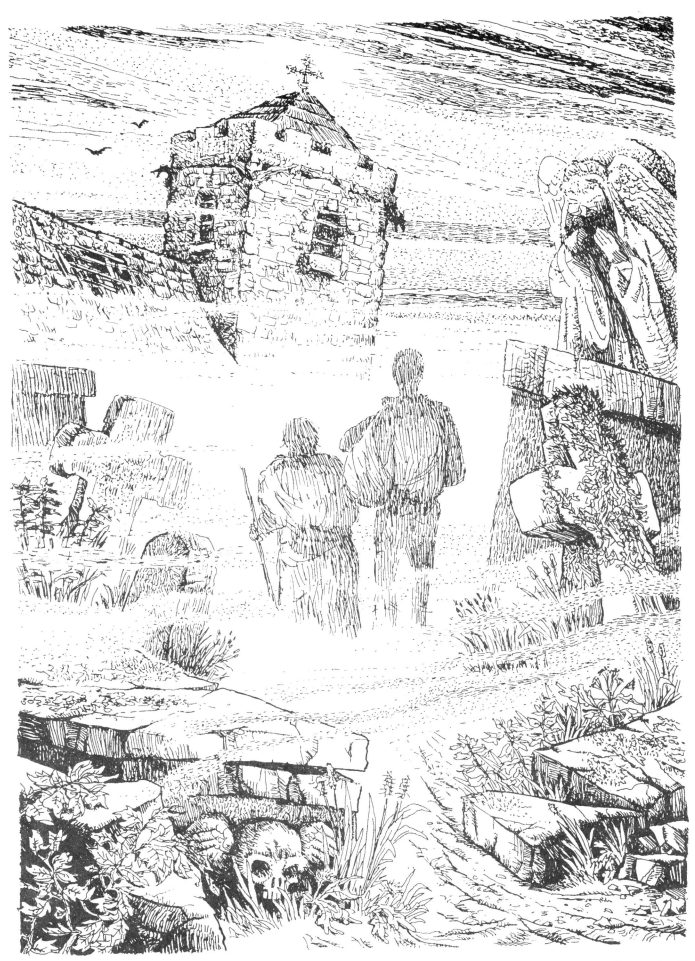

Illustration 3

Extension activities/variations

● *Mood Pictures* – Many pictures evoke emotions and can therefore be used as a starting point for exploring our feelings. Illustrations 1b and 1c (drawn by artist Stella Hender) are provided here as examples. After following some or all of the procedure outlined above, use the information gathered to have children:

  ■ gather other pictures that evoke the same mood
  ■ make a collage representing a mood or feeling
  ■ make links with other events and circumstances that evoke the same or similar emotions (if similar, explore the differences!)
  ■ develop a mime, dance or short play emphasising the mood
  ■ represent a mood in terms of a character, animal, machine, aspect of the weather

● *Music Link* – Prepare some short taped instrumental extracts. Explain to the group that the music you are about to play is a person, a place, an animal, an aspect of weather, a machine, etc. (Perhaps split the class into groups and assign one of these or other categories to each group). Ask the children to write down any impressions that come to mind as the music plays – no matter at this stage about neatness or spelling – spontaneity is what counts. Use the impressions gathered as above.

● *Aromatics* – Aromas are powerfully evocative (which is why the perfume industry works). Use aromatherapy oils to create an ambience in your classroom. Ask children to pretend that the aroma they are about to smell is a person, animal, aspect of weather, etc., as above.

 Literacy Link

All of the above activities can lead towards writing. See the story-making section in *Imagine That...* for further directions.

Music Map

We tend naturally to interpret instrumental music. This activity helps guide children in their interpretations, and points out to them that many interpretations are often possible.

Basic activity

● Select an appropriate instrumental piece and, as you listen to it several times beforehand, write a list of open questions which allow children to focus on specific elements of the music and clarify and elaborate their interpretation. Such questions may be very general:

> What colours do you imagine as the music plays?
> If you could touch the music, what would it feel like?
> What feelings do you have as the music plays?
> What stays the same through the musical piece?
> What slow changes do you notice?
> List some things that suddenly change.

- or questions could focus on certain sequences within the music:

> Imagine two people are talking now (in the music). What might they be saying to each other?
> What do these people look like?
> How are they feeling right now?
> They each have something in their hands. What could these things be?

● You can also use music as a 'primer' to gather ideas for storymaking (see *Best Guess*, p.28). Tell children that the music they'll hear suggests a map or landscape, and that the details of the music represent things they can put on the map. Emphasise that they can only draw something on the map when they've 'heard it in the music and know it's there'.

Extension activity

Prepare a selection of short musical pieces and poems and/or story extracts. Invite children to match these up on the basis of what similarities they perceive between the music and story.

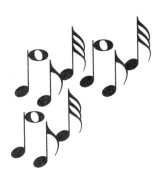

GROUPING	Whole class
TIME	5-20 minutes
EQUIPMENT	Pre-recorded music selection
SKILLS DEVELOPED	Listening, visualisation, interpretation
AGE	7+

Book and Cover

GROUPING	Whole class initially, then smaller groups can work independently
TIME	20 minutes onwards
EQUIPMENT	Suitable book covers plus extracts from the stories
SKILLS DEVELOPED	Observation, comparison, discrimination, evaluation, questioning, discussion
AGE	7+

One aim of this activity, besides the cluster of skills which are sharpened by it, is to raise awareness that artwork embodies the artist's *interpretation* of a story's elements. This idea can be extended by showing the class photographic representations – the camera may not lie, but the person behind it makes sure it's selective with the truth.

Basic activity

● Pick a book where a section or sections of the story are interestingly depicted on the cover. Read (or allow the children to read) the extracts(s), then invite comments about how – and how well – the cover visuals portray the ideas, people and incidents in the story.

● Conclude by asking groups or individuals how they would have designed the cover.

Extension activities/variations

● Read an extract from a book and describe what you think the book's cover would be like.

● Compare covers from similar stories or genres, or by the same or similar artists, and look for similarity of theme, motif and style.

● 'Match' extract with front cover art and back cover blurb.

● 'Match' cover art with pieces of music.

● Do a *Best Guess* activity (see p.28).

● Examine more closely elements of cover art such as font styles, positioning of words, catch-lines ('The world would never be the same again', etc.).

NOTE Authors, anthologists and editors often negotiate the final appearance of a book's cover, which may go through several versions. It would be worth writing to authors and publishers to ask about this: certainly most authors have strong opinions (positively and negatively!) about the way their books are represented.

The Unfolding Story

A story as a finished product is a linear thing, having the well-known beginning – middle – end structure with which children are so familiar. The process of thinking up a story is not quite so straightforward, however, as this activity aims to demonstrate.

Basic activity

- Read/show/tell your group an extract from a story, preferably from the middle section.

- Invite the children to come up with ideas about how the characters could have reached that point.
  Similarly, invite them to speculate about what could happen in the story from this point onwards.
  (At this stage emphasise that all ideas are useful, and that no judgements are being made about them.)

- Vary the activity subsequently by asking how the story might progress if the extract itself were different in some way. You can use a story tree template to map out possibilities (see *Story Tree* in *Imagine That...*, p. 168-9).

> The pool of ideas could be represented visually like the roots of a tree – again, see *Story Tree*.

- The next stage of the activity would be to put ideas into some sort of order – of complexity, realism, upbeat versus downbeat, etc.

- Conclude *The Unfolding Story* by asking groups to summarise one possible version of the narrative based on their own or others' ideas, including the extract.

Extension activities/variations

- Instead of a written extract, use cover art or an internal illustration.

- Explore the emotions of the characters in the extract and/or the situations invented by the children.

- Link in with *Dice Journey* (see *Imagine That...*, p.177).

- Discuss the reader's emotional involvement with stories (text, film, etc.) and explore the children's emotions as they listened to the extract, using any of the self-intelligence techniques you know about.

GROUPING	Whole class
TIME	15 minutes onwards
EQUIPMENT	Extract from a story (in text and / or picture form)
SKILLS DEVELOPED	Listening, retention /recall, brainstorming, discrimination/ choice, questioning, deconstruction, negotiation, speculation, judgement
AGE	Across the range

The Eyes Have It

GROUPING	Whole class demonstration, then groups of any size
TIME	15 minutes
EQUIPMENT	Drawing materials
SKILLS DEVELOPED	Observation, discrimination, interpretation
AGE	Across the range

This activity is linked with *Circle Faces* (p.47), but can be used as a separate exercise.

Basic activity

● With your help, have children express emotions facially – anger, shock, mirth, etc.

● Extend the repertoire of emotions by using pictures from magazines, comics, video clips.

● Put names to the emotions, drawing out whatever distinctions seem appropriate (between mirth and joy, envy and jealousy, for instance).

● Go through the repertoire again, this time asking children to notice the eyes and eyebrows. Get the groups to draw as accurately as they can what they observe.

● Collect in the pictures and then use them in various ways:
 ■ have children sort the pictures into sets, an anger set, an embarrassment set, etc.
 ■ guide children towards more general conclusions about how eyes and eyebrows look when certain emotions are being expressed, i.e., that eyebrows lift in surprise, get drawn together in puzzlement, that the eyes become narrowed in mirth...
 ■ introduce eye-pictures of emotions not covered initially and work with children to put names to the emotions they suggest

Extension activities/variations

● Have groups mime a short story or scene using only facial expressions, with emphasis on using the eyes and surrounding musculature.

● Using a variation of *Circle Faces*, deliberately mismatch eye configuration with the rest of the facial expression. So, for example, put a pair of angry eyes-and-eyebrows on a laughing circle face. Invite children to discuss how and why this looks strange.

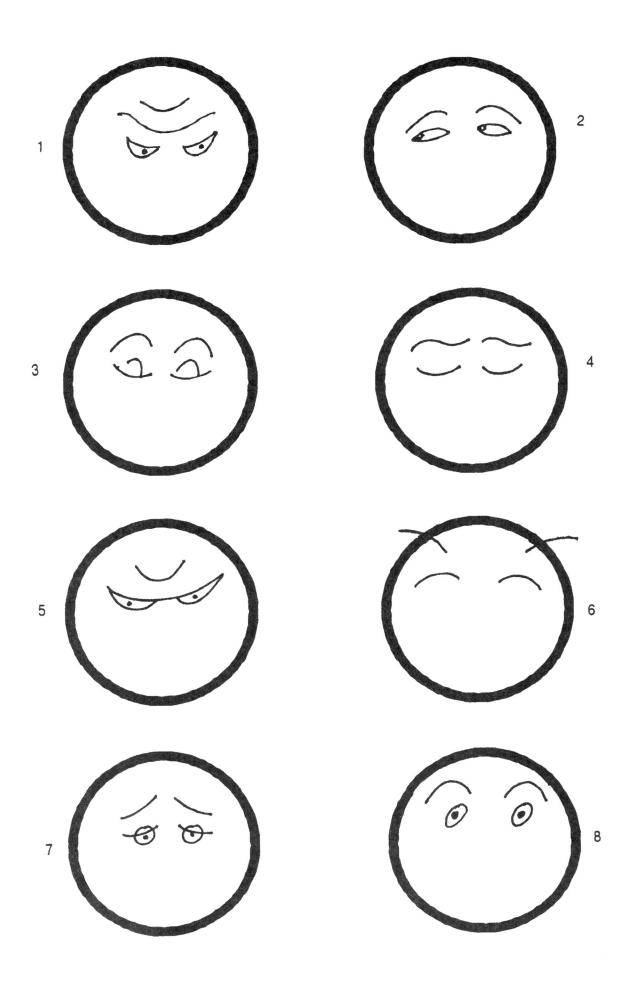

Aliens from Outer Space

This is a light-hearted activity which begins to raise children's awareness that what's 'real' for them largely has to do with their perception of what they experience, that we see things not as they are, but according to how we look at them. This exercise focuses children's attention while allowing their imagination free rein.

GROUPING	Whole class initially, then smaller groups can work independently
TIME	30 minutes
EQUIPMENT	None needed, though various interesting items may be used
SKILLS DEVELOPED	Observation, free association, negotiation
AGE	7+

Basic activity

● Ask children to pretend that they have travelled from another planet and have just landed on Earth. Because this is their first visit they don't know the names of many things, but they are able to speak our language and have an understanding of some Earthly ideas. Their job is to notice what's around them and to send a brief report back to Home Planet...

● Provide some examples of what you mean. Someone crying, for example, might be seen as 'crinkly wet face' - but so would somebody laughing, so further description is necessary. A car could be a 'noisy no-legs big bug', a train a 'chuggy worm', a house a 'dwell-box', and so on. Once children have the idea, gather up a list of such terms for general use. Guide groups carefully through the game, because you are asking children to do something quite unfamiliar in detaching the reality of a thing from its name.

● Conclude the activity by inviting groups to read out their reports, perhaps asking what the 'aliens' found most interesting, funny, shocking, puzzling, about Earth.

Extension activities/variations

● *What If* (see *Imagine That...*, p. 86-8). 'What if' scenarios invite brainstorming and open questioning. Used in the context of *Aliens from Outer Space*, starting-points might include:

> What if the aliens saw our thoughts in think-bubbles above our heads?
> What if the aliens had a machine that forced people always to tell the truth?
> What if the aliens had a kind of chewing gum that allowed us to change our moods whenever we wanted, into any emotion we liked?

Literacy Link

Mood-words and **Nonsense Words** – Take some nonsense words, such as those found in *Jabberwocky*, and work with children to tease out possible meanings. Focus on moods or emotions suggested by the words: 'mimsy', for instance, sounds far less sinister than 'slithy'. Invent more nonsense words that convey meaning before being understood!

Snapshot

This is a variation of the old memory game where players attempt to memorise items on a tray and recall them afterwards. In *Snapshot*, children work in pairs, taking a turn each.

Basic activity

● One child closes her eyes and is led by her partner to a preselected spot in the classroom or elsewhere in the school. Upon arrival, the 'subject' opens her eyes and is asked to look around carefully, noticing as much detail as possible in, say, a minute.

● After this, both partners return to their starting point. The subject attempts, verbally or in writing, to describe the recalled location. As appropriate or necessary, the partner helps to reconstruct the impression. Subsequently, the team can return to the location to check up on details missed (or added!).

Extension activities/variations

● Begin to raise children's awareness of preferential thinking styles and/or eye accessing cues for memory and imaginative reconstruction.

● Begin to raise awareness of different strategies for recall. This is a wide field, beyond the scope of this book, but see Bibliography, notably Tony Buzan's work.

● Allow children the opportunity to create impressions using senses other than the visual – as, for example, in *Imagine That...: Sound Journeys, The Spice Trail, Sounds of Silence*, pp. 55-57.

Literacy Link

Have children make the letters of the alphabet out of various materials: clay, balsa wood, paper, foil, card, sandpaper, etc. Use the tactile and auditory properties of these 'texture letters' as part of the menu of strategies for recalling letter shapes and sequences.

GROUPING	Pairs
TIME	10-15 minutes each way
EQUIPMENT	Writing equipment
SKILLS DEVELOPED	Visual acuity, retention/ recall, imaginative reconstruction, trust
AGE	5+

Sound Mobiles

GROUPING
Individual, pairs, small groups

TIME
1 hour or more (plus teacher preparation time)

EQUIPMENT
Resonant objects/ materials, thread, scissors

SKILLS DEVELOPED
Sensory acuities/ dexterities, teamwork, negotiation, discussion

AGE
Across the range, with appropriate support

The aim of the activity is to have groups create a cross between a mobile and a wind chime. Ask children to help in gathering suitable materials – anything that makes a sound will do: old cutlery, shells, plastic, etc. Materials will need to be prepared in various ways, including, not least, perhaps, the drilling of holes in shells. Obviously this should be done by adults prior to running the activity.

Basic activity

● Before construction begins, encourage children to explore sounds by tapping items together – wood on wood, metal on metal, wood on metal. Emphasise that the selection of the items and sounds is an important part of the process.

● Guide children through the construction of their sound mobiles. When completed, spend some time focusing the class's attention on each mobile:

■ ask children to describe the sounds they hear, inventing new words if necessary (jinkly, clocketty, tep-tep-tep). 'Pencilly-plastic' was one example I was given!

■ ask children what else the sounds remind them of. You don't need to have made a mobile to do this exercise, just scrunch up some cellophane or rattle a plastic necklace for the same results.) You'll be given a wide range of impressions. Keep the emphasis on sound - 'So the sea-shell reminds you of the beach. Good. What other sounds might you hear on a beach? What if you were by yourself on that beach on a stormy day. Are there seagulls? What sounds do they make?' (See *Imagine That...*, *Ten Questions*, pp. 53-4).

Extension activity

Mood Mobiles: Make mobiles to reflect certain emotions, using Circle-Faces (or just mouths, eyes-and-eyebrows), colours, fragments of cut-out pictures, objects that carry associations, etc.

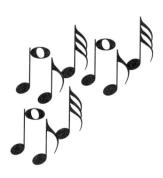

Texture Badges

'Kinaesthetic kids' especially will enjoy this simple activity designed to raise awareness of textures and surfaces, and to discriminate between them.

Basic activity

Using various textured materials – sandpaper, cotton wool, artificial fur, crepe paper, tinfoil – cut out suitable shapes and glue them to peel-off stickers or old button badges.

Split the class into small groups and have group members identify themselves by name and badge: John – sandpaper badge; Helena – fur badge, etc. Each child takes it in turn to sit blindfold or with eyes closed while a partner guides his fingers to the badges of the other group members. The aim is to develop recall through tactile cues.

Extension activities/variations

Brainstorm/speculate associations between textures and emotions. We've all heard about people being 'abrasive' or 'in a prickly mood'. Develop the concept by having children discuss what mood could be represented by, say, crepe paper (emphasising texture, not colour), cotton wool, or tinfoil. This idea can be linked with more sophisticated activities such as *Landscape of the Day* (p.117).

GROUPING
Individual, pair, small group

TIME
About an hour (+ preparation)

EQUIPMENT
Textured materials, glue, sheets of blank stickers and/or old button-badges

SKILLS DEVELOPED
Kinaesthetic awareness

AGE
Across the range, with appropriate support

Multisensory Thinking

| | GROUPING | Whole class initially, small groups subsequently if preferred |

GROUPING — Whole class initially, small groups subsequently if preferred

TIME — 5 minutes upwards

EQUIPMENT — Selection of sounds, textures, colours, tastes, aromas

SKILLS DEVELOPED — Sensory awareness, flexible thinking, awareness of other people's preferred thinking styles, and by extension provides a powerful tool in defining and describing emotions.

AGE — 7+

The aim of this activity is to describe one sensory stimulus in terms of another. This leads to more flexible thinking, raises awareness of other people's preferred thinking styles, and by extension provides a powerful tool in defining and describing emotions. You can limit the exercise to the five senses of sight, hearing, touch, smell and taste.

	1 Sight	2 Sound	3 Touch	4 Taste	5 Smell	6 Feeling
1 Sight						
2 Sound						
3 Touch						
4 Taste						
5 Smell						
6 Feeling						

> **TIP** Use the table and a dice. (I never say die.) Roll the dice twice (or throw two dice) to cross-match two senses in the table.

Basic activity

● Explain the concept to the group, and give a couple of examples: 'The tinkling sound of this bell is silvery. The rattle of this tambourine feels gritty.' If the children fail to grasp the idea, come at it from another angle. Take, say, a sound. Make the sound. Ask, 'If this sound was (or had) a colour, what colour would it be?' or 'If you could touch this sound, what would it feel like?' Emphasise that there are no wrong answers, so whatever responses are made allow everyone to develop the skill and do the exercise better.

● Continue to draw out responses until you're satisfied that the group is familiar with the idea. Keep guiding the children until you feel they can work independently: 'This sound smells like ...? This smell feels like ...? This texture sounds like ...? This colour tastes like ...?'

● Spend some time discussing and comparing responses. You might favour more in-depth responses: if a child says,'The feel of this piece of wood is like the taste of coffee,' ask why. If the child says he doesn't know, invite other people's ideas about why wood might be like coffee. Or, in response to 'I don't know', you might say,'Well, pretend you do and pick the best three ideas that pop into your head.' (This ploy often works wonders!)

Extension activities/variations

● Extend the activity by showing the group increasingly detailed colour pictures and generating group descriptions in terms of sound, for instance. Or play pieces of music and have the children describe them in terms of 'texture maps'.

> **NOTE** The power of this activity becomes more apparent when used in conjunction with other self-intelligence activities which address emotions. Compare, for instance, with *Dealing with Feelings* on p.103. If you want to add the component of 'feeling' or emotion, then it's advisable that you do some other, preparatory, emotion-based work with your group first.

Strike-a-Pose

One of the ways we convey meanings to other people is through our body position. The idea of body language is not new (but *Strike-a-Pose* offers another spin on the idea). However, by learning to 'read' physical posture we become more interpersonally literate, and come to have greater awareness of what our own nonconscious body positions may indicate about ourselves.

Basic activity

● Explain to the group that one of the ways we let other people know how we're feeling is through the way we use and position our body. This might be a whole-body position, or a smaller aspect of it, such as a gesture.

● Go through some obvious examples. For instance, if someone is annoyed she might plonk her hands on her hips, or lean forward and point. Or if someone is surprised he might hold up his hands, lean away, etc. You might want to work from pictures or video clips, or by miming body positions yourself, or by having the children generate examples. (Concentrate on body posture rather than facial expression for this activity).

 You might like to record observations by drawing stick figures and/or taking notes.

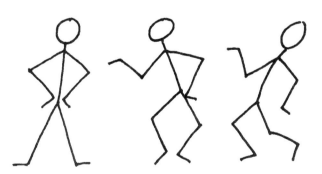

Keep the exercise going until the idea becomes familiar and a range of emotions have been expressed. There is no need to return to the activity often, or to spend too much time on it: children (and adults, actually) can become self-conscious about body position, and may try to strike deliberate poses for one effect or another. It is sufficient to raise awareness of the idea and subsequently incorporate it into other activities.

GROUPING	Any, as appropriate
TIME	15 minutes onwards
EQUIPMENT	Sheets of stick-figure drawings, as explained
SKILLS DEVELOPED	Observation/ interpretation of body position
AGE	Across the range

Extension activities/variations

● Use a collection of body positions generated by one group to explore the idea with another.

● Prepare a sheet of stick figures and ask children to suggest what moods or emotions the postures represent or express.

● In groups, using stick figures, ask children to suggest conversations that might be going on, based on the body positions.

● Use video clips without sound and ask children to suggest conversation and what the scene might be about. (Link in with facial expression work as appropriate).

Literacy Link

● Use extracts from stories and have children suggest what body postures the characters might be adopting at that point.
● Using short plays, have children map out a scene with a series of stick-figure tableaux.

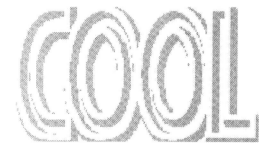

Body Language

GROUPING	Whole class initially, then as appropriate
TIME	20-30 minutes
EQUIPMENT	Body outlines (see illustration)
SKILLS DEVELOPED	Awareness of language related to the body
AGE	7+

Because body posture is such an important component in our ability to communicate, it is widely reflected in the language we use, in both a literal and metaphorical sense. Our own use of body-focused language can tell us a great deal about ourselves, reflecting the deeper structure of our beliefs, attitudes and perceptions about reality. (See 'Brainscapes, mindscapes, wordscapes' in the Introduction). This activity raises awareness of the function and importance of body-oriented language in our interactions with other people, and can lead to greater insights both inter- and intrapersonally.

Basic activity

- Explain to the group that lots of phrases and sayings we use refer to our bodies. Give some examples, including both literal and metaphorical uses:

  We don't see eye to eye.

  I have a nose for this kind of thing.

  I smell something fishy going on here.

  Keep me in touch with what's going on.

  You're a pain in the neck!

  I can't stomach the situation any longer.

  She gave me the cold shoulder.

- Brainstorm a wider selection of sayings, using reference material as necessary.

- Ask children to pick what they think are the most striking examples and to map them, using a template like the one provided.

Extension activities/variations

- Incorporate ideas from the group in a life-size body template for a wall display.

- Discuss the emotions evoked by the situations suggested by various phrases and sayings. For instance, how do you feel when someone gives you the cold shoulder? What mood or emotions are you experiencing if you suddenly smell something fishy going on?

- Help children become more aware of other people's body-focused language. Explain as appropriate that this says a lot about how they think and see (hear/feel) the world.

Literacy Link

Comb through stories and poems for body oriented phrases. What do these also have to say (reading between the lines) about the characters or situation?

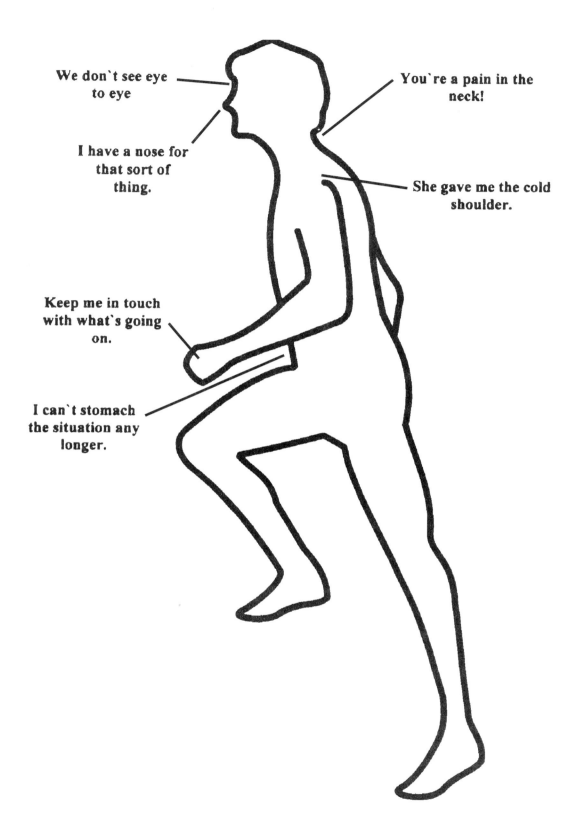

We don`t see eye to eye

You`re a pain in the neck!

I have a nose for that sort of thing.

She gave me the cold shoulder.

Keep me in touch with what`s going on.

I can`t stomach the situation any longer.

Body Language

Circle-Faces

Much of the meaning of our communication is conveyed through facial expression, the effectiveness of mime being one indication of this. We 'read' the complex signals of facial expression in a largely nonconscious way, and react equally automatically. One element in self-intelligence is the ability to recognise emotions in others. The use of circle-face templates helps develop this skill.

Basic activity

Use the circle-faces below in various ways:

● Ask children to put names to the expressions/emotions featured.

● Give out a limited selection of expressions as examples and then have groups draw expressions not featured.

● Arrange the circle faces from positive-to-negative, everyday emotions to uncommon ones, etc.

● Use the faces to allow children to discuss the concept of emotions:

When are certain emotions experienced?

What purposes do different emotions serve?

What does it actually feel like to experience different emotions?

What goes on in the body (i.e. physiologically) when we feel emotions?

What control do we think we have over experiencing our emotions?

What reactions do our emotions prompt in other people?

● Discuss how else emotions are expressed (through voice tone, body language, 'surface structure' language, etc.).

● Have children mimic circle-face emotions.

● Use circle-faces as resource anchors. (Combine with techniques like *Stepping Stars* (p.138), *Badgemaker* (*Imagine That...* p.18), and others.)

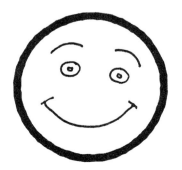

GROUPING	Whole class initially, then as appropriate
TIME	Variable, depending on task
EQUIPMENT	Circle-face and blank circle templates (illustrated)
SKILLS DEVELOPED	Observation, visual acuity, discussion
AGE	Across the range

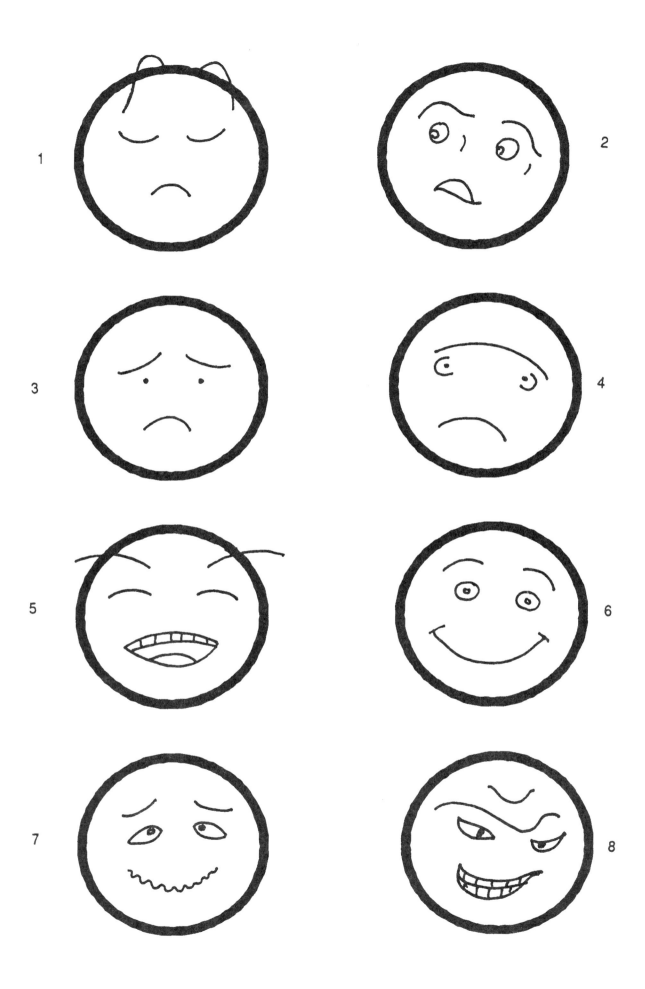

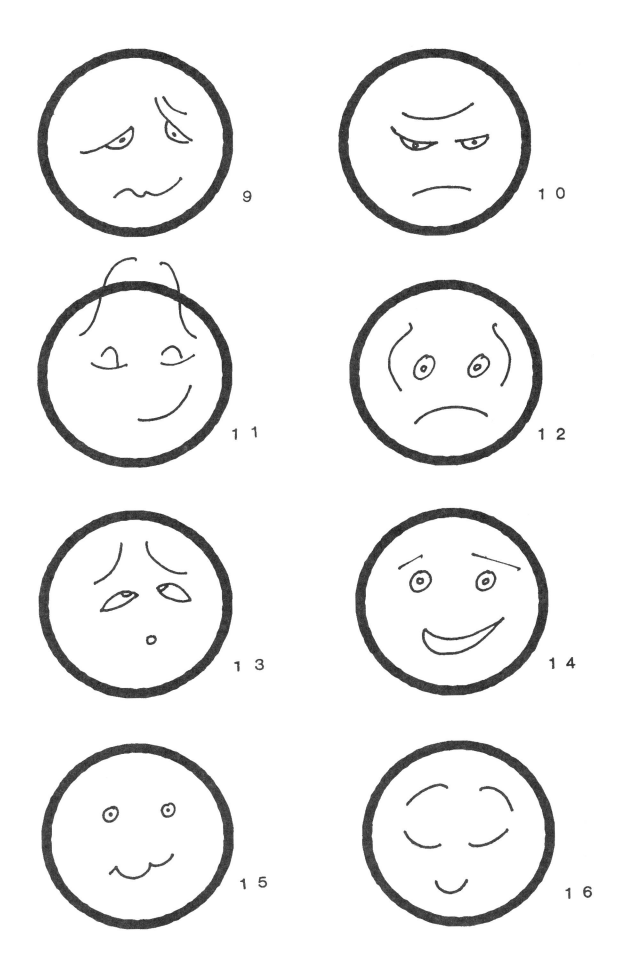

Active Listening

This activity is linked to *Body Language*, although it has a different emphasis and timescale.

People tend to represent (re-present) reality and their understanding of it in sensory terms, often favouring one sensory modality above others. If asked to imagine 'apple', for instance, visual thinkers might see an apple or associated imagery in their mind's eye, or perhaps the word itself. More auditorily oriented people would hear with their 'mind's ear', perhaps the crunch of an apple as it was bitten, or maybe the sound of the word being spoken. Kinaesthetic thinkers would more likely gain an impression based on imagined tactile impressions of holding and eating an apple.

Actually we all employ all modalities in recalling and constructing impressions, but it is well known that most individuals will favour one sense. This preferred modality will be reflected in the person's language. Visual thinkers will express themselves in visually oriented terms - 'I see what you mean', ' I like the look of that', etc. Auditory thinkers might more readily come up with 'I hear what you're saying', 'That sounds fine to me', and so on. Kinaesthetic types will place emphasis on tactile language - 'Keep me in touch with your plans', 'This idea feels right to me...'

Active Listening initially is a way of raising children's awareness of this idea, together with the understanding that people perceive the world differently (in these general sensory terms, and individually through our own unique filters of belief and attitude). Subsequently, children will learn that by making a deliberate effort to match the 'language sense' of others, a powerful rapport is created which makes interactions more effective and beneficial for all parties.

Basic activity

- Begin by collecting examples of sensory language such as those above. Ask individuals to tick the phrases they would normally use (thereby allowing children to identify their own preferred thinking style).

- Suggest that children, during the course of the day, week, or whatever, pay attention to the way people speak. Where appropriate, ask them to note down examples they come across.

- Begin to point out that by matching someone's preferred modality in language, you allow that person to feel more comfortable in talking with you.

Return to this exercise periodically to refresh the group's memory.

GROUPING	Individual, pair
TIME	Ongoing activity
EQUIPMENT	None needed
SKILLS DEVELOPED	Active listening
AGE	7+

The Ten-Minute Chocolate

GROUPING — Whole class

TIME — 20 minutes

EQUIPMENT — Writing equipment and enough chocolates for one each!

SKILLS DEVELOPED — Sensory awareness

AGE — 5+

Raising sensory awareness requires us to pay attention to whichever sense(s) we are working on. This activity is a useful and fun way of consolidating many of the sensory acuity learning points covered so far. Be prepared for children to grumble (usually good-naturedly) when you explain that they are going to take ten minutes to eat a chocolate!

Basic activity

● Use a chocolate selection with bright and varied wrappings. Give a chocolate to each member of the group (whether at random or by letting children choose their favourite is up to you!).

● Ask children to spend two minutes simply looking at the sweet without touching. Invite them to notice shape, colour, lustre and any other visual details. They may write down their observations and impressions at each stage, or right at the end of the session.

● Children now spend two minutes handling the wrapped chocolate, feeling the shape and weight, noting the texture of the wrapping and any sound the wrapping makes (crackling of cellophane, etc.).

● During the next two minutes, children can unwrap the chocolate – not hurriedly, and noticing anything else about the feel and sound of the wrapper. They may smell the chocolate, and are allowed to take a first taste with the tip of the tongue only.

● Now the children can eat the chocolate properly, taking at least two minutes over the task. Ask them to focus attention on the texture of the sweet in the mouth, and of course on the flavours.

● Finally, have the children reflect on their experience. They may remember other occasions when they've savoured eating, or perhaps the taste of the sweet reminded them of something.

● Conclude by giving children time to jot down and share their impressions.

Extension activities/variations

● Taking time to gather detailed sensory impressions often makes a welcome change from the bombardment of information we're subjected to today. Ten-minute 'noticing sessions' can be used as break states and refreshers in between other, longer tasks. Vary the sessions to cater to all senses:

   ■ notice the details of a picture

   ■ tease out the separate instruments in an orchestral piece

   ■ give out interesting objects for the children to handle, with their attention focused on size, shape, weight, temperature, texture...

Literacy Links

● A noticing session makes a useful home assignment. Suggest to children that they notice some new and interesting details about their home, garden, neighbourhood. As a preliminary to this, ask them to recall what colour the exterior paintwork is on a neighbour's house, or where certain things are in their own kitchens. Children might well be able to do this, of course, but will often be surprised to discover how little they have noticed about places and people they encounter every day.

● When studying text, take time to 'open out' extracts by extrapolating other sensory impressions. For instance, if a story describes what a place looks like, ask children to imagine what sounds, textures, aromas you might also find there. When a character speaks, discuss what her voice is like – fast or slow, high pitched or low, etc. When characters eat, gather up impressions of what the meal consists of (if you're not told), and children's recollections of such meals.

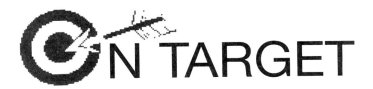

ON TARGET

Fill up the Senses

GROUPING	Individual, pairs, small groups, or the whole class
TIME	Around 15 minutes
EQUIPMENT	As required, see below
SKILLS DEVELOPED	Sensory awareness; language skills in describing experience; interpersonal skills in taking a non-judgmental approach to others' ideas
AGE	Across the range

This activity, a follow-on from the *Ten-Minute Chocolate*, creates opportunities for learners to pay attention to various sensory experiences, allowing them to better understand and appreciate their ability to see and hear, touch, taste and smell. The value of such an activity is the experience itself, though the educational spin-offs as children's sensory acuity becomes more acute are numerous. This is an individual experience, but working in pairs, small groups, or the whole class enhances the activity.

Basic activity

Explain to the group that the activity is all about enjoying the sound of something, or its appearance or smell, etc., for its own sake. In a world where we tend to rush through our lives and where instant gratification seems to be the norm, simply slowing down and noticing things makes for a refreshing change.

> **NOTE** Decide beforehand which sense experience is to be enjoyed and arrange for a state of quiet anticipation in the group. Aim to spend at least ten minutes on the work, and explain to the children that the whole point of the exercise is for them to *take their time* and simply notice the details. Describing what they saw or tasted or touched comes later, and constitutes a separate activity.

Ideas for *Filling up the Senses* include:

- eating a piece of fruit very slowly, savouring every mouthful
- listening to music
- going outside and listening to the sounds all around
- smelling a range of interesting spices – slowly, taking a minute for each
- listening to the notes made by different musical instruments (have someone other than the 'experiencer' play the note)
- feeling a number of different textures – metal, cloth, wood, liquid soap, sand ...

Extension activities/variations

Have children suggest their own ways of filling up the senses. The only groundrule is that the tendency must always be away from the I-want-it-all-I-want-it-now syndrome. Focusing on single-sense experiences develops sensory awareness generally, of course. Eventually *Filling up the Senses* can take the form of 'noticing-walks' around the school grounds, or whenever trips are arranged.

Hand on Shoulder

Besides developing kinaesthetic acuity, *Hand on Shoulder* combines 'informed guessing' with the enhancement of self-esteem and confidence.

Basic activity

● Children take it in turns to sit with their backs to the rest of the group (of three or four others).

● One at a time, the other group members each speak their own name as they place a hand on the sitter's shoulder. The sitter has previously been asked to notice precisely how each friend does this – heavy- or light-handed, tentative, confident, etc. Let each group member go round a few times.

● The second phase of the game consists of group members placing a hand on the sitter's shoulder without speaking their names. The sitter tries to guess the other's identity each time (again paying close attention to the qualities of the touch). Children will be delightfully surprised at how many 'right answers' they get, as their powers of kinaesthetic discrimination develop.

Extension activities/variations

● In the early phase of the game, ask group members to say something positive about the sitter as they place hands on shoulders. So:

> 'This is John... I like the colour of your sweater, Sarah.'
> 'I'm Chrissy... Your hair looks nice today.'
> 'This is Jane... You seem to be in a really happy mood this morning.'

● Ask children to notice the particular qualities of the sitters' clothing as they place their hands on shoulders – not just colours and kinds of materials, but details of what they feel like. So:

> 'Sarah's sweater is dark blue, it's a heavy thick material, soft to touch.'
> 'John's jumper is bright red with blue diamonds in a pattern. The stitches in the wool are big and sort of open.'
> 'Chrissy's blouse is white. It's cotton. It felt really smooth. I noticed a spot of blue ink on her collar!'

GROUPING Small group at first, then larger groups once skill has been acquired

TIME Sessions of 15-20 minutes

EQUIPMENT None needed

SKILLS DEVELOPED Sensory acuity (kinaesthetic, auditory); 'emotional intelligence'

AGE Across the range

Mirror and Pace

GROUPING	Pairs or threes initially
TIME	Ongoing awareness
EQUIPMENT	None needed
SKILLS DEVELOPED	Observation/ awareness of body posture, facial expression, voice qualities; building rapport
AGE	7+

Whether or not it breeds contempt, people feel comfortable with what's familiar. We tend to respond positively when others share our preferences, views and tastes. Similarly we are put more at ease when the person to whom we are talking reflects our body posture, breathing pace, voice tone, and so on. When this occurs – when the 'chemistry' seems right – then rapport has been established and mutual positive feedback occurs.

Such 'mirroring' of one person with another happens naturally, of course, and goes on largely at a nonconscious level. Usually neither party realises (makes consciously real) the process that's unfolding; it just feels good to be with the other. But it is a technique that can be employed quite deliberately to engineer more effective communication and ease of communication.

> **NOTE** As with any technique, *Mirror and Pace* could be used manipulatively. It is important to point out to children that the ethos of self-intelligence is one of respect for and consideration of others. Although there is an element of fun and light-heartedness in acquiring greater emotional capability, the techniques offered here are not tricks or games; they are powerful ways of coming to know oneself and other people. In learning to appreciate this, children will of course by definition be displaying the greater maturity and resourcefulness which is the primary aim of this book.

Basic activity

- Raising awareness of mirroring and pacing might best be done by having children observe others, in the playground, working together in class, and so on. Get the group to notice body posture, breathing rate, voice qualities. Link the idea of how these vary depending on the emotion that's being expressed. Point out examples of mirroring and pacing occurring naturally.

- Let children practice first in simulated situations. Have one member of the group chat with you, the teacher, about something of interest: keep your partner involved by asking questions. Gradually mirror that person's posture, breathing and some voice qualities. Do this elegantly, a little bit at a time. Although everyone in the group knows it's just a demonstration, don't be tempted to rush the process by immediately adopting the other's pose.

- Now let children work by themselves in pairs or threes. If three, the roles are: subject (the one who's being mirrored), operator (the one doing the mirroring) and observer. Each child should experience each role.

- Run these sessions perhaps in conjunction with other ongoing work. Suggest that children practise their newly acquired skill outside the classroom – not constantly, at this stage, and in line with their level of self-confidence. Gradually children will build the technique into their repertoire of self-intelligence skills: they will become 'nonconsciously competent' as the mirroring behaviour becomes automatic.

Extension activity

- An idea associated with mirroring and pacing is 'leading'. This is where the operator reflects the subject's state and then gradually changes it a bit at a time by altering his own breathing, posture and voice qualities. The technique works very well, for example, if someone is angry or upset. Mirror the behaviour – not fully, of course, but in certain key aspects – and then begin to change the parameters. Most times, the subject will follow your lead and find the unhelpful emotion more readily resolved.

Pinch yourself
and know how

others feel.

Japanese proverb

No bird soars
too high if he soars
with his own wings.

William Blake

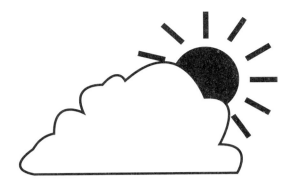

Section Two

UTILISING RELAXATION & BREAK STATES

*O*ne of the most unhelpful suggestions I've ever heard is 'Just try to relax', since effort is the antithesis of relaxation. And let me point out immediately that true relaxation, profound tranquillity, comes from mental quietude as well as physical stillness.

Many people find it hard to relax, given this definition. They might sit down and put their feet up, but their minds are spinning with ideas, problems to be solved, decisions to be made, fears, memories and anticipations. Thus they are anything but relaxed.

The state of relaxation is therefore important per se: it is by definition a pleasant and positive state. I like to call it 'quiet consciousness' or 'settled alertness', and therein lies the clue to its deeper usefulness. When relaxed, the conscious point-of-attention swings easily, like a compass needle. And so the mind can be drawn to ideas coming from the outside, which can then be assimilated without conscious intellectual effort being the main component of that process. That is, meanings are allowed to be made also at a subconscious level, based on previous knowledge and experience.

Similarly, in a relaxed condition, the quiet conscious mind is more open to insights and intuitions rising up from subconscious realms. Being receptive to these ideas is a fundamental component in the art of creative thinking. Since a vast number of ideas are created 'at the back of the head', we need consciously to be sensitive to them in order to understand them. Then begins the more intellectual work of evaluation and verification.

In large measure, and in my opinion, the core of learning and creative thinking lies in this key state of 'systematic daydreaming'.

In gaining more control of ourselves in the sense that self-intelligence implies, we need not only to create resourceful states in ourselves, but also to modify or stop unhelpful states. Techniques for doing this are called 'break states'. They act like full stops at the end of a sentence, indicating that one 'packet of meaning' has ended and that another is about to begin.

We use break states naturally – how often have we tried diversion-of-attention as a tactic to take a child's mind off a grazed knee?

The easy and elegant use of break states, coupled with the ability for yourself and your group to relax, enhances all of the other techniques and activities in this book, helping to create the ideal learning environment, which is one of high challenge and low stress.

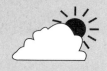

Settling

GROUPING
Any group size

TIME
5-10 minutes

EQUIPMENT
None needed (though you may want to use a diagram of major muscle groups)

SKILLS DEVELOPED
Body awareness, relaxation, understanding links between mood and physiology

AGE
Across the range

Mind and body are fundamentally linked. By deliberately changing posture and relaxing major muscle groups we can reduce tension and raise awareness of where tension accumulates in the body.

Basic activity

● Have children seated, feet flat on the floor, hands resting palms down on thighs.

● Explain that we can learn to relax and feel better by noticing the muscles in our bodies and deliberately relaxing them. Demonstrate this by making a fist and squeezing it tight, then slowly relaxing the fingers. Have the children copy you, first with one hand, then the other.

● Begin with the head. Have children frown in an exaggerated way, then relax the forehead muscles. Do the same with 'mouth muscles'.

● Move on to shoulders. Tell children to make a big shrug, then let their shoulders drop and be heavy. Lots of tension can develop here and in the neck. Relax neck muscles by gently tilting the head side-to-side, backwards-and-forwards, around in a circle.

● Progress down the body, paying attention to each major muscle group: clench – unclench, flex – relax.

NOTE This is a good opportunity to name parts of the body, muscle groups, and other related vocabulary. See, for example, Hewitt: *Teach Yourself Relaxation* and other relaxation texts in the Bibliography for more detail.

Extension activities/variations

● Associate this or any other relaxation activity with a picture and/or sound. Calming background music works well. An 'anchor' such as this works like a shortcut: in future, simply by having children notice the picture, or by playing the music, you'll allow them to access their relaxation state quickly and effortlessly.

● Incorporate a visualisation. After a muscle relaxation session, have children imagine a hollow glass ball filled with a soothing liquid. (They don't need to have their eyes closed for this, and can choose the colour of the liquid!) Explain that when each child imagines the ball cracking like an egg, the soothing liquid will flow down over them and through them, relaxing muscles, soaking away tension, taking away any aches and pains, stresses and strains. The liquid will trickle and run down through the body, pooling at the feet, where it will evaporate away. Use your anchor music/sound as you run this visualisation. (An example script is given in the Appendix.)

Cat Waking Up

Legend has it that the original twelve postures (or *asanas*) of Yoga were based on observations of cats stretching, grooming, and so on. Special attention was paid to the effortless ease of the animals' movements and positions, and the sense of cats being comfortable with their own bodies.

Basic activity

● If you have appropriate visual materials, have the children notice and describe the way cats move, and the positions they assume.

● Use this as a lead-in to the children mimicking and improvising these postures and moves in a calm and gentle way.

● Emphasise particularly that children should be aware at all times of the way their muscles are flexing and relaxing, any 'pools of tension' that have accumulated in certain areas, and the pleasant sensations of relaxation.

NOTE   This activity is not Yoga, but may be introduced as a precursor to Yoga. In using *Cat Waking Up*, it is advisable to liaise with the school's P.E. specialists for hints and tips in encouraging children to undertake such exercise. It is also very helpful if you have some experience of Yoga yourself. Note also that some people object to the philosophical/historical roots of Yoga, and so you may wish not to make any connection between this and the present activity.

GROUPING	Any group size
TIME	5-10 minutes
EQUIPMENT	Any pictures, videos, etc., of cats stretching, grooming, waking up
SKILLS DEVELOPED	Body awareness, development of suppleness, observation skills
AGE	Across the range (older children may be self-conscious)

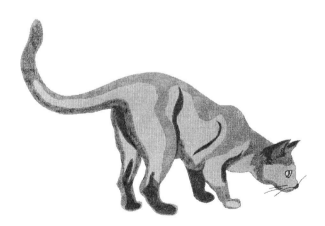

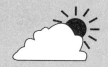

Like the Back of your Hand...

GROUPING
Any group size, though with individual tuition as appropriate

TIME
5-15 minutes initially, then in smaller time-chunks as an ongoing activity

EQUIPMENT
None specifically, although pictures and videos of people's posture, gait, etc., can be useful

SKILLS DEVELOPED
Body awareness, improving stance and posture, understanding of links between physical and mental states (attitude)

AGE
Across the range

We say 'I know this town like the back of my hand', but how well do we know ourselves? Many people develop a posture and gait that reflects their attitude and world picture. Reciprocally, the way we stand and walk can influence our moods. This activity raises awareness of the idea and allows children to begin to influence their own body posture and 'landscape of moods'.

Basic activity

● Begin by having children notice their own hands. Are there any details they've never noticed before? Encourage children to describe, compare and contrast their hands.

● Move on to asking children to notice how they habitually sit, stand, walk. This must not be done in any judgmental way, so you would not say, 'Do you notice that you're slouching, John?' Rather, describe the posture in neutral language: 'Do you notice, John, how your shoulders are dropped and forward, and how you're staring at the ground with your head bent forward?'

● At first some children are likely to 'sit up straight' or similar, as they recall past admonishments from parents, teachers and significant others. The aim is not to force children to assume a posture that is incongruent with the way they are thinking or feeling, but rather to help them be aware that body posture and attitude are linked. Particular cases provide useful feedback to you and to the child herself, leading perhaps to appropriate interventions to modify moods.

● Develop the activity by noticing body posture in more detail, taking care to have children describe examples in a non-judgmental way. ('Look at Jenny – she walks like a duck!' is unacceptable). Guide subsequent discussion into how posture and outlook can be linked. Mention phrases and sayings we use, such as:

> He's down in the mouth.
> She has the world on her shoulders.
> He's walking on air.
> She holds her head up high, etc.

Extension activity

● Encourage children to notice their own postures, using a full-length mirror. Mirrors can also be used to explore facial expressions – what you might call *'Reflection on Reflection'*!

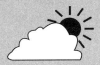

Relaxation Is -

This simple 'talk around' activity broadens children's awareness of what relaxation amounts to and how it may be achieved.

Basic Activity

- Begin the discussion with a few questions, such as:

    What do you think relaxation means?
    How do you know when you're relaxed?
    Do you know ways of becoming more relaxed than you've ever been before?
    Do you know people who never seem to relax? (Why is that, do you suppose?)
    Do you think you can be relaxed while you're running, for example, or doing homework, or swapping opinions about something important?
    What do you think is happening inside you while you're feeling relaxed?

- Continue by offering some examples:

    For me, relaxation is just sitting and watching the clouds go by.
    For me, relaxation is being curled up in a big armchair with a good book.
    For me, relaxation is watching the stars on a quiet night...

- Invite further ideas from the children, framing them with the qualifier 'For me'. Avoid differences of opinion at this stage. The aim of the activity is simply to collect a wealth of examples of how people relax.

Extension activities/variations

- Have children create an individual relaxation scale of 1-10. Invite them to position their own ways of relaxing on the scale. They might then 'try out' other children's ways of relaxing and enter them on the scale.

- Create a relaxation area in your classroom or school. Incorporate ideas from the children – calming pictures and objects, comfortable seating, appropriate colours, suitable music. Encourage relaxation time as a whole-school policy. Use the relaxation area as a powerful anchor for accessing that state of calm.

- Link relaxation with visualisation/guided fantasy work. A sample guided relaxation/visualisation is given in the Appendix.

GROUPING	Any group size
TIME	10-15 minutes
EQUIPMENT	None needed
SKILLS DEVELOPED	Discussion, listening, increasing awareness of relaxation states and situations
AGE	7+ (with younger children more discussion and guidance might be necessary)

Thinking Back

GROUPING
Any group size

TIME
5-10 minutes

EQUIPMENT
None needed (optional stimulus picture, sound or scent as a starting point)

SKILLS DEVELOPED
Increasing ease at accessing information, understanding that mental and physical states are linked, concentration, developing sensitivity to one's thoughts and feelings

AGE
7+

Ironically, while we require children to use their memories and imaginations constantly at school, we tend to castigate them for daydreaming and indulging in reverie. (How clearly I remember being caught often 'gazing into space' and, when asked, 'Just what do you think you're doing?' replying 'Nothing Miss', because this got me into less trouble than admitting that I was having a daydream.)

The ability to relax – an important component in creating learning environments of high challenge but low stress – depends upon increased control over one's mental and physical states. This means accessing internal information, which we do by the use of memory and imagination. The creative process itself might well be called 'systematic daydreaming', and here we are using it to reach and anchor resourceful states of relaxation.

> **NOTE** Leech and Hall: *Scripted Fantasy in the Classroom* (see Bibliography) gives a clear and well-researched account of how 'systematic daydreaming' can be used flexibly and powerfully in many areas of the curriculum.

Basic activity

● Begin by talking about daydreaming:

> How many of you daydream?
> Do you like doing it?
> Why is that?
> What do you think (some/most/all) adults think about daydreaming?
> What's the difference between daydreaming and, say, making up a story?
> Or between daydreaming and thinking about your last holiday?

● Explain (or at least, as the teacher, realise yourself) that daydreaming can be passive, just following the drift of your thoughts as they come into mind, or an active process in which you consciously connect thoughts and ideas arising spontaneously in your mind. It's important, too, to know that what we think about and how we think about it can affect our moods and how we feel.

Extension activity

A basic exercise is to ask the children to 'think back'. Specify what you want them to think about...

> Think back to something pleasant you did last weekend.
> Think back to a time when you were much younger and really enjoying yourself.
> Think back to any time when a friend really proved to you that (s)he was a true friend.
> And so on.

● Follow-up discussion (i.e. reminiscence) might be appropriate, and will certainly be enjoyable.

● Once children are at ease with recalling specific times, ask them to notice how good they feel as they think back in this way. Encourage them to be aware of and make distinctions between the good feelings they recall ('call back') from, say, a holiday memory and a party memory. Draw from them descriptions of these feelings in as much detail as possible.

Anchoring

When you have raised children's awareness of the good feelings they can access at will, you can begin to teach them to anchor these resources. There are many ways of doing this. For example, invite children to link a small physical movement ('I touch my left thumb and left little finger') with the good feelings they remember. This movement will be an anchor for these feelings insofar as it 'holds them in place'. Say, 'As you think back to this time/these times, make your movement and notice how those feelings hold steady.' This is a powerful suggestion that children will find helpful in future.

Other anchors include having children draw pictures of good times, etc., and then represent all the details of each picture in a simple way – say, as a bright yellow sun. These symbols can then be used in a number of ways:

- Make button badges for the children to wear.
- Create a collage incorporating all of the children's 'resource anchor symbols'.
- Enlarge the visuals to create posters, flash cards, etc.
- Use the symbols in conjunction with *Annotated Notebooks* (see p.91), for you or the children to use for work well done.

 You might find that some children have difficulty in remembering good times and/or that unpleasant experiences surface spontaneously. If this is an issue which concerns the child and/or her parents, specialist help is always available through NLP practitioners or other therapies.

TIP Use thinking-back techniques in conjunction with *Stepping Stars* (p.138).

Attention to Breathing

Breathing, like blinking, is one of those physical processes that usually remain subconscious ('it happens by itself'), but can easily be noticed and consciously controlled. Because the breathing mechanism is connected to the rest of our physiology, intervening to modify our breathing can create states of calmness and relaxation very swiftly.

Basic activity

Begin by having children sit comfortably. Ensure shirt collars, ties, etc., are loosened. Ask children to notice their breathing – not to do anything to change it, just notice it. You might follow up by asking them to describe what they've noticed.

Presumably the atmosphere as you run this activity will be relaxed anyway. Draw out the idea that when people are relaxed, their breathing tends to be even and unhurried. Discuss the way other emotions, pleasant and unpleasant, can affect breathing depth, rate and rhythm.

Make the point that because we can control our breathing, we can use it to change our moods. Gather up phrases and sayings which link breath with mood and emotion – for example, 'Take a breather', 'give yourself breathing space'.

NOTE
The common advice to 'Take a deep breath' or even 'Take a deep breath and count to ten...' before embarking on some significant activity is unhelpful, as it triggers 'emergency' breathing and is an anchor for anxiety and apprehension. A good, deep exhalation, or a sigh or yawn for that matter, is a far more useful break state: it helps release anxiety, tension and/or fatigue.

Follow this basic noticing activity with one of the following breathing exercises.

GROUPING	Any group size
TIME	5-10 minutes
EQUIPMENT	None needed
SKILLS DEVELOPED	Body awareness, increasing control of tension or anxiety states
AGE	7+

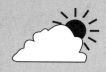

Basic Breathing Techniques

The Whole Breath

Take a few normal, deep breaths. At the 'bottom' of the breath, fully exhaled, hold the breath out for a few seconds. Now pace the breathing in, slowly and deliberately, to a count of six. At the 'top' of the breath, fully inhaled, hold the breath in for a few seconds. Now pace the breathing out to a count of six. This is one cycle of the Whole Breath. Repeat several times.

White Light/Blue Light Breath

Combine the Whole Breath with a visualisation: as you breathe in, imagine a white, invigorating light pouring in to the lungs and cascading through the body. As you breathe out, imagine a blue light flushing away all the aches and pains, stresses and strains of the day ('breathing out the blues'). Imagine different sounds and/or suggest the white and blue light have different textures. This satisfies children with predominantly auditory and kinaesthetic learning preferences.

Group Breath

Have the whole group breathe together, once you have established a calming and relaxed atmosphere. Combine with the Whole Breath if you wish. This technique is a powerful relaxant and helps enhance group rapport for other activities.

Pacing Breath

Have children in pairs or small groups match each other's breathing (like a mini Group Breath). Begin with this when you want small groups to work co-operatively and creatively together. Extend the activity by having children notice how people breathe when they're angry and upset. Practise with children the art of pacing the breath of someone in such a state, and then gently modifying one's own breathing to lead the other into a calmer and more resourceful state.

NOTE Keep a close eye on children as they practise these or other breathing exercises. Explain that gulping too much air in too quickly can cause hyperventilation, leading to dizziness.

GROUPING	Any group size
TIME	5 minutes
EQUIPMENT	None needed
SKILLS DEVELOPED	Body awareness, increasing control of tension or anxiety states
AGE	7+

The Smallest Sounds

How often we tell children to 'pay attention' as a general command, usually without giving them practice in how to use or develop this faculty. Our conscious point-of-attention is narrow anyway, like a slim beam of light that can easily wander away if not properly trained. This activity allows children to develop the duration and focus of their concentration auditorily, though similar exercises can be devised for sight, smell, taste and touch.

Basic activity

- Begin by explaining the difference between active and passive listening. When we listen actively we seek out sounds and meanings; we are searching for something particular. Passive listening is simply to sit back and detach, and let sounds wash over you. It's the difference between being involved and just being there.

- Ask the children to settle themselves and simply become aware of the sounds going on around them. There's no need for them to do anything other than notice. You can also suggest that just sitting back and doing nothing can allow them to drift deeper into a lovely state of relaxation...

- After a couple of minutes (this time can be progressively increased if the activity is used repeatedly) ask the group to pick out nearby sounds – not talk about them, just be aware of them. Then ask the children to notice sounds farther away – and farther away – until they're listening to the farthest, smallest sounds of all. Build in the suggestion that the smaller the sound, the more wonderfully calm and peaceful the group can become.

Extension activities/variations

Work with the children to gather up 'sound' words. Make these up if you like! Make a 'sound map' of concentric circles where children can record the sounds they noticed in relation to themselves (see example).

GROUPING	Any group size
TIME	5 minutes
EQUIPMENT	None needed
SKILLS DEVELOPED	Auditory acuity, concentration, attention to detail
AGE	Across the range

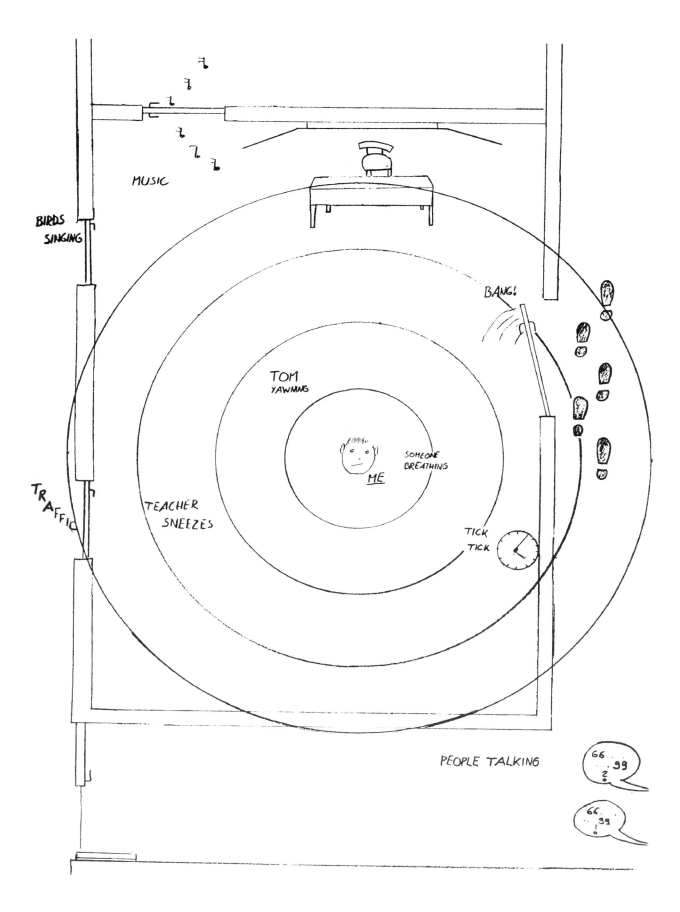

Sound Map

Literacy Link

When working with shared texts, take any scene and discuss with the children what sounds you might hear if you were to 'step into the book'. (Answers will be a mixture of deduction and speculation.)

Music Link

Play extracts of music. Ask children to pretend that an extract is a person, or a place, or something happening. As the music plays, have the children jot down ideas as they come to mind.

NOTE

Research suggests that playing Baroque music 'stimulates receptivity and perception'. See, for example, Colin Rose's book *Accelerated Learning*. (See Bibliography.)

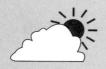

Air-Writing

Air-Writing is one among many spelling strategies that children can employ to give themselves feedback to improve spelling. As a young boy, if I wasn't sure how a word was spelt, I used to write it out in the air. This gave me a clearer sense of the pattern of the letters. (I still do this sometimes before using the spell checker!)

Lazy Eights

Imagine a big figure 8 in the air in front of you. Lay it on its side (make it lazy). With your right forefinger, trace the shape of the 8 ten times. Then retrace the shape the other way. Repeat with left forefinger.

Extension activities/variations

● Have children air-write affirmations to themselves and upbeat messages to each other. Get them to use each hand in turn and not just the dominant hand.

● Have a child 'draw' an object in the air and encourage others in a small group to describe what they think they see, and then to guess the object.

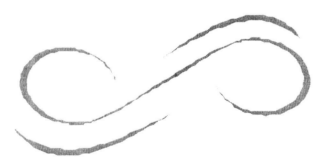

GROUPING	Any group size
TIME	5 minutes
EQUIPMENT	None needed
SKILLS DEVELOPED	Numerous, see text
AGE	Across the range

Brain Gym

Air Writing has strong connections with the large and growing field known as Brain Gym. This includes a programme of movements where limbs cross the mid-line of the body; the thinking behind it is that repeated 'cross-lateral' movements encourage the flow of electrical impulses across the *corpus callosum*, the bundle of nerve fibres connecting the right and left cerebral hemispheres of the brain. This helps equalise the part each hemisphere plays in the thinking processes the individual employs to solve problems – what you might call cross-lateral thinking. Much is made of left-brain-dominant thinking in today's society; Brain Gym seeks to redress the balance.

Cross-patterning

Stand upright, easily balanced and centred on both feet. Lift your left leg, while simultaneously bringing your right hand across the mid-line of your body. Slap the right hand down on to the left knee. Return to base. Then lift the right knee and bring the left arm over to slap the left knee. Increase the pace to an easy, swinging rhythm. Continue for a minute or so.

 Air-Writing and related Brain Gym activities also act as 'break states' (see below).

At any given time we are embedded in a state of thinking – feeling – reacting. Such states may be pleasant and resourceful, or unpleasant, unhelpful or detrimental. Any break state intervention acts like a full stop at the end of a sentence, indicating that one 'unit of meaning' has ended and another is about to begin.

Sometimes just a simple distraction can be enough to shift a child out of a 'downstate' into an 'upstate'. Another easy and effective technique is to raise the individual's awareness of the state (s)he's in and encourage them to reflect on it. 'Why are you angry?' for instance, can be exactly the right thing to say when a child has got himself 'into a state'. Similarly, 'I can't understand what you say when you're crying' can instantly shift a child who's upset to a more resourceful level.

Relaxation techniques may sometimes need to be preceded by break state interventions. Those relaxations themselves can become break state techniques once they've become more familiar.

NOTE For details on a powerful toolkit of spelling strategies, see Dilts and Epstein: *Dynamic Learning*. For more on Brain Gym try Dennison and Dennison: *Brain Gym For Teachers*. (See Bibliography for details.)

Anchoring States

One of the ways our brains make sense of the world is through association: a network of links can be made both consciously and subconsciously (and often subconscious networks result in behaviours that the conscious part of the individual does not understand, or which seem 'contextless'). We are talking here about 'meaning making'. These constructed meanings create our perceptions of the world, but are also coloured by those perceptions. And so our personal 'map of reality' becomes increasingly self-referential as it drives our patterns of thinking, feeling and reacting.

These patterns constitute the states we find ourselves in as we move through life. Obviously, some of our mental / emotional / physiological states are negative, unpleasant and unhelpful. Others are positive and empowering. The concept of 'anchoring' or holding states in place owes much to the field called NLP, Neuro Linguistic Programming. There is a vast and growing literature on this subject, which has been described as 'a methodology that leaves behind it a trail of techniques'. Many of the activities in this book coincidentally hold hands with NLP thinking, or derive directly from it.

Powerful associations are created in the classroom, and these may be negative or positive. Reflect for a few moments on when you were a child at school, and on how you felt about particular subjects, classrooms and teachers. Even a fleeting recollection can bring back feelings and associated physiology, an echo of how you felt at the time.

A basic premise of self-intelligence is that raising awareness will lead to increased understanding (stabilising the ground on which we make our meanings), and that in turn will lead to greater control through choice. If the only tool you have is a hammer, you'll regard every problem as a nail. If the only response you have is anger, you'll regard every situation as a conflict. Self-intelligence is about equipping children with an emotional toolkit, and giving them the skills to pick the right tool for the job.

- Something as simple as a smile or other nonverbal expression of approval as you give praise creates an anchor: consciously or subconsciously the child links your gesture with the good feelings (s)he gets on being praised. Subsequently, the good feelings can be recalled and the state held by repeating the gesture. (You will of course recognise this as simple common sense and good practice. Good teachers have always drawn out the best in children instinctively. All we're doing here is raising awareness of what comes naturally, in order to more fully exploit its power.)

- Another effective technique is to mark out mentally certain areas of your classroom for different purposes. And so you might stand in a particular spot and/or assume a certain body posture when you deliver praise to the class. Use another position to deliver straight information, another when exercising discipline, and so on. There's no need to explain to the children what's going on, since they'll pick up the meanings subconsciously. The point is that those particular parts of the classroom will become associated in the children's minds with praise, attending to information, being told about behaviour, etc., so that eventually you need only drift towards your chosen spot to achieve the desired effect. You can also 'mix and match' anchors. So, for example, you might combine the spot-for-giving-information with your body position for offering praise.

Once the concept of anchoring states has been grasped, the possibilities for its use become endless. Look back at what we've covered so far in this book and notice how many of the techniques can be used to access and anchor positive states. Similarly, keep the idea in mind as you read on...

NOTE More detailed discussion of anchors and other NLP techniques is beyond the scope of this book, but you will find useful references in the Bibliography.

Most people are
as happy as they make up
their minds to be.

Abraham Lincoln

Section Three

ENHANCING EMOTIONAL LITERACY

*L*iteracy in the usual sense means the ability to read and write. Emotional literacy means the ability to 'read' one's own emotions and those of others, and to express one's emotions in positive, useful and meaningful ways.

I first came across the term in Daniel Goleman's inspirational book, *Emotional Intelligence*. In it he makes key points which are monumentally obvious, but which somehow our educational system has lost sight of and fails to cater for. These include the notion that systems are composed of people; those people are the reason for the system's existence; without those people's needs and requirements being attended to and fulfilled, the system is meaningless; so that

- children learn more when they are happy, engaged and positively challenged (and teachers in this state teach better too!)
- children learn better when course content is meaningful to them, and
- a key element of learning lies in positive relationships

All of these ideas, and many more, confirm again and again one of the greatest pieces of wisdom I ever heard applied to the educational system: that equality of opportunity is not the same as identical opportunity. If that aim of identical opportunity were ever achieved, both teachers and pupils (learners all) would automatically become more emotionally literate.

Meantime, until education comes of age (perhaps by entering its second childhood), there are things we can do to allow children to become more resourceful within the system as it exists. If you can't change your circumstances, at least you can change your responses to them. That's what this section is designed to facilitate.

Resource Cards

I mean, of course, emotional and other 'inner' resources. It's easy for any of us to drift into negative patterns of thinking, where a single setback or criticism can outweigh an accumulation of praise for things done well. This kind of thinking is also selective: once that pattern has established itself, we tend to notice only those things that reconfirm the emerging unhelpful belief.

Resource cards can come in any size or shape, and may record anything we find useful, interesting, enjoyable or inspirational. Standard file cards are pocket-sized, but have limited space – though a picture, a quote, a design and a keyword can have plenty of meaning attached to them.

Reminders of what we can do and have achieved are useful at any time. In reminding us – bringing back to mind – our successes, the simple device of these cards helps counter negative thinking and strengthen positive self-beliefs.

What a strange machine man is!
You fill him with bread, wine, fish and radishes, and out of him come sighs and laughter and dreams.

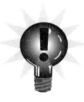

Beware the ghosts that haunt you
And the demons who will taunt you –
Always there but never seen.
They are the spirits of despair
And the wraiths of couldn't-care.
The phantoms of perhaps-I-will.
The shades of might-have-been.

Hugs and Handshakes

We use an 'x' as the symbol for a kiss (and, oddly, to indicate an answer that's wrong). One simple way of allowing and helping children to express how they feel is to devise with them other symbols of friendship, affection and positive encouragement.

Here are some suggestions:

(	=	smile. The number of brackets tells you the size of the smile, so:
(((((	=	'I'm really happy'.
/	=	**looking forward to seeing you**
*	=	**handshake**
( )	=	**hug**
!	=	I understand how you feel.
^	=	I enjoyed reading this piece of work.

Symbols like these are useful and significant 'mini-anchors': think how a tick or a cross on your work at school made you feel[!]. Use them with other self-intelligence techniques such as *Annotated Notebooks* (p.91), *Air Writing*, *Texture Badges*, etc.

Extension activity

Home-made symbols are a useful tool when marking work, and/or in allowing children to consider their own efforts. Such symbols can express a subtle or complex blend of emotions, and an awareness of them will help children to reflect on their work.

What information or impression do you suppose is conveyed to a child who, in a spelling test, writes 'seperate' and has it marked X? What effect is created – or intended – by a cross next to, say, three-quarters of the answers in a quiz? The child knows it's wrong ... and wrong again ... and wrong again ... But the usefulness of such feedback is limited. Extend your and your children's repertoire of responses with a menu of feedback symbols. Make a chart of them for your wall.

~	=	You're almost there. Let's talk about it.
#	=	This is an interesting answer. Come and tell me how you reached it.
+/+	=	I'm especially pleased with the effort you've made. I bet you feel really good about this work.

And so on...

This is Me

GROUPING	Whole group demo, then individual work
TIME	15 minutes
EQUIPMENT	None needed
SKILLS DEVELOPED	Noticing and self awareness, further understanding of self, reflection and self assessment
AGE	7+

Although it is simplistic (and inaccurate) to separate what goes on inside a person from what goes on in the world, there is an important distinction to be made between external circumstances and internal responses. Even if we have no influence over circumstances, we can all develop greater control over how we react to what happens. This activity allows children to begin to make these understandings.

Basic activity

● Draw a circle or whatever shape/design you feel best represents you. Anything you put inside it is something about you – something about how you think, feel or behave. Anything you put outside the circle is going on externally – circumstances, events, situations. (See two examples provided. In the second example James, who loves Warner Brothers films, has chosen the Warner Brothers shield as his shape)

TIP Initially you can do this as two separate activities. That makes the distinction clear, and makes the technique simpler.

● Explain to children that they can write in the circle, make drawings, stick pictures, or whatever. They are creating a kind of collage of themselves, noting down things they like, things which are part of their personality, ideas which are important to them. The collage can be added to as time goes by.

● At first have children focus on the positive aspects of themselves. You will realise, however, that the technique also allows for exploration of negative issues. These could be broached as and when you think appropriate, and certainly not before you and your group have experience of a range of self-intelligence techniques.

NOTE This activity has profound and powerful implications when combined with other ideas. See also *Circle Diagram* (p.131) and ideas relating to metaphorical thinking in the section 'Encouraging a Creative Attitude'.

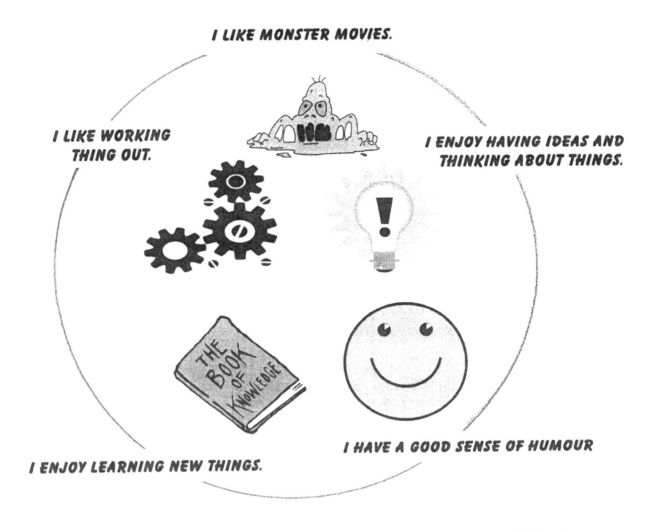

I LIKE MONSTER MOVIES.

I LIKE WORKING THING OUT.

I ENJOY HAVING IDEAS AND THINKING ABOUT THINGS.

I ENJOY LEARNING NEW THINGS.

I HAVE A GOOD SENSE OF HUMOUR

This is me

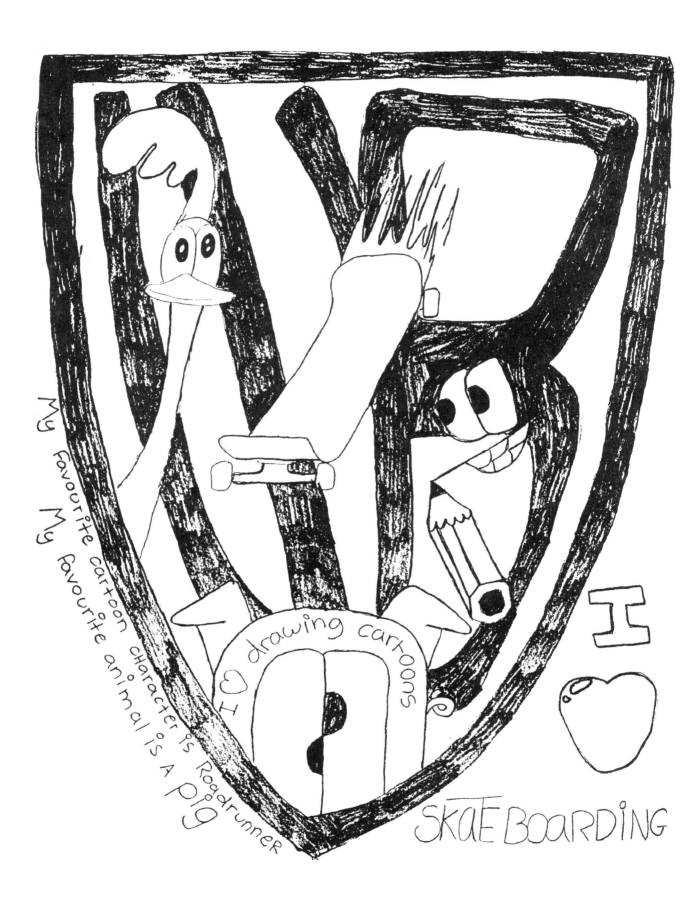

The 'But' Button

What we say connects with what we believe, obviously. Words are like the fruit of a tree directly linked to the roots of how we feel about ourselves. Often we are not fully aware of our habitual speech traits, or that they're telling us something important about our personal world picture.

For example, 'Yes, but' is a door that opens, then slams shut. ' OK, James, let's have some ideas for writing a story, shall we?'– ' Yes, but I don't know if I'll be able to do it / I'm no good at writing stories / I like writing stories though my handwriting lets me down', etc...

Raising awareness of such limiting speech patterns allows children to modify them, and eventually, therefore, to modify the beliefs they represent.

Suggested activity

- In the example above, make a badge that says, 'Yes but' and ask the child concerned – James in our case – if he'll wear it. (If he says, 'Yes, but', persevere!) Instruct his classmates or work group to notice when James says 'Yes but', and have them touch the badge to remind him of it. Emphasise that this gesture should be friendly and encouraging, not judgmental.

- Provide James with an alternative - 'Yes, and' is a good one. Once James begins to correct his own speech trait, give him a 'Yes, and' badge to wear for a while to anchor this new way of speaking, thinking, feeling and believing.

Extension work

Patterns in our language can have pervasive and cumulative effects. Small interventions usually have the same snowball effect. For instance, if you ask a child to do something and she says she can't, respond with 'Well, pretend you can and let me know when you've done it'. Something as simple as that can work wonders: what children can't do for real, they feel safe to pretend they're doing. And in the same example, the subtle use of 'when' presupposes a successful outcome.

Similarly, when you specify an outcome to children, the addition of a sentence like 'I don't know how many good ideas you'll come up with, maybe only six, or perhaps many more' says a great deal about your positive expectations of the group's high standards. Used in conjunction with, say, spatial anchoring in your classroom (see p.74), this simple device can be very powerful.

> **NOTE** For more detail on how language clues us in to people's realities try, for example, O'Connor and Seymour: *Introducing Neuro-Linguistic Programming* (see Bibliography).

GROUPING	Any group size
TIME	The time taken to make the badges
EQUIPMENT	Badge-making kit, or pre-bought badges or stickers
SKILLS DEVELOPED	Awareness of speech patterns, and how 'unconsidered' speech traits can affect and reflect our self-image and self-beliefs
AGE	Across the range (with variety of use)

Positive Strokes

A 'stroke' is a unit of attention that one can give or receive. It is usually verbal – although how effectively have we as adults developed the glare to control our children's behaviour! A stroke may also be positive or negative, real (sincere) or feigned (plastic).

POSITIVE	NEGATIVE
REAL	PLASTIC

Strokes can also have conditions or limitations attached to them. Consider 'I'll be really pleased when you've finished your work'.

Whether or not this unit of attention is real or plastic (both the teacher and the child will know!), the pleasure the teacher promises is conditional upon that child finishing the work. It may be perfectly true that the teacher will be pleased with the finished product, and how much more encouraged the child will feel if the teacher says, 'I'm really pleased with the way you've worked so far. I'm looking forward to seeing the finished piece.' If this is accompanied by a hand on the shoulder (positive kinaesthetic anchor) the effect of the words is enhanced.

NOTE Obviously the most beneficial strokes are positive, real and unconditional, used as part of an ongoing context of encouragement, backed by sincerity which is reflected in one's whole behaviour. Since expectations determine outcomes, when you truly expect your group to shine, your whole attitude will say so loud and clear.

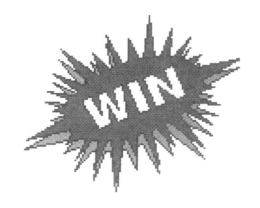

Affirmations

Affirmations appear time and again in the literature of personal development, and may be considered as focused and repeated positive strokes, often 'self-administered' - and frequently ineffective for a number of reasons. However, when used congruently they form a powerful instrument in the toolkit for enhancing emotional resourcefulness.

The Doubt Factor

Perhaps the most famous affirmation is Emile Coué's 'Every day in every way I am getting better and better.' Imagine standing in front of the bathroom mirror one morning and repeating this to yourself, possibly in a serious tone or maybe frivolously – but with great determination. Next day you reaffirm that you are getting better and better in every way... Though perhaps you check yourself to find whether in fact this is so, and in what particular ways. Do you notice any improvement? Yes? Or are you kidding yourself?

Day three goes by; day four; day five... By now you're quite likely wondering if any improvements are the result of 'mental reprogramming' or just a random run of good days. Day six – and how come that disagreement with the boss seems to undo all of the good work you've put into your affirmations?

If you conclude that no real change has occurred – if the doubt factor creeps in – then you'll have created a negative feedback. Future repetitions of 'Every day in every way I'm getting better and better' are likely to be accompanied by the sly thought of 'Oh, no, I'm not!' - in which case the affirmation will be neutralised or even reversed.

It is self-evidently (though also demonstrably) true that what and how we think determines what and how we feel and behave. Affirmations are not simply a product of New Age mystical flimflam, but constitute a powerful modifier of extant negative thinking patterns. Coué's framing is limited because of its very nature; it fails to satisfy all the criteria of the most effective affirmations, namely that they must be:

- positive
- precise
- present-tense
- determined
- personal
- unconditional
- direct
- sincere

The 'As If' Principle

Once an affirmation has been framed according to the above criteria, it must be acted upon as if it has already worked. This principle is similar to (but not exactly the same as) the pretend-you-can strategy mentioned on p.83. It is a kind of reframe, taking you out of the thinking – feeling – reacting of your present state and associating you with your desired state. Expectations determine outcomes – and to behave as if your expectations have already been realised enhances this empowering technique.

> **TIP** Clearly, affirmations can be applied to oneself or the children in your class. They may be used overtly – you can explain to the children what they are, and help your class to frame various affirmations to set any number of goals. Or you might employ them more subtly and implicitly, in conjunction with *Annotated Notebooks* (p.91) or *Watermark Worksheets* (p.86), for instance.

Once the idea of affirmation has been established as part of the classroom environment, many of the devices and activities in *Self-Intelligence* can be seen to utilise its principles and processes.

Watermark Worksheets

A 'reminder' - a re-minder – is something that 'brings back to mind'. It can be as obvious as a comment or a photograph, as insubstantial as an aroma or a faint and fleeting sound. Some reminders are so subtle that we fail to recognise them as triggers – we are reminded, but don't know how, in which case the reminder is subliminal: it creates a response below the threshold of our conscious awareness.

There are many ways of using subliminal reminders in an educational context. One technique is to use peripheral displays – posters placed around the walls above the children's eye-level when seated. Such displays will be glanced at often (when children daydream, for example!), but rarely consciously noticed. Nevertheless, the child will be repeatedly exposed to the information, with the increased possibility that it will be meaningfully connected.

Watermark Worksheets employ faintly printed background material, over which is printed information to be learned, or a framework on which the child is required to write. Faint watermarking can barely be seen, and indeed may not be consciously noticed if the child is engaged and involved in the task at hand.

NOTE Watermarks can be text and/or graphics, and can come in the form of a statement, question or affirmation. Some software packages include a watermarking facility. Three watermark worksheets are provided here for immediate use.

I am relaxed and confident in my work

Having good ideas is easy and fun
Having good ideas is easy and fun
Having good ideas is easy and fun
Having good ideas is easy and fun
Having good ideas is easy and fun
Having good ideas is easy and fun
Having good ideas is easy and fun
Having good ideas is easy and fun
Having good ideas is easy and fun
Having good ideas is easy and fun
Having good ideas is easy and fun
Having good ideas is easy and fun
Having good ideas is easy and fun
Having good ideas is easy and fun
Having good ideas is easy and fun
Having good ideas is easy and fun
Having good ideas is easy and fun
Having good ideas is easy and fun
Having good ideas is easy and fun
Having good ideas is easy and fun

I feel good about myself

Annotated Notebooks

Teachers have annotated pupils' notebooks for as long as teachers and pupils have existed! The basic principle of Annotated Notebooks in the context of self-intelligence is that

- children write their work on the right-hand page
- the left-hand page is left free for annotations

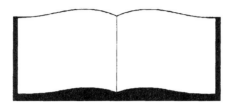

ANNOTATE   COMPOSE

The annotations can be inserted by the teacher, the child or (with the child's permission) anyone else. Pages may be annotated before work is done, during composition, afterwards when the child looks back – or at any stage in the preview – do – review process.

TIP
Pictures, icons and other graphics act as shortcuts to positive memories and emotional resources pertinent to the writing process. A range of appropriate sticker sheets can be bought at most good stationers. Alternatively, preparing your own takes relatively little time.

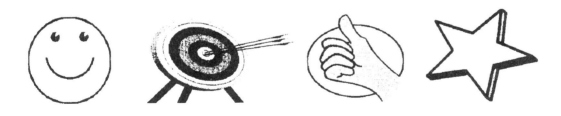

Suggested activity

1) At the preview stage, annotations serve to 'prime and prompt' the child to keep ideas, techniques and points in mind as she prepares to write. Prompts need not refer only to technical aspects of the work ('Remember full stops.' - ' Take time to form your letters neatly.'), but can apply directly to useful emotional states ('I was so pleased with your last piece of work, and I'm confident this one will be even better!' - ' Remember how much you enjoy writing stories – think of the time you did a story really well, and as those feelings come to you now, begin writing...').

2) During the composition phase, annotations help to keep the child focused, interested and 'self-sufficient' by offering pieces of information, asking questions, suggesting resources, giving reminders and re-anchoring positive feelings. It's important to realise that some children will pay careful attention to most or all of the annotations, while others will give them barely a glance. Neither way (or anything in between) is right or wrong, but rather more or less useful as a strategy for the individual. Support this ethos by reassuring children that anything entered on a left-hand page can be used if, when or how they please.

3) In the review phase of the work – the looking back time – annotations can help consolidate the hows and whys of work well done, and may pinpoint areas or points for development. Here the left-hand page can also be used for the child to record her feelings about the work, for self-marking, to be awarded/award herself feedback stickers (see next page), and for many other purposes.

NOTE

The intention of annotated notebooks is not for teachers to blanket-bomb the child's work with corrective statements and marks. The technique should be used within the ethos of self-intelligence. Children improve their skills from a sound platform of high self-worth, confidence and self-esteem. All annotations should directly or indirectly support that primary aim.

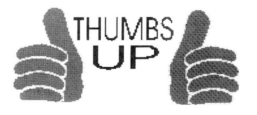

Self-Marking / Feedback Stickers

There are three phases to the successful completion of creative work:

- the thinking time
- the doing time
- the looking-back time

Self-marking and the use of feedback stickers are useful strategies children can employ when they review what they have done.

Children's self-marking of work is not a substitute for a teacher's comments. On the contrary, the two are complementary. Nor is it the case that children will give themselves top marks for very little effort. It's been my experience that when children appreciate the ethos within which they work, and are given the opportunity to evaluate their output, they do so honestly and perceptively, picking out strengths and weaknesses together with valuable insights for improvement.

Self-marking can make use of all of the techniques you currently employ, although for the purposes of developing emotional resourcefulness comments, signs and grades should relate to the child's own capabilities and potentials rather than being comparative judgements within a competitive frame. Also, emphasis should be placed on children's emotional response to their work and annotations referring to its technical aspects. This means that feelings of pride, pleasure, achievement, confidence and self-worth should be drawn out, gathered and anchored. (Feelings of disappointment, frustration, apathy, anger, etc., need to be addressed and resolved. Activities throughout this book suggest ways of doing this.)

Basic activity

Consolidate children's self-marking by evolving with them an agreed set of icons they can use subsequently as a shorthand way of summing up their feelings about aspects of their work. This idea is mentioned in connection with *Annotated Notebooks* (p.91).

> **TIP** Shop-bought stickers add colour and interest to a work-page, but in the long term will be expensive. Desktop-published labels or made-to-order rubber stamps are viable alternatives. Cheaper still, use sheets of clip art: print them on coloured paper (or have the children colour in the visuals), cut out and paste into books. This works especially well with younger children, who generally take great pride in the colouring-and-pasting part of their review!

Some ideas for self-marking.

Use a star rating for a child's perceived quality of her work and/or portions of the work:

 I don't feel very pleased about this work. Here are my reasons why...

 Overall I quite enjoyed doing this work. Here are the different feelings I have about it now...

 I feel pleased about this work, and I enjoyed it. Here are the things I did which gave me these good feelings...

 I am pleased and proud of my work. I have learned new things about how to do the work / about myself. Here is what I learned...

You can also combine icons for children to give a star rating to different aspects of their work.

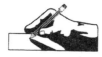 handwriting

 thinking and preparation

 research

 effort

 achievement (how far I reached my targets)

Also encourage children to sum up what they feel they've learned from a piece of work, and how they can use these insights in subsequent assignments.

Positive Reframe

Beliefs about ourselves shape our feelings and reactions, and are reflected in the language we use. There are therapeutic techniques which take a 'bottom up' approach, addressing limiting beliefs and the history of incidents which gave rise to them so that they can be reviewed and modified, and the issues they represent resolved.

A 'top down' approach, and one that is much easier to apply in a day-by-day classroom situation, guides children towards changing a negative outlook by changing the language they use about themselves. This positive reframing can filter down to deeper levels and have a cumulative effect in shifting limiting beliefs and resultant unpleasant and unhelpful feelings. Really, it's a question of engineering a change of perspective from the glass being half empty to it being half full.

Positive reframing through language can be done in many ways, and has generated an armoury of powerful and elegant techniques (many within the field of NLP – see Bibliography). Challenging unresourceful perceptions and feelings isn't simply a matter of disagreeing with a child: 'Please sir, I can't do this.' - 'Why, of course you can Darren!' - Rather, it's a question of allowing the child to become aware of the language he's using, and to go beyond it to more positive ways of seeing.

Suggested activities

Simple reframing devices include the *But Button* and the 'Pretend-you-can Technique' (p.83). Others you might consider using are:

The Can't Barrier

'I can't do this.'
- You can't do this because? (List reasons, then work on them.)
- What stops you?
- What might happen if you did?
- How, exactly, can't you do this? (Break the behaviour down into smaller pieces. Work with the child to draw out its various aspects. Use other 'Big Question' words as appropriate: Why, exactly, can't you do this? Where? When? With whom?

The Always/ Everything Distortion

Challenging generalisations allows children to 'buy out' of their extreme thinking. Look out for 'all-or-nothing' words like 'all, always, never, everyone, no-one, every time/place/thing':

'People are always yelling at me.'
- Which people?
- People are *always* yelling at you? (Challenge 'always').
- People are always *yelling* at you? (Challenge 'yelling').
- People are always yelling at *you?* (Challenge 'you').

'Oh, everything's going wrong!'
● Everything?
● How are things going wrong?
● What would need to happen for them to go right?

Similarly, other extremes - 'couldn't, mustn't, shouldn't, have not, unable to', etc. - can be challenged and changed:

'I couldn't do that.'
● What stops you?
● What would/might happen if you did?

The Mind-Reading Distortion

'She's not talking to me now, so I know she hates me.'
● How does her not talking to you mean she hates you?
● How (else) do you know that she hates you?
● What do you think 'hate' means?

The 'Teach Me How To Do That' Technique

'I really get upset when she's late!'
● That's interesting. Teach me how to be upset by her being late.

And get them to do it! At the very least this allows the child to become more aware of how his 'being really upset' behaviour is constructed. It also gives you useful feedback {like the child's body posture, eye position, etc.) that could lead to useful insights for other interventions. Combine modifiers as appropriate: in the example above, challenge 'she'. Ask 'How late does she need to be before you get really upset? ... What does really mean?' And so on.

Outcome Thinking

When a child presents you with a behaviour that's limited, unhelpful, unresourceful, help to reframe by focusing on outcomes:

● What would *you* rather have?
● How would you prefer to feel?
● What will you be doing to make sure this happens?
● Let's think of four things we can do right now to help...
● When you have changed how you feel, what will be different inside and outside of yourself – how will you see/hear/notice/think/feel differently?

> **NOTE** If linguistic interventions like these have a minimal effect, combine them with other techniques given in this book. A particularly lucid and practical guide to this subject is Lewis and Pucelik: *Magic of NLP Demystified* (see Bibliography).

Winnability Stickers

How well I remember treasuring a gold star for work well done at school! It summed up all the things I had done right and remained a powerful token of a teacher's pleasure in my achievement.

Winnability Stickers takes that good idea further, although here the emphasis is on social and emotional qualities shown by the children, rather than the technical merits of their work.

It is important to realise that the whole enterprise is one of raising awareness of desirable personal qualities, and a recognition that these are also useful and beneficial skills in life's business of dealing with others. A Winnability Sticker represents a positive stroke rather than a sign that you have done better than your classmates.

Basic activity

To save overcomplicating the system, choose a number of attributes that you and the children value – kindness, sensitivity to others, co-operation – and award tokens on that basis.

TIP A spin on the idea is to identify a desirable quality and award stickers without telling the children what they represent. This encourages children to notice closely their own and their friends' behaviour in order to solve the mystery and earn a token.

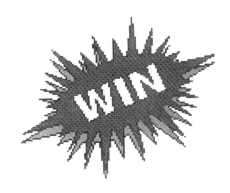

The Happy Coat

The Happy Coat forms an unusual and colourful record of the class's progress through the year.

Basic actvity

Take an old coat and, over time, cover it in badges. The badges can incorporate affirmations; children's names plus positive personal qualities; signs and symbols; quotes; interesting or useful facts (in visual or shorthand form); intriguing questions, and so on. Spend some time each day or each week allowing children to review the badges on the coat, add new ones, borrow badges to wear in class, discuss their content, etc.

> **TIP** Have children wear the coat for special occasions, or as part of the ritual of having the group absorb its contents.

Extension activities/variations

You can use the badges as a basis for writing, drama, or as a starting-point for work in other subject areas.

PowerBox

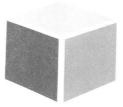

PowerBox combines elements of 'Let's Pretend' and the 'As If Principle'. Like many of the activities in this book, *PowerBox* focuses, enhances and gives direction to resources the children already have inside themselves.

Basic activity

Take an ordinary shoe box or similar, and wrap it in decorative paper. Use it as a resource anchor for various purposes:

- An ability/quality/good feeling I want is in that box. When I hold the box I will understand more of what I want and how to get it.

- Three answers (or maybe more) to my problem are in the box...

- Four or more ways to make my writing better are in that box. When I hold the box these ideas will come to me...

A-Mazed

'How do I know what I think until I see what I say?' is a phenomenon which occurs at any age or in any context. The very act of articulating our ideas verbally or in written form can bring us to new understandings.

A basic activity of this sort is to decide that you wish to recall incidents or gain general impressions from a certain time in your life. Take a pen and paper and begin writing - 'I remember ... I remember ... I remember ... I remember ...' Eventually memories and impressions will come. Just let them flow without trying to direct them. In fact, put no intellectual effort into this activity at all. The work is being done mainly by the subconscious mind. Your writing hand knows what it's doing.

NOTE
If ideas suddenly dry up, go back seamlessly to 'I remember ... I remember ...' - and if you find you can't remember, simply begin writing 'I can't remember ... I can't remember ... I can't remember ...'

This reminds me of a lovely story I was told, of a little boy whose Grandma was trying to teach him to say 'chrysanthemums'. He tried very hard, but couldn't do it. So Grandma told him to go and report this to Grandpa. So the little boy hurried over to Grandpa and said, 'Grandma told me to tell you that I can't say the word "chrysanthemums".'

Basic activity

A-Mazed is a variation of this basic activity of 'effortless writing'. Provide a maze template and work with the child on the issue to be explored – a feeling she wants to understand or change, a memory she wishes to have, an idea she'd like to explore.

Find the exit of the maze and suggest that by the time the child 'writes her way' to that point, she'll know much more about the topic she's exploring. (This engages the phenomenon of pre-processing, where the mind subconsciously anticipates reaching a goal and will begin gathering information).

Allow the child to enjoy finding her way through the maze, tracing the route faintly in pencil. Then leave her to write her way through it - 'I remember ... I remember', or 'I understand ... I understand.'

NOTE
If ideas don't come forward on this occasion, run the activity through a few times as appropriate before leaving it for a more effective technique. Always have extra paper handy, because the child might produce nothing in the maze, but right at the end will begin to generate insights.

GROUPING	Individual work
TIME	10-15 minutes
EQUIPMENT	Maze templates
SKILLS DEVELOPED	Ease of expression of feelings, self-understanding
AGE	7+

The task here is to recall an experience that reinforces self-confidence:

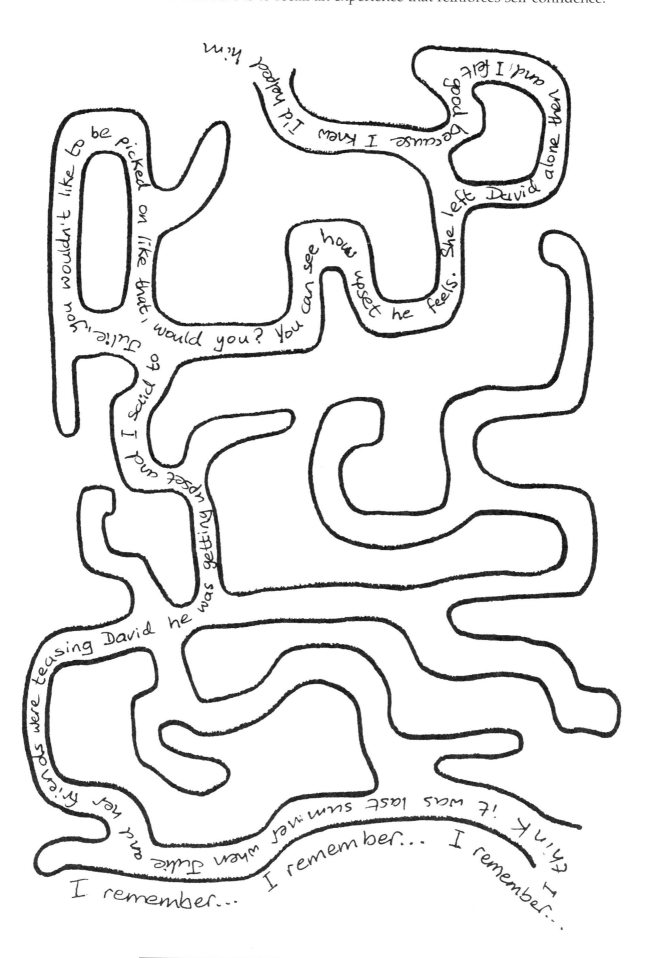

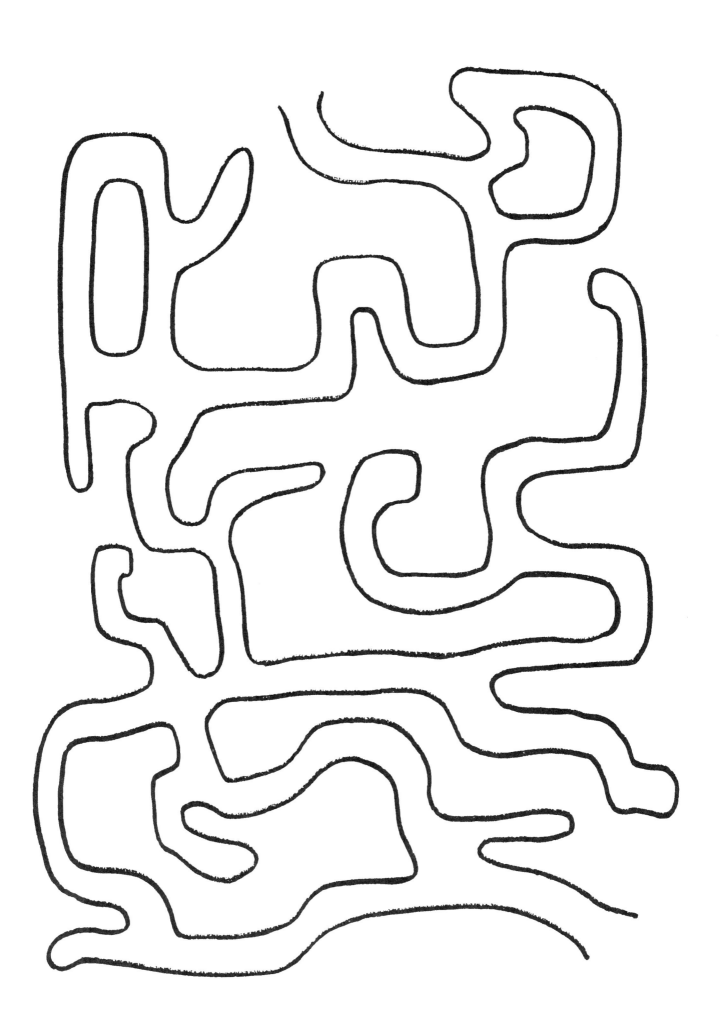

well done

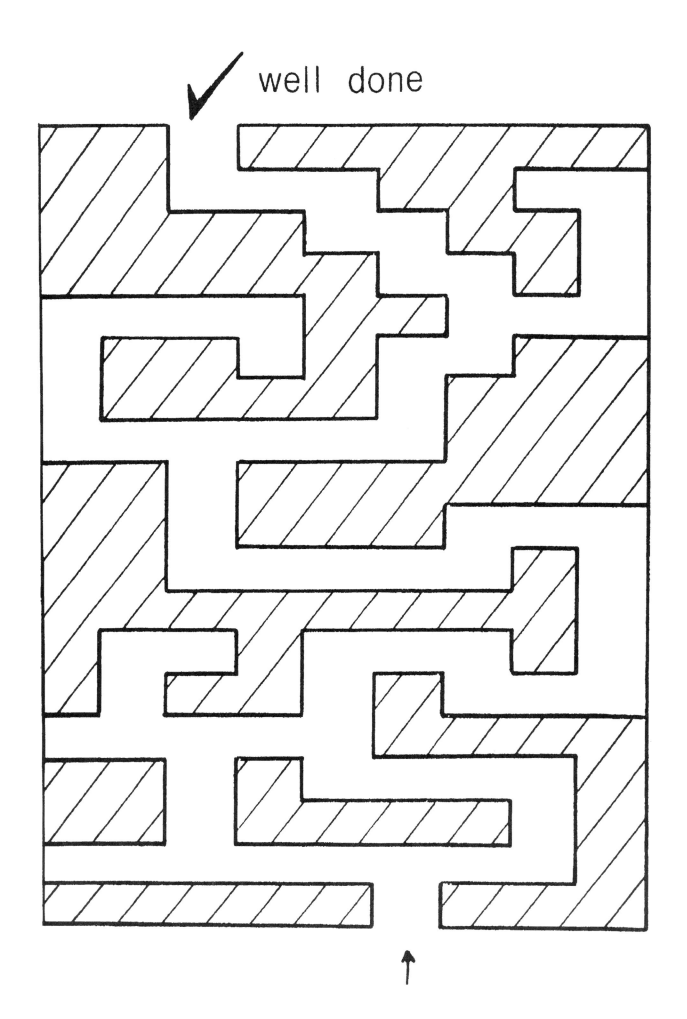

Dealing with Feelings

Often a sense of helplessness and frustration accompanies the experience of unpleasant emotions, a sense of not being able to control them. Either that or, especially with children, one is too wrapped up in the emotion itself to think to intervene.

Basic activity

When a child displays anger or whatever, or is simply upset, sit down with him and go through the following process. Let's use anger as our example:

Teacher: If this anger had a colour, what colour would it be?

(If the child says 'I don't know', reply with 'Well, just pretend. Make it up as you go along – the first thing that comes into your head.')

Child: It's red.

Teacher: What kind of red?

(Go after more detail as you think necessary or appropriate.)

Child: Very red – deep red.

Teacher: And what shape is the anger?

Child: Round, and spiky. Like a curled-up hedgehog.

Teacher: OK, fine. What size is it?

Child (moulding hands in the air): About this big, football-sized.

Teacher: And if you were to hold it in your hands, how would it weigh – heavy? Light?

Child: It's heavy, really heavy.

Teacher: Is it hot or cold?

Child: Um... It's warm – warmer. Getting warmer.

Teacher: If you tapped it with, say, a pencil, what sound would it make?

Child: I'll tap it with a spoon... It makes a kind of clunk.

Teacher: Nice sound?

Child: Dull sound.

Teacher: And whereabouts in your body is this anger?

Child: It's in my chest, but the spikes are sticking through to other places – through into my stomach and in my eyes.

Teacher (feeding back the impression): Right, so your anger is deep red, football-sized and spiky. It's really heavy, getting warmer, makes a dull clunking sound, and it's in your chest with spikes sticking through to other places... Now, do what I say right away, just the first thing that comes into your mind, and then tell me your answer – change the colour now.

Child: Now it's light blue.

Teacher: Change the shape.

Child: It's going to a rugby ball shape, flatter...

Teacher: Change the texture – what it feels like – do it now.

Child: It's smoother, like leather.

GROUPING	Teacher-pupil one-to-one works best
TIME	5-10 minutes
EQUIPMENT	None needed
SKILLS DEVELOPED	Awareness of emotions and how emotions can be accessed and modified, control over emotional states and responses
AGE	Across the range

> *Teacher:* All those spikes gone?
>
> *Child:* Yes.
>
> *Teacher:* Change the size.
>
> *Child:* It's going smaller, but not much.
>
> *Teacher:* That's OK. Weigh it in your hands now and change the weight.
>
> *Child:* Lighter and lighter.
>
> *Teacher:* Change the temperature.
>
> *Child:* It's cooler.
>
> *Teacher:* Tap it with a spoon, and -
>
> *Child:* It's a nice ringing sound, chiming. Like a wind chime.
>
> *Teacher:* Shift the whole thing somewhere else now.
>
> *Child:* Well... I want to bring it out and kick it away like a ball.
>
> *Teacher:* Go on then. Do it in your mind or for real! (In this case the child kicks away an invisible ball).
>
> *Teacher:* So now we have a light blue, rugby-ball shape that feels like leather. It's smaller now, growing lighter and cooler, and it makes a nice chiming sound. And you've kicked it away!
>
> *Child:* Yes.
>
> *Teacher:* (breaking state for the child): Oh, by the way, how's your short story coming on?
>
> *Child:* Oh, um. Fine.
>
> *Teacher:* Check with yourself now. How do you feel?

In most cases, the feeling will have diminished, changed, or disappeared.

> **NOTE** It may be necessary to do more than 'dismantle' an unpleasant emotion. If so, ask the child to remember a pleasant feeling. Watch for a change of facial expression and/or body posture and/or breathing as the memory comes, together with the good feelings that accompany it. As this happens, ask:

Teacher: So what are you feeling strongest of all just now?
Child: Just, well, happiness really...
Teacher: And if this happiness had a colour, what would it be? ...

Go through the parameters with the child (size, shape, texture, etc.) and tell the child to enhance them, to make them more. Feed back the enhanced feeling and anchor it with a touch on the arm, a smile and 'Well done', drawing the child's attention to some appropriate visual. Then break state again (ask the child the time, for instance).

Often, emotions feed on themselves. We experience a feeling and that colours our conscious thoughts and behaviours. A feedback loop is set up and the emotion rolls on unchallenged. In *Dealing with Feelings* we have a way of defusing unpleasant or unhelpful emotions and replacing them with more beneficial ones – although with the proviso that even unpleasant emotions can be driven by underlying positive intentions (see *Positive Intentions*, p.113).

TIP In a group situation, *Dealing with Feelings* works best with pleasant emotions. For each parameter you may need to reach a general agreement with the group. Build in the chance for children to make individual changes to the impression you create collectively.

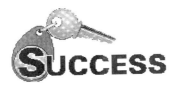

Scrunch!

Scrunch can be used to round off a *Dealing with Feelings* session, or as a variation of *Flipping the Coin* (p.120).

Basic activity

If you are experiencing an unpleasant emotion, once you have learned as much as you can from it and why it's there, modify it in one of the ways suggested elsewhere in this book. Then

1)   express it on paper as a word, sentence or drawing

2)   scrunch up the paper and throw it away

This acts as a signal to the subconscious and symbolises your conscious wish to be rid of the feeling.

Extension activities/variations

There are any number of variations.

William Schutz in his book *Joy* describes how he would project his anger and frustration into a heavy stone, really psyching himself up to pump the feelings into the rock. He would then carry the rock up a hill near to his home, using the carrying time to think through the causative issues to come to decisions about how he wanted to change. At the top of the hill, he'd stand with the rock held ready, and when the moment came to let go, he would hurl it as far away from himself as he could.

Outcomes

This is a speculation game designed to show children that there are many possible emotional responses to situations. It also demonstrates that you needn't be locked into the same habitual response – if you always do what you've always done, you'll always get what you've always got!

Basic activity

● As group leader begin the discussion by focusing on an emotion, say, anger. Discuss situations, imagined or from the group's own experiences, that evoked the response of anger.

> **NOTE** Work with one situation at a time (using as many situations eventually as are appropriate, or as time allows). If the situation is imaginary, encourage ideas from the whole group about what was said, people's facial expressions and body postures. If the situation is real, collect details from the child concerned.

● Now say, 'What if you'd felt [for example] patience rather than anger. How would things have been different?'

● Ideas might well come thick and fast, but if not, then spend some time 'teasing out' the components of patience:

> Is it made up from other emotions, or is it an emotion in itself?
> How do you know that you are feeling patience?
> How do you know when someone else is feeling patient?
> When is patience normally used?
> When is it most useful?
> Are there times when it's inappropriate?

Then go back to the scenario in which patience replaces anger, and see what comes out of it. You may subsequently use the same scenario and talk through several emotions replacing anger, or you might pick a different scenario each time.

Extension activities/variations

One way of encouraging ideas to come forward without too much intellectual effort is to use a dice.

● Select six negative emotions and six positive emotions that might replace them:

1) anger	1) amusement
2) apathy	2) composure
3) bitterness	3) delight
4) contempt	4) eagerness
5) disappointment	5) encouragement
6) distress	6) optimism

Sidebar

GROUPING Small groups work best

TIME Open-ended

EQUIPMENT None needed

SKILLS DEVELOPED 'Ongoing' self-intelligence strategy

AGE 7+

- Now roll the dice twice to select the emotions you'll work with. So, 4 and 3 – contempt replaced by delight. What might be the outcome in a situation where you replaced contempt by eagerness?

You and the children will swiftly realise that not all of the scenarios selected are realistic or likely. Maybe eagerness can't usefully replace contempt (though check the validity of 'can't'). But it will quickly become apparent that emotional responses are not set in stone, and that it's possible to have increasing flexibility over the way we react.

Control Panel

One-to-one teacher + pupil works best

TIME

Open-ended

EQUIPMENT

Non needed

SKILLS DEVELOPED

'Ongoing' self-intelligence strategy

AGE

7+

This visualisation is another way of modifying emotional states by direct intervention. As with many activities in this book, *Control Panel* is just a game of the imagination, but its effects are real: thoughts, feelings and behaviours are connected, so what we do on a mental level has emotional / physical consequences.

For some people it works better than the *Dealing with Feelings* technique, since they prefer the familiar idea of a control panel provided for them, rather than 'making it up as they go along'.

TIP You can invite the person you're working with to draw the panel as a preliminary to running the activity. You can, of course, add details as you go.

Basic activity

Before drawing the panel, discuss which emotion you want to change and decide if the issue actually amounts to one emotion or is a compound of several. Let the basic 'controls' reflect this.

> *You:* OK, so you think these feelings you have about Abby are jealousy and anger?
>
> *Pairworker:* Yes, she's always boasting about how good she is and what she can do...
>
> *You:* Always?
>
> *Pairworker:* Well, sometimes.
>
> *You:* And that makes you angry and jealous. Why is that, do you think?
>
> *Pairworker:* Well, I suppose I wish I could do as well as she does. Sometimes I do, but when I don't I get – um, frustrated.
>
> *You:* All right. Do you mean you get frustrated with Abby?
>
> *Pairworker:* No, I get frustrated with myself.
>
> *You:* And what about the anger?
>
> *Pairworker* (smiling sheepishly): I think I'm angry with Abby for making me jealous and frustrated.
>
> *You:* OK. Which one do you want to put on your panel first?
>
> *Pairworker:* The frustration.
>
> *You:* And how will you show it?
>
> *Pairworker:* I'll have it as a big control knob that I can turn down.
>
> *You:* And the anger?
>
> *Pairworker:* Two buttons, 'on' and 'off'. I don't want the anger really, not for this.
>
> *You:* And the jealousy?

> *Pairworker:* Hm... Like, a little lever that I can slide up or down.
>
> *You:* Why would you want to slide it up?
>
> *Pairworker:* Um. I don't know really... Well, sometimes – yes – being a bit jealous can make you want to try harder.
>
> *You:* All right, that's fine. Start to draw the box now.

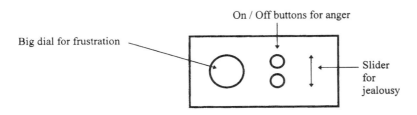

You may find that, although you discuss further refinements to the control panel, your pairworker will 'internalise' these and not need to draw them out on paper. Also, as she becomes more involved, her hand movements will reflect the fact that she's associated with the process.

> *You:* OK, so what do you want to do first?
>
> *Pairworker:* Well I'll turn the dial down for frustration. I think, because all the controls are wired together, once I've done that it will be easier to set the rest.
>
> *You:* Go ahead then – you can draw it, or do it in your head, whichever is best...
>
> *Pairworker* (looking at the drawing, but making hand movements): All right, I'm turning the frustration dial down – I've done that now.
>
> *You:* Fine. What next?
>
> *Pairworker:* Anger off! (pushes the button).
>
> *You:* And now?
>
> *Pairworker:* The jealousy's a bit high. I'm going to slide it down now... That's it.
>
> *You:* How will you know that these settings are right for you?
>
> *Pairworker:* Well, if I need the jealousy to be a bit higher, I can always slide the lever up...
>
> *You:* Yes, and how will you know it's time to do that?
>
> *Pairworker:* Hm, well I can have a kind of light near the slider. That will come on when the control panel thinks the settings are wrong.
>
> *You:* Good idea. Go ahead then... OK, and now how will you know when that light comes on?
>
> *Pairworker:* I'll just feel it. I'll just know it's there.

Further discussion identified this feeling as 'anticipation', and modified it to be 'positive anticipation' - that the pairworker's encounters with Abby would now be more fruitful, incorporating pleasanter emotions.

Once you and your pairworker decide the procedure is complete, have her draw out the finished version of the control panel and then anchor it for immediate access later, as required.

'Best Use'

In the same way that we can become more emotionally resourceful by assuming that all emotions have meaning and are underpinned by positive intentions, so we can more effectively utilise the resource of our feelings by giving some thought as to the best use that we can make of them. An emotion's best use can be explored in anticipation by discussing possible future situations (although children may have past experiences of them).

The point is that if we assume humiliation (or whatever) is simply unpleasant and has no purpose or meaning other than to make us feel bad, then the emotion controls us instead of the other way round. This attitude also leads to a 'hardening of the categories' - to use a phrase coined by Postman and Weingartner – a sense that things will always be like this because they always have been.

> **NOTE** This idea is related to *Positive Intentions* (p.113) and is an extension of it. It might be used as a teacher-led group activity, although when children become more familiar with the notion, then periods of quiet individual reflection are also appropriate.

Let's suppose that in some other class a child has been humiliated in front of his friends by doing some work badly:

Basic activity

● Take time to discuss the 'ingredients' of humiliation: what does it feel like inside, how strong might it be in this situation, how do other people react to it? etc. In other words, construct a profile of that emotion.

● Now ask:
  ■ What is that feeling telling the child concerned?
  ■ What meaning does the feeling have?
  ■ What lesson does the child learn from that feeling?
  ■ What is the best use the child can now make of that experience?

● Whether you use 'hypothetical' and general scenarios like the one above (so that children don't feel vulnerable and exposed), or whether you work with small groups or one-to-one on real situations, pinpoint best uses and write them down. And so, the meaning and best use of humiliation might be:

  ■ to make me do and check my work more thoroughly before presenting it
  ■ to make me realise that in the past the reactions of other people have caused me to feel like this
  ■ to make me realise that the humiliation is far stronger than it needs to be when I do something wrong
  ■ to make me realise that it's part of me putting myself down. I don't feel much pride or pleasure when I do things right, only a sense of relief that I didn't do them wrong!

> **NOTE** This exercise can lead to obvious conclusions, or might throw up some deep and powerfully useful insights. *Best Use* is a high level skill that is best used when children are familiar with self-intelligence work.

GROUPING
Various as appropriate

TIME
Open-ended

EQUIPMENT
None needed

SKILLS DEVELOPED
'Ongoing' self-intelligence strategy

AGE
7+

Recipes

Basic activity

- Begin by looking at the language of recipes. Note that in cookbooks we are given a list of ingredients and their quantities, then the method of preparation, and then the method of cooking.

- Now take a situation (begin with positive ones), such as a birthday party. Ask the group what happens at parties and what feelings you'd find there. (You might wish to refer to the *Emotions / Feelings / Moods checklist* on p.168.) Write down the emotional ingredients of a typical birthday party and gather up words that refer to quantities of things: a pinch, spoonful, dollop, lashings, a trace, plenty of, just a dash, etc.

- Now write the recipe.

'Take a kilo of excitement, plenty of anticipation, and a large spoonful of happiness. Mix these thoroughly and flavour with a little satisfaction. Allow to stew for a time in a hot room and keep simmering with generous quantities of music until all the guests are perspiring and red. Remove from the heat. You may find a little irritation or envy floating about on the surface – in this case, do not stir! Instead, set aside to cool. Return the whole pot to a gentle simmer. You may find that a dash of attraction and a liberal dollop of delight will improve the look of the dish. Any bitterness might spoil the outcome'... and so on.

Extension activities/variations

Once this game is familiar to children, use it as a variation of the *Outcomes* technique (p.106) by asking what the party or whatever would be like if other ingredients were added or removed.

GROUPING	Whole class initially, then varied groupings
TIME	20-30 minutes
EQUIPMENT	None needed
SKILLS DEVELOPED	Awareness of a range of emotions, understanding of the emotional elements of social situations
AGE	7+

Emotions Collage

Raising awareness of emotions and addressing unpleasant or unhelpful emotional responses is an ongoing challenge. Keep positive emotions in mind with an emotions collage: a display board including

- children's symbolic representations of emotions
- facial expressions
- evocative pictures
- badges

  ... and so on.

TIP If you can, place your collage strategically in the room where it associates positively with some other aspect of your self-intelligence strategy. (See, for example, notes on spatial anchoring, p.74.)

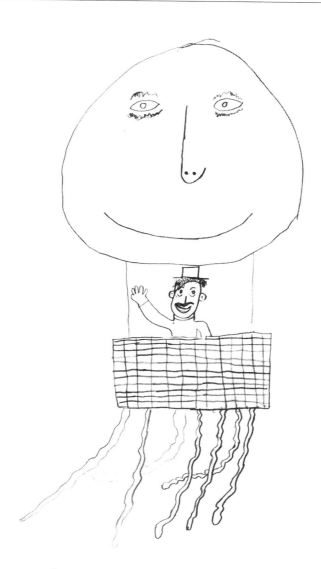

'Joy is a big yellow balloon that shines like the sun, with rainbow ribbons tied to its string'
Words by Sarah (age 9), interpreted by Julian (age 7). Colour it in yourself!

Positive Intentions

Think about putting your hand inadvertently on hot metal – it hurts, and you snatch your hand away. The pain itself was unpleasant, yet the positive intention behind the pain was to prevent further damage to your hand. Now consider the idea that even unpleasant emotions have a positive intention behind them. This is a powerful notion (although it is easy to doubt).

> **NOTE** *The Emotional Hostage* by Leslie Cameron-Bandler and Michael Lebeau explores this concept in great detail, and offers a toolbox of techniques based upon the premise

Boredom, for example, might serve the purpose of alerting you to the fact that nothing useful is going on. Apathy could allow you to realise that deeper down you feel helpless and/or hopeless within a situation.

The key formula here is that

awareness + understanding = control

There's little use per se in just being bored, or wallowing in an apathetic state. The trick is to find out what the emotion means and what you are going to do about it. (Finding out, by the way, often means 'looking in'. You can assume that your emotional landscape is mapped out in your head, and that the signposts are there, if you will but notice them.)

By assuming that 'emotions are feedback' you are primed to read their message in yourself and in your children. A feeling of guilt, for example, can mean that some part of you feels you have violated a personal standard. If this is the case (one can't make a general assumption) then you are a step away from knowing which standard has been violated, and what your future actions might be.

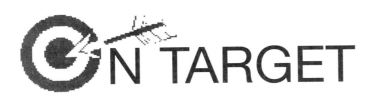

Basic activity

Asking precise questions of the kind outlined in *Positive Reframe* (p.95) can draw out an understanding of the message behind the emotion. Obviously, calming a child down by whatever means would be a useful preliminary to having him look at the emotion himself. Asking why he is angry, for example, should never be rhetorical, interrogative or judgmental. If he says, 'Because Jamie snatched my pen,' follow the trail:

Teacher: How does Jamie snatching the pen make you angry?

Child: I don't know.

Teacher: Pretend you do, just mention whatever comes into your mind.

Child: He took it without asking. He should have asked me!

Teacher: What is it about Jamie not asking you that made you angry?

Child: I wouldn't do it to him. He ought to treat me better.

Teacher: OK, so do you feel, then, that Jamie should have shown more respect for you?

Child: I suppose so... He should ask first, shouldn't he?

Teacher: Of course he should. So, let's think of some things we can do about it...

Of course, not every case would be as easily resolvable as this. It may be, for instance, that deeper issues are involved: perhaps the child has modelled his anger or aggression response from a parent, or maybe the anger represents a deeper sense of frustration, or hides an underlying fear.

NOTE
Teachers are not child psychologists, nor am I suggesting that you should be an explorer in the world of Pastoralia. At the end of the day we all go home to our own lives. But at the very least I feel that teachers (and in an ideal world, all adults) should be, and be seen to be, caring presences to whom children can turn when they are in difficulty.

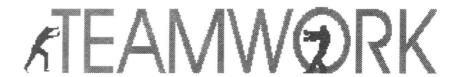

What Does It Remind You Of?

All of us sometimes find it hard to talk about emotions – not just because the emotion is unpleasant or extreme, but often because we somehow don't seem able to find the words to express ourselves. Indeed, we may not have a word to describe how we feel at the time.

Basic activity

- The epigram that you can measure a circle by starting anywhere is profound. If a child presents an emotion that causes this difficulty, have her look around the classroom. Say, 'What can you see here that reminds you of how you feel?'

- If the child tells you that nothing reminds her of the way she feels, pick a few things at random and ask which one is least like the way she's feeling. Get her involved in the game of selecting an object that most reminds her of how she's feeling.

- When an object has been selected, ask what it is about the thing that reminds her of her feeling. Keep her focused on the task. Encourage her to say whatever first comes into her mind – this helps prevent the tendency to consciously construct ideas, which may have little to do with the message behind the emotion. The item the child chooses is helping her to work at a metaphorical level, yet in a concrete way.

Geraldine, a therapist friend of mine, works with a sand tray and a bookcase full of toys (with adults as well as children). On one occasion, a businessman client pushed all the sand into a pile in one corner of the tray. Then he selected a small toy soldier and buried it up to its neck. Geraldine asked what this meant. 'I don't know,' said the client. ' It just feels right...' Then he picked a large rubber spider and, as he lowered it over the soldier, he said with a flash of realisation, 'Oh my God – it's my mother!' It turned out that the man's mother used to call him 'my little soldier', and he now understood that his present emotional difficulties were caused by his sense of being 'smothered ' by his mother.

NOTE Just as teachers are not psychologists, we're not therapists either – nor, it can be argued, should we be. The aim of this book is to show you how to allow children to move more capably through their emotional landscape, to use emotions actively and flexibly by understanding that we need not be helpless and at the mercy of unpleasant emotions, and can 'gather up' good feelings and have access to them at will. When this is done collectively, within an environment of encouragement and support, it drives educational achievement and fuels the joy of learning.

Landscape Metaphor

GROUPING	Whole class or large group initially; can then subsequently be used by individuals
TIME	Up to 30 minutes
EQUIPMENT	None needed
SKILLS DEVELOPED	Awareness of emotions and their inter-relationship, understanding the usefulness of metaphorical thinking
AGE	7+

We have already come across techniques for discussing emotions in more concrete terms (*Dealing with Feelings, What Does It Remind You Of?*), **and this activity takes the idea further.**

The practical relevance of *Landscape Metaphor* **is that it develops work already done on raising awareness of emotions and emotional states by naming, describing and exploring them, rather than suppressing, denying, or being a helpless 'victim' of unhelpful emotional responses. As adventurers in the landscape, children can move from one location to another, implicitly (at first) realising that movement between states is not only desirable sometimes, but possible.**

Basic activity

Explain to children that you are going to enter a 'world of feelings' and map them out. Things in the landscape will stand for different emotions. Give a few examples:

● Sorrow might be drawn as mountains, because both are hard to get over.
● Fear could be a dark forest, because you're reluctant to go inside and explore.
● Happiness might be a grassy hill, because you enjoy looking at the world from the top.

It's important to have a reason why a feature of the landscape should represent a feeling. Similarly, the relative positioning of emotions is significant. Envy might be a stone that's heavy to carry, drawn near jealousy, a bigger rock with sharper edges that can easily hurt you. Loneliness might be a single tree outlying the forest, both placed in the north where it's cold – and so on.

Because people perceive and experience emotions differently, you may have to work to reach consensus on how the collective map should look. Once it's been established, however, and children are more familiar with the concept, suggest to them that they can redraw the landscape to fit their own ideas.

NOTE Confronting and understanding emotions as emotions can be daunting. With *Landscape Metaphor*, once the initial work has been done, you needn't mention emotions much at all, but can talk in terms of physical geography – so that when a child tells you she's 'had an avalanche inside that's blocking the river', you know it's time to help her by pulling more tools out of the toolbox.

Extension activities/variations

Landscape of the Day

Once children have become easier and more familiar with the idea of metaphorical thinking, you can encourage them to keep a kind of diary-map of how they have been feeling through the day, the past week, etc. This is a shorter version *Landscape Metaphor*, for which you should allow 10-15 minutes. You will need drawing materials.

Have the children use emotional metaphors they've already encountered, and make up new ones as needed. Draw a map that blends symbolic features with actual ones – one child might draw his house on a hilltop; another might draw the school surrounded by a dark forest, and so on.

The feedback you get from these maps (should children decide to show them to you!) will help you to support your group's emotional development and will help them to know that within the framework you've established, expressing and discussing emotions is OK, and to be encouraged.

Positive Personal Pyramid

GROUPING	Individual work, once the idea has been explained
TIME	Up to 30 minutes
EQUIPMENT	Pyramid template (see next page)
SKILLS DEVELOPED	Consolidation / anchoring of good feelings; enhancement of the ethos of individual achievement and group support and co-operation; confidence and self-esteem
AGE	7+

It's easy for any of us to remember selectively against a backdrop of fragile confidence and low self-esteem. In this state we almost automatically gravitate towards the bad things that have happened: the disappointments, the quarrels, perhaps the rejections and perceived failures. An unchallenged accumulation of such recollections can trigger the habit of 'catastrophic thinking', where we inevitably think of the worst case scenario and replay it in our heads again and again, suffering all of the concomitant bad feelings. A Positive Personal Pyramid (or PPP) helps to prevent this slow slide, and redresses the balance of our thinking.

Basic activity

- Give out the pyramid templates and explain that this is a useful way of recording and summarising children's good qualities and personal achievements. You may want to have some brief general discussion to remind the class of the kinds of things they'll be looking for, and to explain that writing down successes is not bragging.

- Go through the levels of the pyramid, perhaps using yourself as an example to illustrate what the children might record. Emphasise that the pyramid is not about other people's opinions, but what you think about yourself. Explain that by 'thinking good' about ourselves we can feel good about ourselves, and that this will allow us to achieve even more in the future.

- Once children are working, look out for individuals whose feelings of self-worth are low. Help them to recall past achievements and successes, and perhaps offer your opinion about qualities you've noticed in them. Being sincere in this is essential.

TIP PPPs can be added to later. Through discussion you may decide to display the results, or children may want to file the work in their personal development folders.

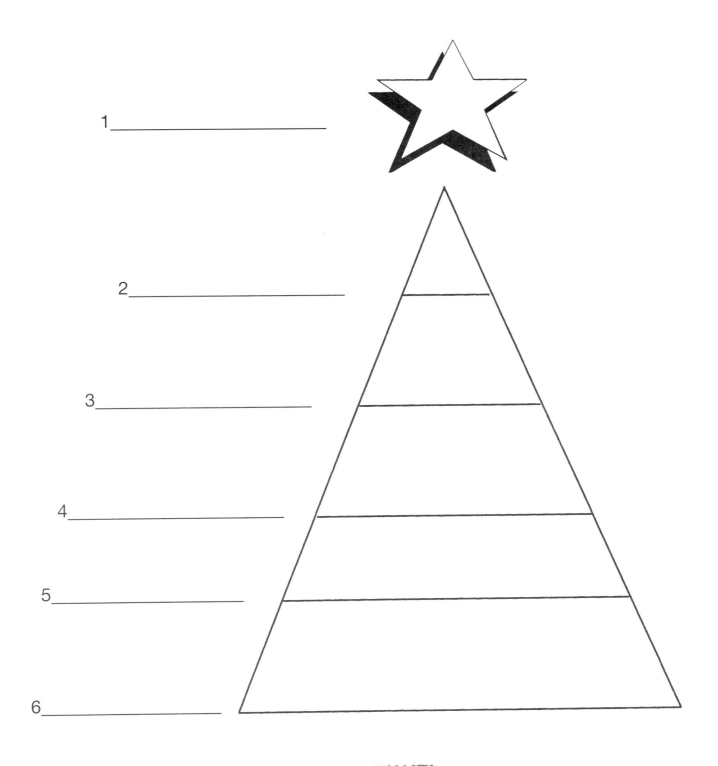

1 _____

2 _____

3 _____

4 _____

5 _____

6 _____

1) STAR QUALITY
2) ONE UNIQUE DETAIL
3) PHYSICAL APPEARANCE
4) PERSONAL QUALITIES
5) PAST ACHIEVEMENTS
6) FUTURE AIMS AND PLANS

Flipping the Coin

A useful rule of thumb is that action follows thought, habit of action follows habit of thought, compulsion of action follows compulsion of thought. Thinking patterns can develop quietly and insidiously, almost without us noticing. In a very real sense we can create our own lack of self esteem and confidence. *Flipping The Coin* helps to redress the balance: saying and 'seeing' are connected, and when children get into the coin-flipping habit of admitting there's a positive to every negative, they will be able to assess their own self-opinions more fairly.

Be aware of how children talk about themselves. When you catch them doing something right, mention it.

Basic activity

When you catch children saying something unhelpful about themselves, encourage them immediately to say the opposite. So, for example:

> *Child* (in frustration): Oh it's no good, I just can't do these sums. I'm no good at Maths!
>
> *Teacher:* Look back a couple of pages – you did those sums right.
>
> *Child:* Yes, but I only got four out of ten.
>
> *Teacher:* That's better than three out of ten, don't you agree?

If you get another 'Yes but', choose another technique such as precise questioning:

> *Child:* Yes, but it's still not very good, is it?
>
> *Teacher:* What do you think you need to know or do to be better? / What do you think stops you being better? / In what way exactly do you feel you're no good at maths?

And you can combine this with exploring the underlying feelings:

> *Teacher:* So what's the difference in the way you feel when you know you're doing maths well, and when you're doing it badly?
>
> *Child:* I don't know – I just feel bad when I know I'm struggling.
>
> *Teacher:* How exactly do you feel?
>
> *Child:* Well, kind of nervous you'll be cross.
>
> *Teacher:* Am I being cross with you now?
>
> *Child:* No, but -
>
> *Teacher:* How else do you feel when you're struggling?
>
> *Child:* Well, I think some of my friends might call me thick.
>
> *Teacher:* Have any of your friends called you thick over your maths?
>
> *Child:* Anthony did a couple of weeks ago.
>
> *Teacher:* I see, and so does Anthony's comment actually mean that you can't do maths?

... and so on. At this point some investigative work (a chat with Anthony) is called for. You might also explore the strategy the child is using (what's going on in his head) that leads him to do maths less effectively.

NOTE
Beliefs of inability may well be rooted in unhelpful strategies-for-doing, or there might be other deeper issues going on, which may or may not be within your jurisdiction or control. At the very least, encourage children to adopt a technique like *Flipping the Coin* uncritically, to help counter the negative effects of the limiting beliefs they currently hold.

Other Person's Shoes

This is a powerful technique that allows children to associate with the feelings and perspectives of others. Clearly (and sometimes not so clearly) we carry our realities around with us, and see the world through our own filters. One crucial aspect of emotional resourcefulness is empathy, the ability to understand and appreciate how other people see the world, and how that leads them to feel.

There are many ways of practising this process. When my wife worked at a special unit for children with mental and physical disabilities, she would have her assistants spend a day being pushed around town in a wheelchair, or wearing ear plugs or glasses with painted lenses, so that they could experience to some extent the world as it looked and sounded and felt to the children they'd be working with.

Basic activity

If there's an argument going on, get the participants to swap shoes and argue from the owner's point of view (if the shoes don't fit, use gloves, scarves, etc., or sit each child down and then have them swap chairs).

In your own classroom, have children sit at each other's places periodically. What does the class look like from that position?

Extension activities/variations

POV [point of view] Spectacles

- Collect old pairs of spectacles. Remove the lenses and attach a tag to each pair. On the tag you might write
- the names of the children in your class
- the name of an emotion
- a category of person – old, fat, black, unhappy, young, optimistic, etc.

As appropriate, have children don a pair of spectacles and describe what the world feels like looking through different 'eyes'. How profound is the maxim that you shouldn't judge someone until you've walked a mile in his shoes! Wearing his glasses is just as educational.

The Attitude Seat

This is a useful little technique when you want someone to appreciate another's point of view.

Sitting in 'the attitude seat' means that you must argue or articulate that point of view in the first person, as though you held it yourself. Children (and adults!) might object to saying things they don't believe, so explain that your own position is strongest when you have a clear understanding of the other person's ideas, opinions and arguments.

Devil's Advocate

A variation is to have two seats facing each other. Two people take their seats and express what they think and how they feel. At an appropriate moment, have them change seats – and change viewpoints, each expressing the other's point of view.

Circle of Three

A further, powerful configuration uses three positions in order to allow people to appreciate ideas and viewpoints from different perspectives.

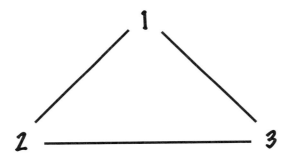

Position 1 involves being associated with your own standpoint (your natural state): seeing, hearing, feeling things through your own eyes, ears and emotions. What you say from this position is based on your own principles and priorities.

Position 2, as in *Devil's Advocate*, involves stepping into the other person's shoes and arguing as if you were that other person and held their beliefs. You speak in the first person with as much conviction as possible, modelling (see p.153) the other person's behaviour as closely as possible.

Position 3 is neutral ground. When you take this position you step back from the argument, detach yourself, become the observer, uninvolved but attentive. By deliberately dissociating from the discussion, debate or dispute you gain an overview of ideas and opinions. This allows you to offer useful feedback and can also provide useful insights into your own thinking with regard to the issue being explored.

Autograph Hunter

GROUPING	Whole class or larger
TIME	15-20 minutes
EQUIPMENT	Sheets prepared according to guidelines given
SKILLS DEVELOPED	Social interaction, self confidence
AGE	7+

This is a good 'ice-breaker' and might be used with a new class, when children from different groups meet, or on similar occasions.

Basic activity

Working with your group, compile a list of positive qualities you/the children would value in one another. These can be very broad such as 'friendliness' or 'always willing to listen', 'good sense of humour', 'sympathetic', 'kind', etc. When you have devised a fairly substantial list that is not open to misuse, format a worksheet/chart for children to use as they approach five or six 'new faces', and run off copies for subsequent use.

If you are working just with your own group, carry out the second stage soon after, before children know each others' names and friendships have 'bedded in'. Give out the lists and let the group 'mill and mix' as children ask each other their names and go through the list of qualities, ticking which ones the questionees feel they have.

Extension activities/variations

Subsequently you might ask your group to write thumbnail sketches of one or two of the people they questioned, emphasising good points, strengths and qualities.

When two groups are meeting for the first time, children might work in pairs to help confidence, later collaborating to write their thumbnails.

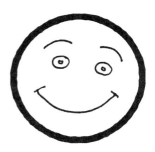

Pat on the Back

This activity is a great socialiser and creates a powerful memento of group feeling. Once children know each other, *Pat on the Back* works well at the end of a term or school year.

Have children fix A4 sheets of paper to each other's backs with sellotape. Then invite them to mill and mix and write brief, positive messages of appreciation on each other's sheet. (Check beforehand that marker pen ink doesn't soak through the paper!)

Criticise Behaviour, not People

A child snatches a toy his friend is playing with. Consider the following responses:
' You are so selfish, Tony.'
' Tony, that was a selfish thing to do.'
' Look what you just did. How do you think that makes Philip feel?'

In the first case the child himself is criticised, making it an identity issue. In the second case, the behaviour is criticised, part of the criticism being implicit in naming the behaviour. In the third case the behaviour is noticed, and Tony's attention is focused on the consequences of his actions – not in terms of sanctions and punishments, but in terms of the effect the behaviour has had on Philip, and more implicitly on the teacher, as disappointment and disapproval will likely reflect in her voice.

All of this is stating the obvious. Yet how easy it is in the heat of the moment to revert to aggressive criticism of the child himself. Cultivating the habit of highlighting behaviour and its effects can pay big dividends. Be assertive about it, of course, and make sure the child realises what's happened. Have Tony tell you what he just did, and how that might make Philip feel. There's little point in your questions being rhetorical, and in any case, if the child doesn't realise what he's done, he can't look ahead to consequences.

Basic activity

Encourage children themselves to take the same approach with each other: eventually the emphasis of their thinking will shift.

Extension activities/variations

Formalise the activity by collecting pictures of negative behaviour and have your children identify the behaviour itself without making automatic value judgements about the perpetrators themselves.

Ripples

This activity extends *Criticise Behaviour, not People*, and works best as an occasional discussion slot. Its focus is the idea that the actions of individuals are cumulative and largely define the ethos and culture of the group – the class, school, community.

Discuss issues from general behaviours, such as crime, to more specific antisocial behaviours like dropping litter or teasing a particular classmate.

In every case, lead the discussion elegantly to explore 'the why behind the why'. Issues are not simply to be disapproved of, but understood. Individuals can then act most positively and powerfully because they are informed.

Hourglass

GROUPING
Individual (perhaps one-to-one with the teacher)

TIME
15-20 minutes (though it may need to be developed as an activity in stages)

EQUIPMENT
Hourglass templates (illustrated)

SKILLS DEVELOPED
Understanding of self, awareness of goal-setting, exploring possibilities for change

AGE
7+

'We know far more than we realise we know. We are therefore greater than we think we are' is a powerful maxim. *Hourglass* allows children to become more aware of blocks to their development and, once that breakthrough point has been reached, to explore the future with a renewed sense of direction and enthusiasm.

Once an issue has been identified, encourage the child to ' let herself learn more about it'. This is a subtle and elegant process of allowing subconscious information to come into conscious awareness. Its success depends upon a number of factors: the child-teacher relationship; how readily the child will 'admit' information into consciousness; how easily she can break issues down into their constituent parts, write about or articulate them, and then expand her thinking to explore possible directions for change.

Basic activity

Explain that the space in the lower half of the hourglass is for jotting any ideas about the issue, why it's there and what it's made of. The more you learn and write, the more you will move towards the breakthrough – represented by the neck of the hourglass. Then have the child begin writing at the bottom of the hourglass template.

Once a breakthrough in understanding has occurred, ideas for 'what I'll do now' spray out into the upper half of the hourglass. The shape of the template is designed to direct thinking, but have spare sheets of paper to hand in case there is a real flood of information.

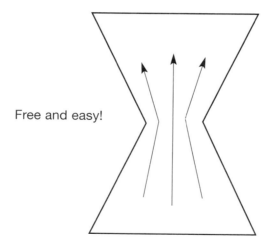

Ideas 'spray out' into upper section.

Free and easy!

Issues are identified and chunked down in lower section.

In the worked example on the opposite page the issue being explored is 'confidence' - more specifically, feeling anxious and embarrassed amongst other people.

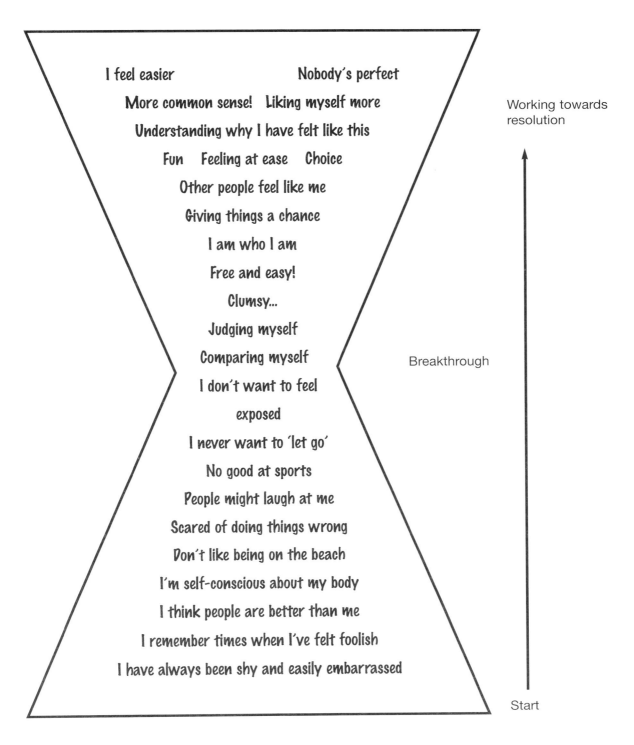

Working towards resolution

Breakthrough

Start

Practically speaking, as you or the person you're working with opens up and admits other ideas pertinent to the issue, what's written in the hourglass segments is likely to be a scribbled outpouring rather than neatly rounded sentences. This is fine, as the activity is based on the idea 'How do I know what I think, until I see what I say?' Outcomes in terms of understandings might be more or less fragmentary or complete, and might be obvious commonsense, or could constitute a more profound insight for the individual.

NOTE Particularly with this technique, it's a good idea to work it through with yourself and/or a colleague before using it with children. Support the will to change with other self-intelligence activities.

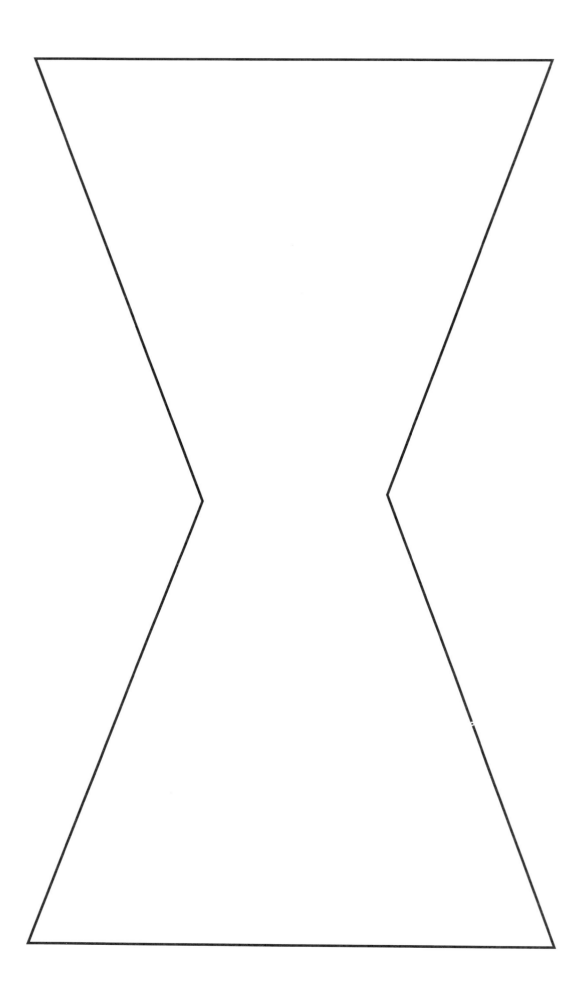

Letters to Myself

Our ability to construct impressions through imagination has both an upside and a downside. Sometimes because we fail to direct our conscious thinking, and sometimes despite our best efforts (because of a subconscious context), we find ourselves anticipating a negative future – with all of the apprehension or anxiety that goes with it. Conversely, we can 'look forward' with pleasure to the possible outcomes and consequences of what we decide to do now.

Run this as a serious activity, perhaps illustrated with your own examples, or letters written by other groups (used with their permission). Emphasise that letters are entirely private, unless individuals want to divulge their contents.

Basic activity

- Begin by asking children if they have ever come across pictures, letters, or other memorabilia of themselves from an earlier time? And did they ever wonder then what they would be like now? Explain that writing a letter to themselves now offers them a chance to 'get in touch' with their future selves.

- Emphasise that this is not a letter-writing activity such as might be done as part of the English syllabus: while neatness, spelling and punctuation are important, these letters are not going to be marked or judged. They need not (and should not) be formal. The children should treat the activity as though they're writing to a friend/penpal – colloquialisms and gossip are allowed – and the focus should be positive, on the individual, and without negative references to others. They can contain a diary element, a record of what's happening now, but also hopes, questions, wishes, and definite plans for achieving outcomes within a timeline – the date on the letter marking the far end of the timeline.

> **NOTE** Using proper notepaper and envelopes gives the exercise greater credibility.

- Once letters are written they should be sealed. Ask the children to write their name and the opening date on the front. This may be weeks or months in the future. Store the envelopes appropriately, in a box or folder set aside for the purpose.

Follow-up activity

When the date for opening letters arrives, allocate some time for the children to read their letters to themselves. Follow-up can be done on an individual basis: failure to achieve goals, changes in circumstances, etc., might need further intervention and help. Or you might make the 'grand opening' a group affair, if the children are comfortable with this. Give some guidance in the form of general questions the group can reflect on:

GROUPING Individual (though may be used with groups of various sizes).

TIME 15-20 minutes

EQUIPMENT Envelopes, letter paper, storage system for letters (file box or large envelope for each month)

SKILLS DEVELOPED Awareness of goal-setting, 'positive future projection', practice of 'As If' principle

AGE 7+

- What are my first impressions now of what the letter says?
- Did my ideas of what I'd be doing and feeling match what's actually happening in my life?
- What did I achieve that I intended to achieve?
- What did I achieve that I hadn't even thought about?
- What did I fail to achieve?
- What are the reasons for this?
- Do I still want to achieve these things?
- So what can I do to make that happen?
- What unexpected things have happened since writing my letter?
- What have I learned about myself from reading my letter now?
- What new things would I like to do in the future?

(Further questions can anticipate another letter-to-myself...)

> **NOTE** This activity is for occasional use. Its basic principles have been elaborated on in great detail by Tad James in *Time Line Therapy and the Basis of Personality* (see Bibliography), which itself is an aspect of the resource-gathering imperative found in NLP.

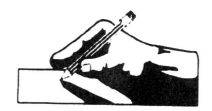

Circle Diagram

This device first appeared in *Imagine That...* as a way of 'getting into' characters created for use in stories. It is also a powerful way of identifying emotions and issues within oneself. Setting up the activity is easy:

- Draw a large circle which represents yourself.
- Subsidiary circles represent emotions, issues, problems, dilemmas, ambitions, etc.
- The larger the subsidiary circle, the more important the issue it represents.
- Overlapping circles represent linked issues.
- Subsidiary circles overlapping the main circle are issues being expressed (outward arrow) or repressed (inward arrow).
- Subsidiary circles outside the main circle are issues approaching (inward arrow) or issues being left behind (outward arrow).

In the example given:

1 = self
2 = a significant issue (person, event, etc.) anticipated for the future
3 = a quite minor issue being expressed (so other people can 'clue in' to it by the way you appear, speak, behave)
4 = a major issue, perhaps not consciously recognised clearly, which is being repressed
5 = a minor issue being expressed, and connected with 4
6 = a minor issue in the past

NOTE It is advisable to undertake this activity yourself before working it through with someone else. This is a powerful technique that may lead to deep insights, but be aware that issues currently recognised (or not) may be negative as well as positive.

Extension activities/variations

- A variation on *Circle Diagram* is to speculate on what your 'map' could look like in the future – after, say, three months, six months or a year. Draw your future self as you intend to be: this mobilises the subconscious to work towards that aim. Similarly, you might combine this idea with *Letters to Myself* (p.129) and *Future Diary* (p.136).

- A further spin on the activity is to personify one of the subsidiary circles. Treat it as a character and set up a dialogue (using the *Attitude Seat* (p.123) works well here). Be that part of your personality and explain what work you do in the life of the whole individual, and what are the positive intentions behind that work.

TIP Remember - 'How do I know what I think, until I hear what I say?'

GROUPING	One-to-one
TIME	15-20 minutes
EQUIPMENT	None needed
SKILLS DEVELOPED	Awareness of emotions and how these relate to oneself and life issues
AGE	7+

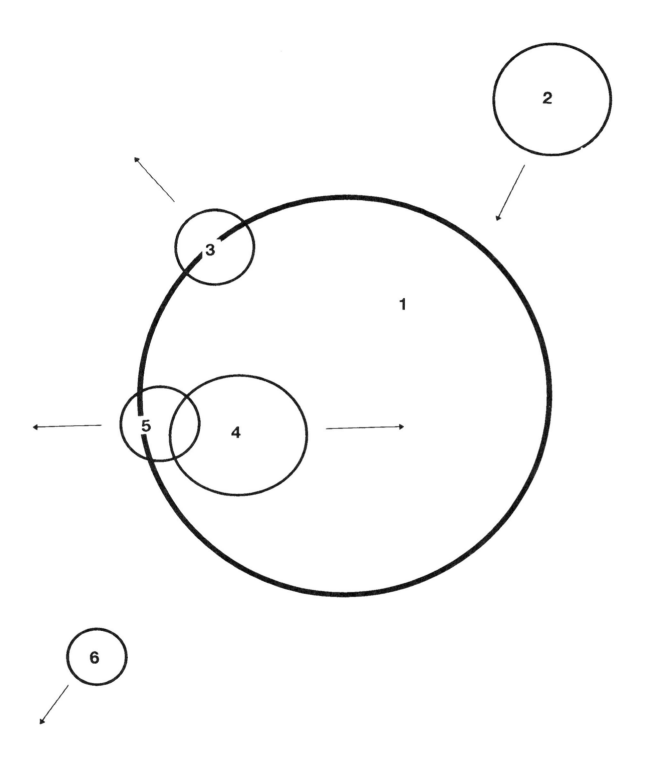

How do I do That?

The issue of taking responsibility for your own emotions is an important one. If you feel that you are the passive victim of unpleasant feelings, or that pleasant ones simply come along at random as circumstances change, then you will not be as powerful as you can be in taking direct positive action to modify the way you feel.

'What you think is what you get.'

Also there is something challenging about the suggestion that other people are not making you feel angry, stressed, frustrated or whatever – but that you are making yourself feel like that in response to other people's words and actions. To be sure, our patterns of response have developed over time and have their roots in our childhood experiences, which is to say, such patterns are anchored in the subconscious and may not be amenable to conscious control instantly.

On the other hand, by accepting the possibility that you can come to understand and direct your feelings, you immediately become more resourceful through enlarging the frame within which you think about yourself.

'Secondary gain'

Another factor which can act as a barrier to change is called 'secondary gain'. This means that even unpleasant feelings carry benefits that may not be consciously recognised. In this case it's easy to use the emotion as an excuse, to blame the way you feel for inaction and maintaining the status quo.

Secondary gains may be on the surface and fleeting – I might snap at someone trivially in order to express anger I feel towards someone else (I'm thinking of specific cases here!). Even a few moments' thought would allow me to realise (to make real, as part of my conscious perception of myself and the world) the misdirection of my anger, and that it stemmed from a larger and deeper issue which needed to be addressed.

But other secondary gains are like currents running deep, and these may only be resolved by specialist intervention once the individual recognises he has a problem. I'm reminded of two cases in particular.

Two case studies

One was a lady who suffered from Crohn's Disease, a form of enteritis. During hypnotherapy she came to understand that this pattern of behaviour had arisen through a constant 'nervous tummy' she'd experienced whenever she was required to meet new people. The pattern had eventually been 'set' - a kind of hardening of the categories – and thenceforward served the purpose of allowing her to remove herself from any unpleasant or stressful social situation. In other words, the Crohn's was the perfect excuse for not visiting the in-laws, or going to that works do, or attending that dinner party. In understanding all this, my client was in a position to make an informed decision over what she wanted to do about the Crohn's – which is to say, she took responsibility for her own behaviour.

Similarly, a male client presented an issue of dyslexia, and indeed had been diagnosed as dyslexic at school. He soon came to understand that the dyslexia was a pattern of behaviour that did not represent a dysfunction within his world view: rather, it was a response he had cultivated as (in his words) 'a cop-out from lessons at school. If you were slow or had trouble with your reading and writing, they put you in a special class where the work was easy. In fact it was a doddle. I hated exams, and because I was dyslexic I got special help, and didn't even need to do some of the tests.'

He was quite sheepish about admitting this realisation, but understood that the programmed dyslexic behaviour had now outlived its usefulness. He didn't gain anything from it currently, and indeed it was making the running of his business more difficult and onerous. In taking responsibility for the behaviour, he also took responsibility for making decisions to change it. After a little more treatment, he let go of the dyslexia and began to read and write more 'normally'.

'Response-ability'

Responsibility equals 'response-ability'. All of us can respond more flexibly to situations once we admit the idea that we are causing our current and habitual responses. Our anger, frustration, stress, nervousness, or whatever, are not written in stone: these and other emotions can be reprogrammed, once the reasons for the original programs are understood.

So when you identify a response that you are not happy with, ask yourself in all seriousness, 'How do I do that? How am I making myself angry? How am I making myself stressed?'

The answers might focus first on the physiology that allows the emotion to be expressed: that increase in heart rate, that tensioning of the shoulder muscles, the leaning forward, the clenching of the jaw. Observation takes presence of mind, the directional use of your conscious attention. Once identified, you can consciously and deliberately take steps to modify some of these features.

And you will also most likely have insights and intuitions (inner tuitions) reflecting the deeper layers of meaning behind the response. Encourage and clarify these understandings through the selective use of self-intelligence techniques. You might like to begin with *Verb It*, the one that follows here.

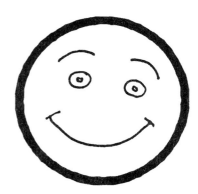

Verb It

An emotion that is named sounds like a state you are in, whereas if it is expressed as a verb it sounds more like a process you are going through. 'I am in a state of worry. I am worrying.'

Active, verb-based expressions sound dynamic; they have energy and movement. By 'verbing' unhelpful states you stop being the passive victim of a feeling and become the active doer of that feeling. This can create the anticipation of using the energy of, say, worrying, in a different way.

Basic activity

Play *Verb It* for yourself before working it through with children. Turn names into actions and see what happens:

- *Take your name and verb it.* What are the implications and connotations of this? - I am Steving. I am going to Steve tomorrow, just like I Steved yesterday, only better!

- *Take a feeling, problem or issue and make it dynamic through verbing* – Are you sadding again? How do you sad? Teach me how to sad? How does unsadding work?

> Today I am happying. Look, I'll show you how to happy. Soon you'll be able to happy better then ever, and then you'll wonder how you never happied!

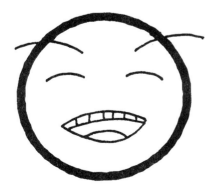

Future Diary

GROUPING

Individual.

TIME

20-30 minutes

EQUIPMENT

A personal notebook or folder for each child to use as a diary.

SKILLS DEVELOPED

Awareness of goal-setting, 'positive future projection', practice of 'As If' principle.

AGE

7+

Future Diary extends and enhances goal-setting work done previously. Its particular impact lies in the fact that children are encouraged to associate with their 'future self', which leads to clearer insights of the resources already available to the individual. This, in turn, clarifies and focuses goal-setting; leads to a more complete understanding of the steps needed to achieve future goals; and gives positive future projection an extra dimension and power.

Basic activity

Explain to children that they are going to pretend to be themselves in the future: have them decide on a particular age, though this not be the same for everyone in the group. Emphasise that this is 'just' a game of the imagination: on that future date individuals can be just who they want to be. A certain amount of wishful thinking is allowed, though the real power of the technique comes through realistic intentions, expectations and goals.

> **TIP** Future Diaries can be in book form, although perhaps a ringplan folder is a more useful format. This allows extracts to be sequenced chronologically, and redrafts and additions to be more easily inserted.

Similarly, when the children write, suggest that they simply imagine themselves as they are in the future (visualisation training will pay dividends here). There's no need for them to try hard to think of what to say. Ideas will flow naturally and freely, and this is to be welcomed, since this is essentially a spontaneous 'first draft' piece of writing. Content takes precedence over form and style: children can always tidy up and polish the work later if necessary.

The act of writing a future diary scenario anchors the impression powerfully in the mind. Subsequently, children can 'revisit' their older/wiser/more mature selves for feedback, to model behaviour, reprogram aspects they aren't happy with, gather up ideas and good feelings based upon future goals now achieved.

> **NOTE** It's an idea to let the group know in advance that they'll be doing this activity. This allows a reasonable period for pre-processing to occur, when the mind consciously, and especially subconsciously, gathers up information pertinent to the task. It's a kind of automatic preparation for the work, requiring little or no conscious intellectual effort. You may want the group to do some preliminary work – brainstorming, *Decision Tree* (see p.192), etc. - before they write their future diary.

Emotion Diary

Whereas most diaries focus on events, people and places, this variation emphasises emotions detached from their context.

GROUPING	Individual work

Basic activity

Instead of writing, for example, 'Last Tuesday Linda pushed in front of me in the dinner queue and made me really angry', take the next page in the diary and say something like:

TIME	Open-ended

> 'This is a page about anger. I remember that the anger came really quickly. It started in my stomach and grew up into my chest, making me feel all tight and sort of closed in. I noticed that my teeth were clenched tight and I knew my face had gone red. Even though one person had caused the anger, it was odd that I felt angry with everybody. It was all really hot and tight and over with quickly, although other fainter feelings hung around and I felt bad all afternoon...'

And so on. A further value of the diary comes in looking back some time later. The pages have no dates, places or names to identify them. It's likely you'll have forgotten the context of the emotions you're reading about: all you'll have are the 'pure' details which serve to highlight the emotion and your perception of it.

EQUIPMENT	Notebooks, writing materials

Extension activities/variations

Annotate your diary retrospectively:

SKILLS DEVELOPED	'Ongoing' self-intelligence strategy

- Jot down ways you've learned of intervening to change unhelpful emotions.

- Make a note of patterns in your emotional landscape ('I notice I tend to get angrier more easily towards the end of the week').

AGE	7+

- Cross-reference pages to build up a detailed profile of particular emotions.

In this way you'll become much more familiar with your emotional responses and the fact that they exist inside you, which is where they need to be dealt with.

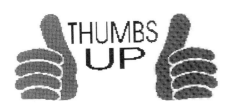

Stepping Stars

GROUPING	Individual / small group
TIME	Varies depending on activity
EQUIPMENT	Large, coloured card stars
SKILLS DEVELOPED	Goal-setting; 'active anticipation'; accessing emotions; emotional flexibility
AGE	7+

This technique combines visualisation, anchoring, the *'As If"* principle and time-line-related ideas.

 Stepping Stars – basic activity

- Use some large, coloured stars (readily available in stationers'). Take one of the stars, place it on the ground and explain to the individual or group that when you step on the star you can experience all over again a wonderful emotion that you've had before.

- Work with children one at a time. Say that when you're ready to have that good feeling (and you'll know when inside), step on the star. Explain that when this happens a pleasant memory will come, or maybe the child will begin to have the memory first, and that will trigger the feeling.

- Explain too that as the feeling/memory starts to fade, the child can step off the star and bring the good emotion with him.

- Watch the child closely for posture and facial expression, which will provide feedback that things are happening. As he steps on the star and the memory or emotions begin to peak, you may want to anchor the state (having agreed this previously) or have the child use his own previously established anchor. You should notice when the experience has peaked. If the child makes no move, invite him to step off the star and bring the good feelings with him.

- Check that the emotion has been 'kept' by asking the child to use his anchor or signal. If he experiences the emotion again, the work has been immediately successful.

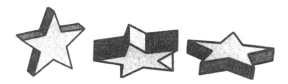

NOTE If the signal fails to work, you can repeat the *Stepping Star* exercise now or later, or invite the child to wonder why the emotion is not there as you both had expected. Possibly there has been some subtle response: in this case use the *Deeling with Feelings* technique (p. 103) and have the child turn up and intensify the feeling. If there seems to be no response even after checking, there may be a block to allowing the positive emotion to come forward. (Other techniques which explore the context of the difficulty may be appropriate).

Extension activities/variations

An extension of the basic stepping star activity is to have several differently coloured stars representing a number of positive feelings/pleasant memories. Working with individual children, have them step on and off the stars in turn so that they gather up a 'package' of good feelings they can take away. Anchor each emotion as per the basic activity.

You might want to consolidate the package by having a final star that represents and sums up all of the emotions to be found on the other stars. A button badge featuring a star of the same colour allows the child to carry the emotions with him in a clearly visible way.

If you want to work with a small group, draw star outlines on the floor in different coloured chalks, and have the children step into the outline as they are ready. This work can be 'content free', which is to say that the children don't need to tell you what they're experiencing: their postures and expressions will let you know what's going on.

 Stepping Stars – Into the Future

This variation utilises the kind of positive anticipation found, for example, in *Future Diary* (p.136). You may wish to work with stars whose colours already have meaning for the children (having experienced the basic *Stepping Stars* activity), or you can use a neutral colour, in which case the stars simply stand for steps into imagined future times.

The aims of this future-oriented technique are several:

- to help neutralise and counteract habitual negative thinking
- to focus attention on desired states and outcomes
- to gain insights into resources the child already has to achieve those outcomes,
- to gain insights into (perhaps previously unsuspected subconscious) blocks to achievement
- to gain insights into what needs to be known / done in order to reach the future state that is being anticipated

> **NOTE** This is not a game of wishful thinking: children are not being encouraged into kidding themselves that they can fulfil unrealistic aims. You are not saying to children that they can be anything they want to be (although plenty of personal development books advocate otherwise). Rather, you are allowing children to become aware of the resources they already possess that will help them to achieve their aims, and to realise the steps that may need to be taken to get there. You are also giving children the experience of associating with – stepping into – their imagined futures, rather than simply viewing those futures from afar, as distant prospects.

Proceed as follows:
- To set up the activity, explain to the individual or group that this is a way of finding out what they think it would be like to have already achieved an aim. Have them think of that aim. Ask them to pretend that the stars you are about to lay down on the floor are steps into the future, towards that aim...

- Place three or four stars down. Tell the children that, even as you do this, they may understand what those steps mean to them – but that it doesn't matter if they don't. It might also be the case that some children will have a sense of needing more stars, some fewer.

Now  *Then*

- If you are using stars whose colours have already acquired meaning for the children, then each child will have to lay down his own path, although it's not necessary for the child to dwell on which coloured star should go where in the sequence. You could, of course, always make use of the 'multi emotion' star used in the basic activity, and have a star path of that colour.

- Say to the children that they are to step on the stars only when they are comfortable to do so, and when they are ready to learn (maybe in detail) what it feels like to be one step closer to their aim. Each child can tell you/the others about their journey as it happens, or they may wish to keep it to themselves.

- Follow the procedure for the basic activity, encouraging children to notice what they learn as they make their journey, and to take that understanding with them.

- As they stand on the final star, invite them to 'look back' and review, however generally, the process of arriving at this spot. Explain that they can now bring back with them all the useful ideas they've gathered: children don't need to retrace their steps, but can bypass the intervening stars to get back to the here-and-now.

 Stepping Stars – Forward to the Past

You can set up a sequence of stars for children to access their memories. It is most easily and immediately of use for getting to pleasant memories.

> **NOTE** Even this early on in their lives, many children have blocks to their development, 'unfinished business', traumatic memories, repressed or denied information. *Stepping Stars – Forward to the Past* is one way of addressing these issues, but should only be used if you feel competent and confident to guide a child through the therapeutic process.

Use the same explanations and rationales as for *Into the Future*. Even as you run through your preface, the children you're working with may well be anticipating the activity and having pleasant memories. Suggest that when they step on to the stars they can have completely unexpected pleasant memories, which they can bring back to the present together with all of the good feelings that go with them.

Then   *Now*

As well as bringing things into the present, children can take present resources back to their 'past selves': pieces of advice, their increased capabilities, reassurances that things are going fine, messages of optimism, strength and positive anticipation...

Stepping Stars – Exploring Possibilities

All of these techniques rely on the principle that we each carry our realities around in our heads, like a 'meanings map', and that those maps can be reconfigured to allow us to get where we want to go more effectively. The mind learns by absorbing information: that information can come from outside, or from the mind itself. Since how we think, feel and behave are fundamentally interconnected, 'thinking games' lead to powerful changes in our emotional responses and subsequent actions.

Our 'meanings maps' also include our perceptions of what our individual futures might be like. These imagined scenarios, created both consciously and subconsciously, can evolve without reflection and deliberation: we can drift into carrying a vision of the future that may not be helpful or in our best interests. In fact, we can actively fuel impressions of dull or dire tomorrows by indulging in the kind of negative thinking that 'drip-feeds' our subconscious mind with images which it feeds back to us as feelings and behaviours. Habits of negative thought become habits of negative action.

Stepping Stars can be used to raise awareness of the fact that the future – and our impressions of the future – are not written in stone. There are many possible outcomes in our lives, and our chances of achieving particular goals are increased when we make deliberate, informed decisions on the way.

To run this activity, you and your group will need to have used *Stepping Stars* in its simpler forms before.

Proceed as follows:

● Work in a big space. Explain now that the stars you will lay down are like stopping points and signposts on a journey into the future, just as if you were following a map with many routes towards the places where you want to be.

● You might choose to do a group activity first. Let's say you want to explore together the aim of 'being successful in life'. Place a star on the floor. This spot represents Now. Ask for what being successful in life means to the children. You may receive plenty of suggestions. If you can accommodate them all, fine. If there are too many (or some are impossible or downright silly), select the ones that are the most workable or useful. So:

■ Getting a job that pays well.

■ Having lots of friends.

■ Living in a big posh house.

■ Having freedom, doing just what you want to do.

Write these on stars and place them some distance away – but with space beyond, since further thinking beyond those aims might occur.

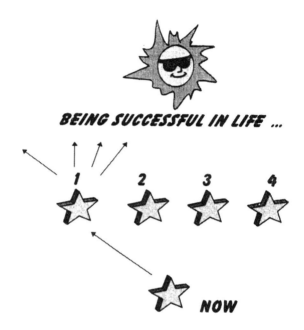

● Take one aim at a time, let's say 'Getting a job that pays well', and ask for ideas on what steps need to be taken to reach that point. You may well find children indulging in 'reactive thinking' (guess the right answer), so expect:

■ Doing well in the SATS.

■ Working hard at school.

■ Going to college.

■ Gaining qualifications.

● Encourage more radical thinking. Suggest that any ideas could be useful in the end, even if they don't seem to be right now. Note down what comes along...

■ Practising something I enjoy and do well (collect examples).

■ Learning how to get on with people.

■ Deciding to do something entirely different.

■ Having good ideas.

■ Not doing what my mother/father/Uncle Fred does now.

■ Doing lots of jobs to gain experience.

● There are different ways of proceeding from here.

a) You can open up possibilities and allow ideas to flow freely (making logical connections between them later) or

b) you can taking one idea at a time and break it down into smaller steps.

A) Open up possibilities...

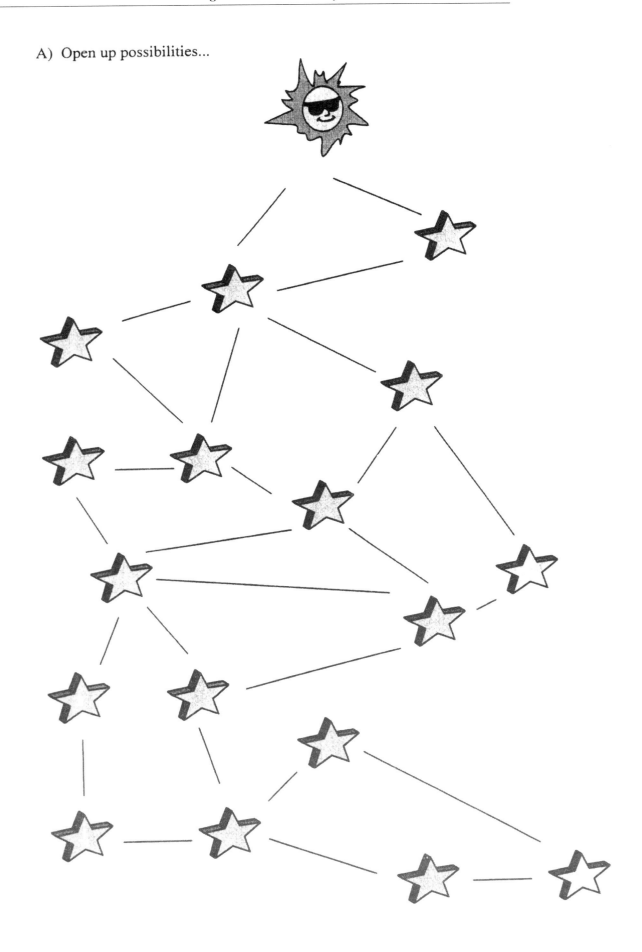

B) Progressively chunk down -

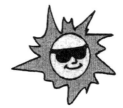

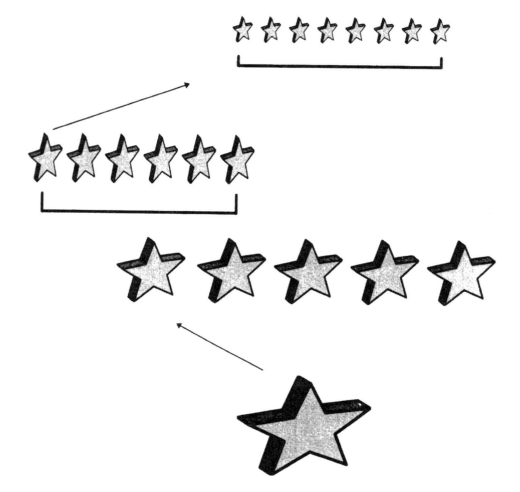

Stepping Stars – Chunkdown Decision-Maker

This variation is effective when you pair-work: one partner identifies her goal, the other steps with her along the way and helps guide her towards achieving that goal. You may wish to use *Stepping Stars* first to open up possibilities, then, from those many ideas, select the best / most appropriate to your present needs and requirements.

Stars are laid down as a consequence of asking questions such as:

- Here I am now. Where do I want to be next?
- What do I need to know to get there?
- (Where do I find out what I need to know?)
- What do I need to do to get there?
- (Where do I find out what I need to do?)
- Is there anything preventing me from taking this next step?
- (If yes, what? And how do I overcome it?)
- What will be the consequences for me if I take this next step?
- What will be the consequences if I don't?

This sounds like a very logical, rational process, but insight is a valuable element in any decision- making. What we decide to do or not often depends on hunches, how we feel, and what I call 'factless knowledge' - that often imponderable, unfathomable sense of just knowing what's right.

Using *Stepping Stars* in this way not only allows our feelings (as well as our reasoning) to play a part in goal-setting; it also gives us practice in noticing and listening to emotions that are frequently wiser than the voice of our intellect, which so often shouts louder and gets its own way

 Stepping Stars – Meeting Halfway

The language of battle often describes and defines differences of opinion, disagreements and arguments. We 'stand our ground', 'defend our position', 'fight for our beliefs', with all of the uncompromising aggression that suggests.

An old Chinese proverb tells us that the angry man has his eyes shut and his mouth open. In our own school situation, children in dispute will shout their cause loudly, armouring themselves with anger, denying fault, loading blame on to the opponent. Listening, understanding and compromise seem miles away in the heat of a quarrel.

Once your group has become familiar with *Stepping Stars* (and the raft of other self intelligence techniques offered here) you can use the activity to help children 'take steps to build bridges' in resolving disagreements.

● Place stars some distance apart, and have each child stand on one. Listen to what each child has to say, without taking sides or expressing any personal opinion.

● Now allow them a few stars each. Explain that the purpose of the game is to let them reach an understanding of (if not agreement with) the other's point of view. Get each child to make a statement which demonstrates that they comprehend why the other feels aggrieved, and/or make some suggestion towards compromise or a resolution. Each time they do this (to your and their satisfaction), have them place down a star and use it to take a step towards the other.

● When they are ready to meet in the middle, give praise and have them step on to stars that have positive associations (previously anchored).

Lucy (crying and angry): Daniel snatched that toy off me! I was playing and he snatched it.

Daniel: (without prompting) You wouldn't let me have it -

Teacher: Wait a minute, Daniel. Lucy, you know we share toys here.

Lucy: Yes, but he just took it!

Daniel: Because you wouldn't share!

Teacher: OK. (Shows stars.) We've used these before. Daniel, take this star – that's it, put it down and stand on it. That's how you feel at the moment. Lucy -

Lucy: I'm not going to. He just snatched it!

Teacher: All right, Daniel you're standing on a star, so I'll talk to you. (Puts star down a few paces away.) Let's suppose this star is Lucy's point of view. Dan, why not take a step towards sorting this quarrel out. We know how you feel, but how can we sort things out?

Daniel: Well... I could ask Lucy to share the toy, instead of just snatching it.

Teacher: That's a good idea. (Gives next star. Daniel puts it down and takes a step towards Lucy's [vacant] star). Lucy's not joining in, so what else can you do to make things better, Dan?

Daniel: Um, well, I could say sorry for snatching.

Lucy: He's always snatching!

Teacher: Wait a minute, you're not joining in, are you? I'm willing to listen to Daniel because he's using the stars like I want him to. (Lucy reluctantly steps on her star).

Lucy: He's always snatching.

Teacher: 'Always'? You mean, whenever you're holding something, Daniel snatches it from you?

Lucy: Yes.

Teacher: Every time?

Lucy: Well, sometimes.

Teacher: OK, he sometimes snatches. He's willing to say sorry this time. Are you willing to listen? (Lucy pouts but nods.) All right, that's fine. Take this star and place it there in front of you. Now step forward on to it... Dan -

Daniel: I'm sorry, Lucy.

Lucy: Don't do it again.

Teacher: Well, Lucy, you're asking Dan to promise something – not to snatch again. He's explained that he snatched the toy for a reason, because you wouldn't share.

Lucy: I do share.

Teacher: Were you sharing this time?

Lucy: No, but -

Teacher: How can you expect Dan to keep a promise unless you keep one too? Do you think that's fair?

Lucy: Suppose not...

Teacher: Dan?

Daniel: I won't snatch if Lucy shares.

Teacher: Sharing means you each have some time with the toy, or whatever. If you both want it at the same time, then I suggest you toss a coin to see who uses it first. Dan, take another star and move a step closer to Lucy... Lucy, Dan says that he won't snatch if you'll share. Is that all right?

Lucy: Well, OK.

Teacher: So now you can make your promise.

Lucy (avoiding eye contact): I'll share if Dan doesn't snatch.

Teacher: Right, you take this star and move a step closer to Dan. Seems to me you're close enough to shake hands now...

This scenario (based on an actual incident) was resolved quickly, although the indications are there that Lucy especially was reluctant to compromise. But at least she was made aware of the principles of compromise, while the use of the Stepping Stars gave a structure to the process, kept it focused, and created expectations that the matter would be settled in a few steps. There was also a symbolic quality to the ideas of moving closer, taking a step towards resolution.

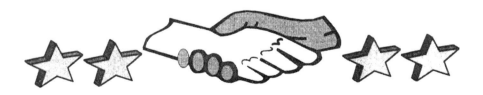

Pole Bridging and Talkthrough

As a writer I well appreciate the wisdom of the saying, 'How do I know what I think, until I see what I say?' By allowing ideas to appear as it were 'through my fingers', I generate the raw material that my intellectual, judgmental self can then evaluate, edit and redraft. *Pole Bridging* and the *Talkthrough* technique are verbal procedures based on the principle behind 'How do I know what I think, until I *hear* what I say?'

Pole Bridging

Pole Bridging allows children to verbally map out their journey as they go along.

As an example of the process, I am reminded of my father, who was a great DIY enthusiast and odd-jobber. If, say, his electric drill broke he would take it down to the workshop and spend weeks fixing it, rather than pay to have it professionally mended. For him the pleasure was in taking the thing apart and putting it back together. If it worked subsequently, that was a bonus. Often, when I took Dad a cup of tea, I'd hear him muttering to himself...'Now, if I ease that spring in there, then that lever can move upwards, so I can fix the screw into that hole and begin to tighten it, so I can slide the casing over like this...' I realise now that Dad was 'Pole Bridging' - working things out as he went along by articulating the process to himself.

Surely as adults we've all had the experience, in discussion, of coming to a new or deeper understanding of our own arguments and standpoint by the very act of explaining what we mean? A restatement of ideas and opinions helps refresh and clarify them in our minds. It is a habit to be cultivated within an environment where children are encouraged to express their own (developing) understanding, rather than feed back unchanged morsels of knowledge we've previously offered. Learning, as every good teacher knows, occurs when knowledge is passed through the 'filters' of children's individual experience. In that vital sense, as Postman and Weingartner say, knowledge is a quest, not a commodity.

Talkthrough

Talkthrough is a version of *Pole Bridging* involving two people. It is a kind of pairworking. Each one of the pair is both a 'sponge' and a 'mirror' for ideas, reflecting and responding to what the other is saying. It is a world away from the 'brighter' child telling the less able one what to do. The relationship is vital, based on mutual respect, self-worth and the urge to find out more, using what you both already know.

> **NOTE** *Talkthrough*, even more than *Pole Bridging*, is a high-level activity best introduced when children have had the experience and benefit of other self-intelligence activities. It amounts to an attitude based on active, careful listening and a preparedness to notice the other person's emotions and be sensitive to them. From that basis a useful dialogue can develop where self-intelligence techniques combine to form a strategy leading to resolution of the issue – as illustrated in the examples in this book.

Visualisation

We all have the mental ability to recall impressions – to call them back from memory – and to construct them through the use of the imagination. My belief is that, practically speaking, constructed impressions rely, too, on our memories, while remembered impressions contain an element of imaginative construction. It is also the case, I feel, that both the conscious and subconscious parts of the mind are always involved in bringing recalled and imagined thoughts to our attention.

conscious	imagination
memory	subconscious

The word 'visualisation' itself, together with 'imagination', 'the mind's eye', 'looking forward', 'picture this', and others, predisposes us to think that our recalled or constructed impressions are primarily visual. Actually, we represent ('re-present') reality to ourselves in several sensory modalities: we hear with our mind's ear, touch with our mind's fingers, feel with our mind's heart. Although we each have our preferred representational modalities and styles, we would be depriving ourselves of a useful dimension of our thinking if we did not pay attention to and utilise the full range of our 'visualisational' capabilities.

In fact, the capacity to use our minds in this way lies at the heart of all of our thinking processes and skills. Each of us makes use of the power we have to move mentally beyond the here-and-now, which is essentially what happens even as we absorb information (formally or informally) and 'make meaning' of it that is relevant to ourselves as individuals. Put another way, without the ability to visualise the world would appear very different to us, and in fact would quite probably be meaningless.

Visualisation is such a huge and diverse subject that it would be impossible to do anything here other than to introduce it as a key component of any self-intelligence work. Broadly speaking we can visualise with more or less focus...

Free visualisation / free association / random daydream

In this state our conscious minds are 'idling'. We are not actively problem-solving or making decisions. Rather, we are watching the largely unconnected drift of our thoughts, snippets of memories, proto-ideas, fleeting connections. Despite our tendency to admonish children for daydreaming, it is a useful state that is full of potential for generating ideas and the mental 'raw material' that can be consciously worked on subsequently.

Guided visualisation

This state feels similar to daydreaming or reverie, although our thoughts are being guided in a very general way by an outside stimulus. A basic guided visualisation activity is to

- relax your group into a daydream...

- mention a single word every thirty seconds for, say, five minutes...

- have the group write down their train of thought and any cohesive ideas produced

This is a bit like supplying some of the dots in a join-the-dots puzzle. The mind puts in more dots and joins them to make the input meaningful.

Scripted visualisation

In this state the attention is caught and led in detail through a richly woven scenario. Defined like this, music, novels, art all count as 'scripted visualisations'. This is not to say that the meanings enfolded in a scripted visualisation are prescribed to the nth degree. Any good music, art or literature is multi-layered and able to sustain a variety of interpretations (individual meaning-makings) supported and informed by the artist's own intentions.

Actually, while our conscious point-of-attention is drawn through the piece, we are working too at a deeper level, connecting up what we are hearing, seeing, thinking to the vast mental Internet that is our subconscious mind. This is why a story, poem, picture or whatever can have a powerful emotional impact on us, even though at the time we can't say exactly why.

Refer to the Bibliography for further reading on visualisation.

Ten Questions

This activity combines the best of guided and scripted visualisations, insofar as the questions themselves are precise but the scenarios and interpretations they evoke are widely variable. You can make up as many sets of questions as you like for different purposes.

TIP The activity works best over a short time span – any more than around ten questions leads to 'concentration fatigue'. You may need to use break states and Brain Gym exercises during *Ten Questions* anyway, to refresh children's attention.

A sample list of questions is offered below. Note how they allow children to operate in all major sensory modalities, and tend to move from smaller to grander responses. Explain to children that you'll leave no more than a minute between questions. Responses can be single words, phrases, sentences and/or drawings. Encourage children to express what comes into their minds without trying very hard. Explain that if nothing at all comes to mind, that's OK: they're not being pressured into answering.

1) You are standing on a shingly beach, listening to the sea splashing up and drawing back down through the pebbles. What sounds do you hear?

2) You are tempted to paddle in the refreshing water. You take off your shoes and socks and walk barefoot towards the water. What does it feel like walking over the shingle?

3) After your paddle, you return to your car. You (or another) try to start the engine, but it won't start straight away. The inside of the car fills with the smell of petrol vapour. Without mentioning whether or not you like it, describe the smell of those petrol fumes.

4) You wind down the windows and wait a few minutes before trying the engine again. As you wait, it begins to rain very heavily. You sit listening to the sound of that heavy steady rain on the roof of your car. Without using obvious words like 'pitter-patter' or 'splish-splash', describe what you hear.

5) You start the car and drive away. Just before you round a bend and the beach disappears from sight you notice something very interesting – right now! Describe what it is.

6) What memory comes to mind right now? Make a note.

7) Describe your own face in a few words. What are the exact colours of your eyes?

8) You meet an alien on the way home from school. He is so fed up with the human race that he's decided to wipe us out in thirty seconds time. What would you say to him to try and stop him?

9) How are you? Note what comes to mind.

10) Note down some pleasant emotions and an object that reminds you of each.

GROUPING	Whole class initially
TIME	20-30 minutes
EQUIPMENT	Prepared sets of questions
SKILLS DEVELOPED	Multi-sensory visualisation, intuition and insight
AGE	7+

Literacy Link

The *Ten Questions* technique can be used as a primer for storymaking, and as a way of allowing children to become more involved in a shared text. Take a scene from a story and construct sequences of questions which will allow the group to explore the wider context of the scene in their imaginations (bearing in mind that we are not looking for 'right answers').

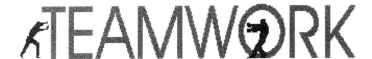

Modelling

Modelling is a kind of visualisation – a powerful kind, where you associate mentally with some other person and/or with aspects of yourself. When we take on different roles and personas in childhood as we play, we are engaging in the modelling process. It is one way in which we rehearse the world, finding out what we are and what we can be by running it through in a 'pretend' way to begin with. Such rehearsal continues to some extent when we identify and empathise with characters in books, films and on TV. In that sense the elaborate embroidery of our complex personalities contains the threads of many other people whom we've encountered, one way or another, throughout our lives.

Of course, we can and do model negative elements of others too. This may result in facets of our selves, in patterns of thinking/feeling/reacting, that we don't like and don't want. It's likely that we won't have consciously and deliberately modelled these behavioural features: they will have arisen in us by default, simply as a consequence of having been so influenced over a period of time. But the fact that these behaviours are in place doesn't mean that they're here to stay. Behaviours are cast in thoughts and experiences, not in stone: they amount to information written on to our map of reality. They give rise to beliefs, attitudes and opinions that can dominate our lives. But a vast range of techniques has evolved to access and modify those that are unwanted, unhelpful or limiting.

The self-intelligence activities throughout this book demonstrate the point. Behaviours that children have modelled by default can be changed. New behaviours, or aspects of a behaviour, can be added to one's own repertoire. Children can

- revisit their younger selves in imagination and 'take back' advice and other resources into the present

- visit their older, more resourceful future selves for the same purpose

- 'make believe' or 'act as if' they can do successfully the things they find difficult

- explore what it would be like to emulate a 'fantastic' (real or imaginary!) role model that they admire

- explore the idea of themselves as role model

- combine elements of these to create powerful new states of thinking, feeling and behaving.

(In this sense, of course, 'make believe' amounts to 'making beliefs'.) Using swift and simple techniques, links between particular situations can be enhanced, added to or erased, so that children no longer need to feel, for example, nervous before a test, or embarrassed and self-conscious in the presence of other people.

Two vital points need to be made here:

1) This kind of work is not 'dabbling', and it is not wishful thinking. Our culture, influenced as it is so much by experts and authority, has led to a suspicion and nervousness about 'delving' into the mind. This is in part a hangover from the Freudian belief that the unconscious (subconscious) mind is a malign pressure-cooker of repressed sexual desires and fears, and that it's all too easy to flip the lid and let the monsters out.

2) The plain fact is that as teachers we are constantly asking children to use their memories and imaginations to help them learn. And also, however implicitly and informally, we are endeavouring to modify children's behaviour according to the standards and expectations that we and society hold.

Beyond this, our aim as educators is surely to allow children to evolve beyond the educational system, by enabling them to become resilient, self-reliant, independent creative thinkers. This aim is much more readily achievable when children are also in touch with their own feelings, and have the capacity to be sensitive to and work with the feelings of others. This is the heart of all self-intelligence work.

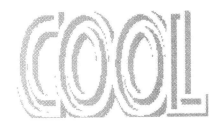

The grand essentials in
life are something to do,
something to love and
something to hope for.

Joseph Addison

Four things do not return:
the spoken word, the
sped arrow, the past
moment, and the
neglected opportunity.

Arabian proverb

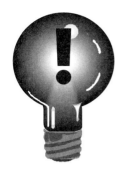

Section Four

ENCOURAGING A CREATIVE ATTITUDE

*O*ne of the very few college books I've kept is Neil Postman and Charles Weingartner's *Teaching as a Subversive Activity*, which is as relevant today as it was over thirty years ago when it was written. Maybe more so now. Some of their chapter headings – *Crap Detecting, The Inquiry Method, Pursuing Relevance, What's Worth Knowing* – are bound to get a reaction from you, of one sort or another.

Postman and Weingartner also deal with the notion of 'meaning-making', which is not just central to any educational system, but a core component of surviving and flourishing in life. We all need to make sense of the world – and this happens anyway at a vast rate, and despite the prepackaged morsels of meaning we offer up to children in the form of a structured curriculum. We all absorb the world, we soak it up! We take in and process (largely nonconsciously) millions of bits of information every second. These we weave together to create our own individual 'maps of reality' - our sum-total understandings of what the world is about, and how we fit in to that bigger picture. Our perception of our environment, behaviour, capability, beliefs, identify and spirituality grows out of the immensely complex network of associations seething in our heads.

Creative thinking and meaning-making are synonymous for me. Thinking creatively means being more in touch with the map of reality and being willing to explore connections to see what results – and in that exploration, to encourage further that process of linking ideas together in new ways.

This is not primarily an intellectual effort, although conscious analytical / judgmental thinking plays its part. And its success depends heavily on the *attitude* one adopts towards the process, and towards the essential function of education (Latin: *educare*, to draw out).

A creative attitude, it seems to me, incorporates curiosity, insight, playfulness, perseverance, independence and therefore self-confidence. These things form the fertile soil from which creative ideas can grow so that the fruits can be picked and utilised.

There is now an extensive literature in this field, and some of the books which have been useful to me are mentioned in the Bibliography.

For our purposes in developing self-intelligence, the activities in the following section focus on the *attitude* one needs to think creatively, which has beneficial effects across the curriculum and beyond.

Personal Coat-of-Arms

This activity is like a full stop at the end of a sentence. It rounds off nicely a programme of self-intelligence work by asking children to think about their own qualities, strengths, abilities and attributes. In short, it invites children to sum up in a positive way their own uniqueness.

Basic activity

● Select examples and a template and explain to the group that they will each be designing an individual coat of arms. (Group designs may come later). This is a good time to refresh the concept of symbols and representations – the notion that colours, shapes, icons and other aspects of design can stand for quite complex ideas. If you have done *Dealing with Feelings* (p.103) and worked on enhancing a positive emotion, the children should be familiar with this.

● Suggest that before work is done 'in best', children should rough out the design of their coat-of-arms, gathering their thoughts about personal qualities and how these should be represented. The outcome need not be drawn as such; a coat-of-arms collage can consist of pictures from magazines, greetings cards, clip art or whatever. Also emphasise that no-one will be required to explain what their design means if they don't want to – the activity Personal Coat-of-Arms means what it says.

● Subsequently group identity can be strengthened by children working together on a class or year-group or whole school design.

GROUPING
Individual initially, then the activity can be run with groups

TIME
30+ minutes

EQUIPMENT
Coat-of-arms template (optional)

SKILLS DEVELOPED
Consolidating positive qualities and sense of self identity, self-review and reappraisal, increasing self-worth

AGE
7+

My imagination   My acting

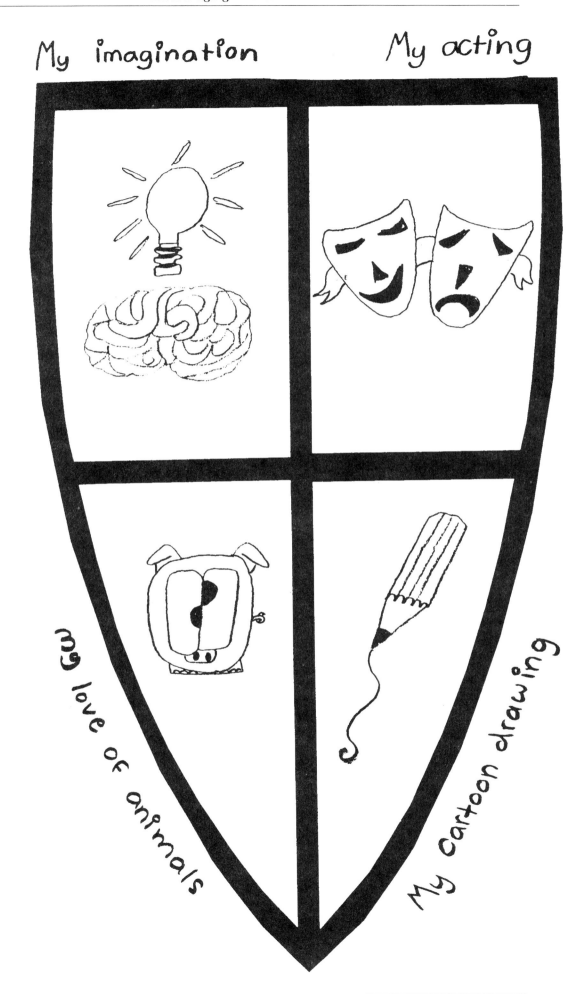

My love of animals   My cartoon drawing

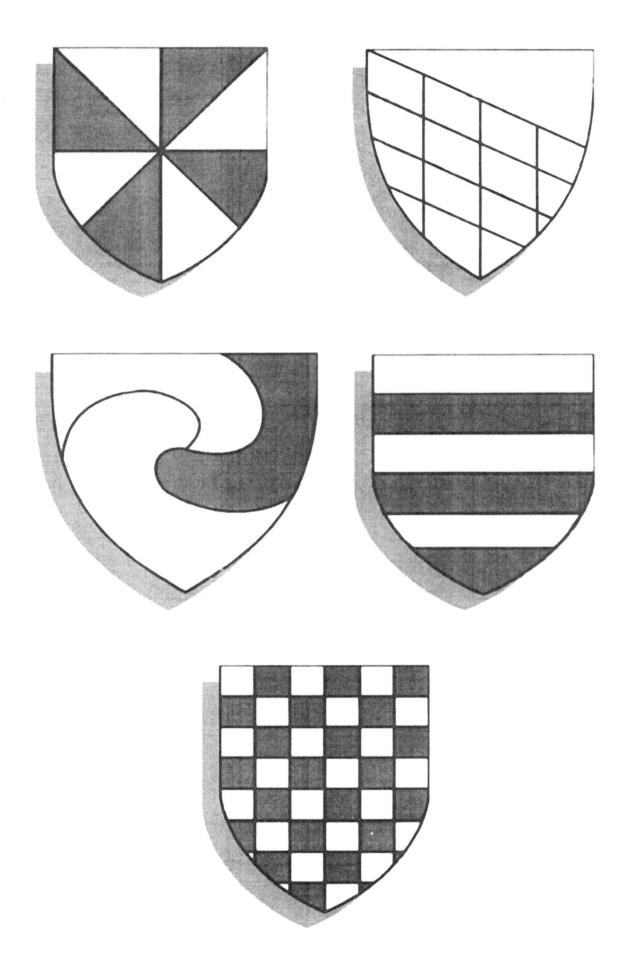

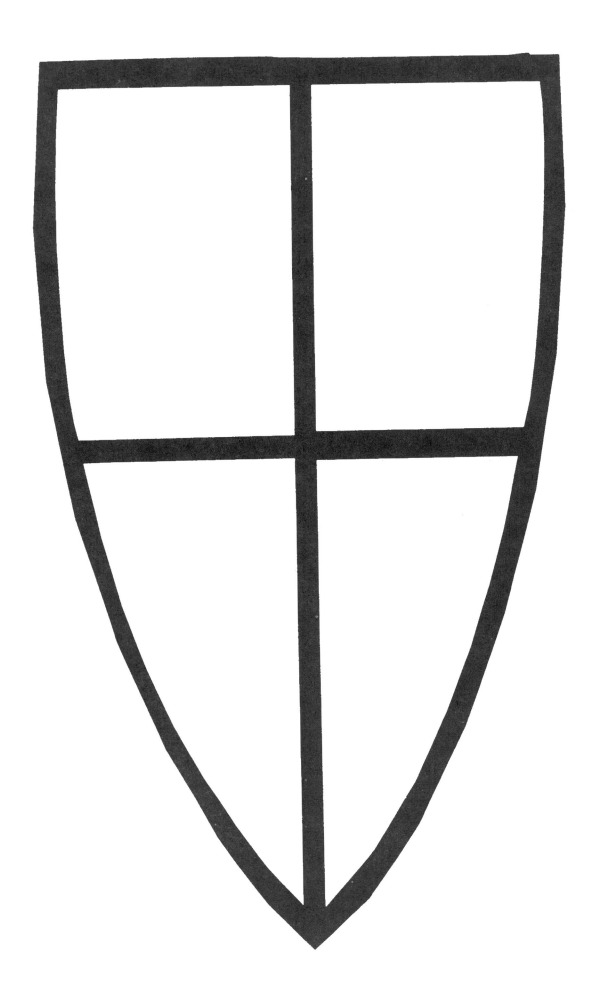

Odd-One-Out

GROUPING	Any group size
TIME	15 minutes
EQUIPMENT	None needed
SKILLS DEVELOPED	Divergent thinking, discussion and negotiation, independent thinking
AGE	7+

We were often given odd-one-out exercises at school as part of our work in English. Lists of words were presented and we would be told to circle the odd-one-out in each case. This resulted in 'reactive thinking'; the assumption that in each list there must be one odd-one-out and to find it was the Right Answer; any other answers, for whatever reasons, were Wrong.

Basic activity

A healthier variation of this activity is to present the class with a list of words:

Split the class up into as many groups as there are words in the list.
Ask each group to brainstorm ideas as to why the word they've been allocated could be the odd-one-out. Suggest that there could be many reasons in each case, and that ideas are not right or wrong, but more or less likely or useful.

Here are some starter lists:

- beech elm oak violet ash apple
- slate gold silver iron lead copper
- tea coffee biscuit cocoa water juice
- river mountain valley glacier road forest
- baker miner barber florist newsagent butcher

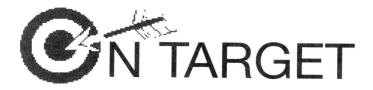

Flashcard and Outpour

This is a variation of classic brainstorming, an activity where ideas are generated and gathered within an environment of mutual respect and encouragement (high challenge, low stress). All ideas are acceptable. Links between ideas are welcomed. No ideas are evaluated at this stage. Information is allowed to flow out from the creative subconscious into a collective 'pot'. This is the raw material that can be worked on further – individually, in pairs, in groups. The activity is useful in story making (see my book *Imagine That...* for more detail and background), and is included here with emotional literacy in mind.

Basic activity

Explain to the group that you will be showing a series of cards. Some will have a picture on, others will have individual words or sentences. Each card will be displayed for only a few seconds. Once the card has been shown, the group has sixty seconds to say anything that comes to mind (within acceptable limits!). Children are encouraged to speak out, or at least to scribble down their thoughts, if these are personal. The cards are not intended to be linked, but if children find links between them that's fine.

It's worth having a tape recorder running since ideas are likely to come thick and fast. Children should also be ready with pen and paper.

Extension activities/variations

This activity is a good warm-up to more extended and elaborate creative thinking exercises. It also allows children to become more at ease with the notion that having 'the right answer' to hand is not the only way learning proceeds. Consider using *Flashcard and Outpour*, then -

- for getting started on stories
- when children get stuck in story making
- to generate ideas for group projects
- to raise and begin to explore issues
- to investigate words that have many shades of meaning
- to explore emotions and issues ('How do I know what I think until I hear what I say?')

GROUPING	Whole class/large group
TIME	5-10 minutes
EQUIPMENT	Prepared flashcards
SKILLS DEVELOPED	Separating the processes of generating and evaluating ideas, stimulating creative thinking, working within a group
AGE	7+

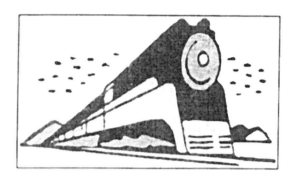

Although they shook hands on the promise they`d made, only Colin was smiling...

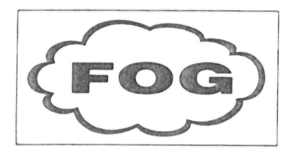

SET

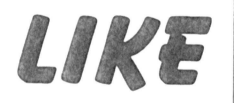

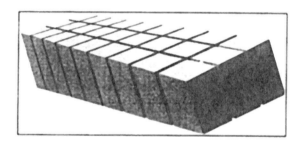

It was a cold and stormy night. Suddenly...

'And Then' Storycards

Because finished narratives are linear structures, children often carry the belief that they must map out their stories in the same way. The rule to remember here is that creation is messy! Ideas around a theme can come in all shapes and sizes and in any order. Even the use of techniques and devices to stimulate creative thinking can result in what I call the 'and then' syndrome. Show children an illustration from a story and ask them what might happen next. Often you'll get 'And then ... and then ... and then ... and then ...' (frequently based on the plot of a current soap opera!).

The storycard technique illustrates literally that stories can be broken down into bits, rearranged, played with and recombined. It helps children to move away from the 'categorical thinking' that narratives begin as linear, logical, predictable structures.

Basic activity

Take a story the children know – a fairy tale would work well – and chunk it down into bite-size pieces. Most stories will break down quite naturally into scenes. If the tale is well illustrated, use the visuals on the storycards, perhaps including some key words also. Use the card set in various ways:

- Shuffle the cards and ask groups to put them in the original sequence.

- Make story variations or new stories using cards in a different order.

- Lay out some of the cards with gaps in between. Ask children to recall and describe the missing parts of the story.

- Combine cards from two or more stories to create new narratives.

- Use storycards with key words (perhaps even those from the national literacy strategy) to explore how they connect.

- Take one story card and have children speculate and describe what might be 'beyond the frame'. Encourage impressions of sounds, smells and textures.

- Combine the above and concentrate on how the characters might be feeling in a given situation. Use this as a focus to review and consolidate other self-intelligence work, or as a springboard to further emotion-related activities.

GROUPING	Whole class/large group initially
TIME	15-20 minutes
EQUIPMENT	Prepared storycards
SKILLS DEVELOPED	Observation and sequencing, manipulation of information, working co-operatively, creative thinking
AGE	7+

Emotion Symbols

GROUPING	Any
TIME	10-15 minutes
EQUIPMENT	Selection of pictures and objects
SKILLS DEVELOPED	Awareness of emotions and the differences between them, ease in talking about emotions, talking at a metaphorical level
AGE	7+

This activity complements others in this book, such as *Hourglass, Dealing With Feelings, Self Marking*, **etc. By comparing feelings with objects and designs, and by being encouraged to speak openly about emotions, children develop an ease of expression which helps them to make distinctions between similar emotions, and to judge the intensity and appropriateness of emotional responses.**

TIP Initially, use *Emotion Symbols* to talk about emotions generally. Later, as necessary, you can use the technique on a one-to-one basis when children have issues to address and resolve.

Refer to the checklist of emotions provided and add to it as necessary. Prepare for the activity by assembling a stock of images and/or objects. Useful categories are:

- animals
- machines
- weather
- natural objects (plants, rocks, other substances)
- occasions and seasons
- household items

Basic activity

Begin by explaining to children that you'll all be selecting a feeling and picking an image or object that represents it in some way. You might choose the feeling, and then help the children reach some kind of agreement about which image suits (or you may choose this also and ask how the image reminds the children of the selected feeling).

For instance, suppose a lion is chosen to represent anger. This could be because both are strong and dominant; they have short bursts of activity followed by periods when they are quiet and dormant, but watchful and ready to pounce. Both are feared and perhaps on occasions respected. Both may express themselves if pride is hurt or threatened.

TIP A variation of the technique is to transform the image / object in imagination to see what effect this has on the emotion it represents. For instance, if you turned the lion into a cub – what emotion would it then become? Working this through as a visualisation can be a powerful way to intervene when emotions seem to be getting the upper hand.

It would also be worth noticing dissimilarities between a chosen emotion and image, in order perhaps to select a more appropriate image.

Match the emotions with the images below and discuss why the pairs are similar...

JEALOUSY

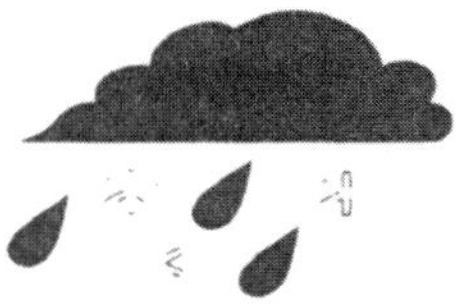

NOSTALGIA

AFFECTION

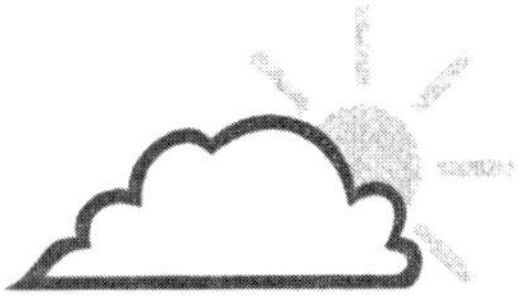

CURIOSITY

WONDERMENT

APPREHENSION

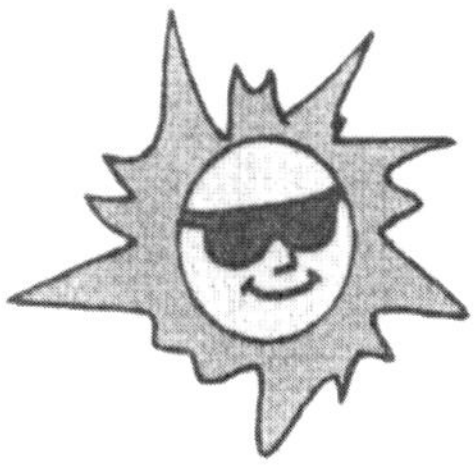

DETERMINATION

DISAPPOINTMENT

HORROR

PRIDE

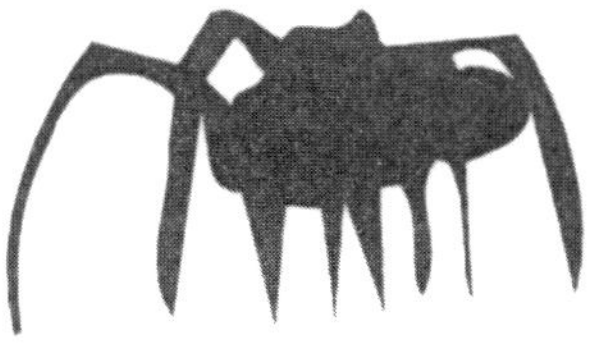

OPTIMISM

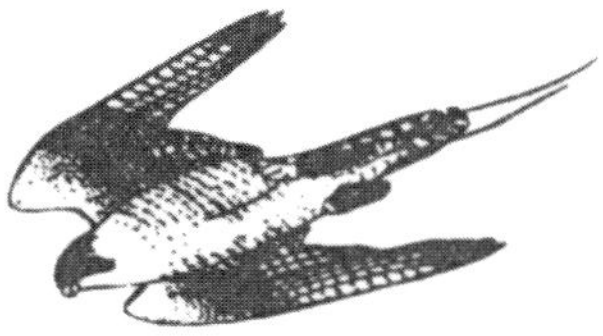

STARTLEMENT

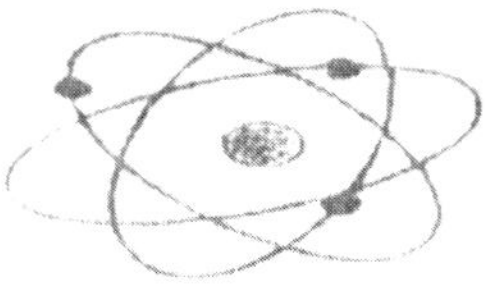

UNEASE

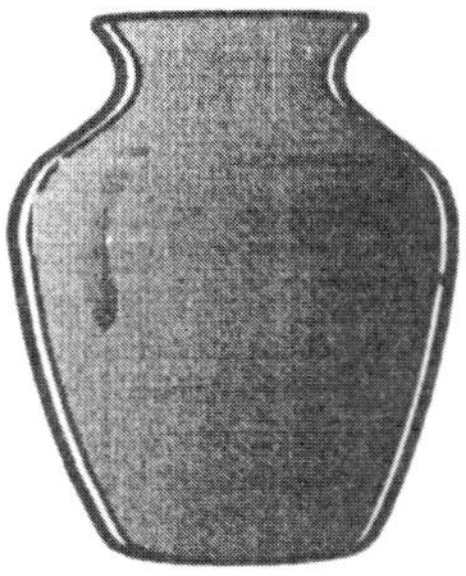

DELIGHT

Emotions/Feelings/Moods Checklist

Purists might wish to separate out emotions from feelings from moods, but for our purposes – because we and our children experience these things – a comprehensive list will do. Refer to *Roget's Thesaurus* **for more ideas, and variations on the emotions included below.**

The term 'emotion', incidentally, derives from the French *emouvoir*, after *mouvoir*, 'motion'. An emotion is a physical / mental state that moves us in some way.

GROUPING Pairs or small groups, then larger groups or whole class for feedback

TIME 10 minutes for activity plus time afterwards for feedback

EQUIPMENT None needed

SKILLS DEVELOPED Observation, visual acuity, discussion

AGE Across the range

acceptance	detachment	hilarity	regret
affection	determination	hope	relief
aggravation	disappointment	hopelessness	remorse
agitation	disapproval	horror	repentant
aloofness	discomfort	hostility	resentment
ambition	discouragement	humiliation	resignation
amusement	disgust	humility	respect
anger	dismay	indifference	responsibility
annoyance	distress	impatience	restlessness
anticipation	dread	impetuosity	revulsion
anxiety	eagerness	impulsiveness	sadness
apathy	ebullience	inadequacy	safety
appreciative	ecstasy	incredulity	satisfaction
apprehension	effusiveness	inferiority	security
assurance	elation	innocence	sentimentality
attraction	embarrassment	inspiration	serenity
awe	empathy	interest	seriousness
awkwardness	empowerment	irascibility	shame
bitterness	enchantment	irritation	shock
bliss	encouragement	jealousy	smugness
boredom	enjoyment	joy	sombreness
camaraderie	enthusiasm	lethargy	sorrow
capability	envy	listlessness	startlement
caution	esteem	loneliness	stubbornness
chagrin	excitement	love	superiority
cheer	exhilaration	melancholy	suspicion
comfort	exuberance	misery	sympathy
compassion	fascination	nervousness	tenacity
composure	fear	nostalgia	tenderness
concern	flippancy	optimism	tension
confidence	fondness	outrage	terror
contempt	forgiveness	passion	thrill
contentment	friendliness	pathos	unease
coolness	frustration	patience	uncertainty
courage	fulfilment	peacefulness	vitality
curiosity	fury	pessimism	warmth
cynicism	gentleness	petulance	wistfulness
dejection	gladness	pity	wonderment
delight	gratification	pleasure	
depression	greed	power	... and so on
desire	grief	powerlessness	
desolation	guilt	pride	
despair	happiness	rage	
despondency	helplessness	reassurance	

Extension activities/variations

Using the list

Apart from the uses explained or implicit throughout the book, you might use the list, or items from it, in the following ways:

- Arrange emotions in terms of how positive/negative, common/rare they are (See 'Emotion Spectrum' in my book *Imagine That...*).

- Make up 'chains' of feelings through discussion of incidents or experiences that can cause one mood or emotion to become another. For instance, waiting in a slow-moving queue might turn tediousness into irritation into frustration into anger.

- Put emotions into 'families': draw overlapping circles and fill them with related emotions.

- Discuss the differences between emotions, feelings and moods.

- Discuss and explore emotion words the children are not familiar with - 'irascibility', for instance, is one they might not have heard of. Increase understanding by using a technique such as *Emotion Symbols*: if anger is a lion, irascibility might be a terrier (find reasons why).

Thought-Bubbles

GROUPING	Whole class initially, then any group size
TIME	20-30 minutes
EQUIPMENT	Visuals such as those illustrated (comic book art, or similar)
SKILLS DEVELOPED	Ability to 'read' emotions based on facial expressions, body postures and contexts; metaphorical thinking in relation to emotional states.
AGE	7+

Emotional literacy means, first and foremost, recognising and being able to deal capably with emotions in ourselves and others. Emotional states arise or are created or 'reconfirmed' through situations we experience. Exploring such situations and the broader contexts in which emotions play a part helps develop our self-intelligence quotient.

The activity relies upon artwork panels from comics, storybooks or graphic novels.

Basic activity

● Blank out the text in the speech-bubble (as in Fig. 1) and invite children to speculate on the words being spoken or thought. Focus attention on what seems to be happening. Ask the group to notice the facial expressions of the characters and their physical postures. Discuss what the characters might be feeling at this point.

● Begin with a single panel, as this creates a large frame for speculation and creative ideas. Move on to sequenced panels (Fig. 2) and talk about how the characters' emotions might change as the situation unfolds.

● Vary the activity by placing icons and symbols in the thought/speech boxes. Use these as springboards to discuss possible text and emotional content of the scene (Fig 3).

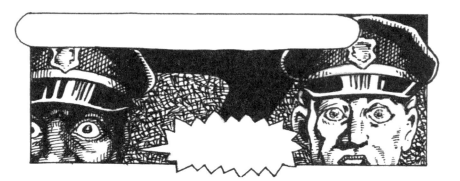

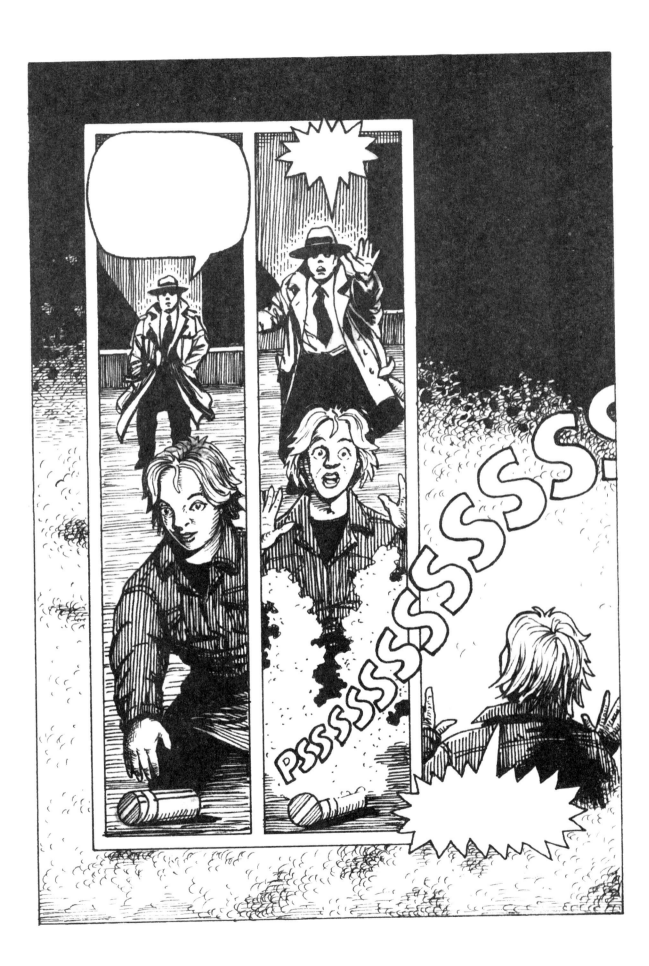

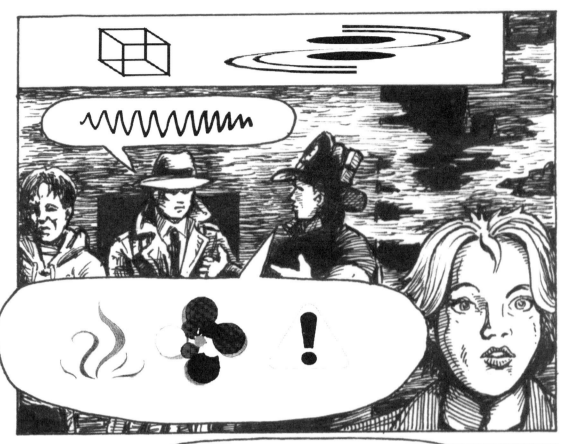
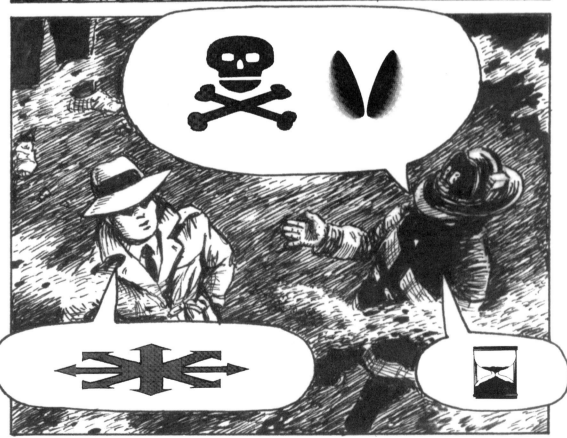

Waterworld

Waterworld can be used simply and primarily as a stimulus for creative thinking and subsequent writing / drama. (See *What If* and *Parallel World* in *Imagine That...* for related writing activities.) For our purposes here the focus would be on exploring and understanding scenarios and emotional responses resulting from them.

Basic activity

Imagine, for example, a series of Earthlike worlds, populated by humans. So we might have:

- **Waterworld** where land is scarce
- **Low Gravity World** where objects have a tendency to drift upwards
- **Nightworld** where the sun shines briefly once a year
- **Fog World** where visibility is limited and wireless communications and long distance travel are impossible
- **No-Memory World** where people recall only what has happened that day
- **Truthworld** where lies don't exist
- **Heart-On-Your-Sleeve World** where people's facial expressions inevitably and truthfully betray what they're thinking
- **Shrinkworld** where children grow until they become adults, then shrink to one inch tall
- **Telepathy World** where everyone's mind is an open book
- **Question World** where learning can only take place by asking questions, and never by being simply offered facts

I'm sure you can think of many other ideas. Repeating the activity allows children to become easy and familiar with discussing imaginary and sometimes quite fantastical scenarios. It also allows you to approach important issues and explore their emotional contexts, since you'll appreciate you can use the various worlds allegorically – as Jonathan Swift did in *Gulliver's Travels* and H. G. Wells in *The Time Machine*.

Begin by choosing your world and gathering ideas about what it would be like there in terms of landscape and climate. Lead the discussion towards what the people there would be like; what difficulties would they face; what emotions would they experience; how would their lives differ from ours, and so on.

Extension activities/variations

Follow-up work might include stories, plays, improvised drama or art. Use other self-intelligence techniques (*POV Spectacles, Other People's Shoes, Stepping Stars*) to have children step into their imagined scenarios.

GROUPING	Whole class discussion, subsequent smaller group or individual work
TIME	15-20 minutes initial discussion
EQUIPMENT	None needed
SKILLS DEVELOPED	Discussion skills, ease in adopting different perspectives, understanding of emotions-in-context.
AGE	7+

New World

This is a variation of *Waterworld.*

Ask children to imagine that ... they can start the world from scratch, leaving out, putting in and changing anything they desire. You might wish to work with the whole class on some basic parameters first:

● Would gravity be different, and if so, how?
● Would water have the same properties?
● Would chemical reactions be different?
● Would the rules that define things as 'alive' be the same?

It might be appropriate to invite smaller groups to work on different aspects of the New World. And so, you might have a 'raw materials group' a 'plants and animals group', a 'human beings group', and so on. In each case, ask them to consider:

● What would you keep?
● What would you leave out?
● What would you change?
● What would be completely new?

The work can be as detailed and extensive as you wish. Feedback would include exploring the children's sense of values behind the decisions they'd made, and discussion of the new creations, inventions and innovations they'd considered.

NOTE
The pool of ideas generated by *New World* forms a valuable resource for subsequent story making.

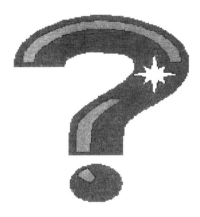

Context Sentences

Basic activity

Jones lay slumped on the sofa.

The use of context sentences encourages group participation and questioning, and is an easy yet effective way of beginning storymaking. The very point of this activity is that it begins with sentences which are out of context, and therefore beg many questions in order to put them into a frame:

- Who or what is Jones?
- How did he or she come to be slumped on the sofa?
- Where is the sofa?
- Under what circumstances or in what condition is Jones 'slumped'?
- What happened to bring Jones to this point?
- What might happen next?

Extension activities/variations

- In developing self-intelligence, link the activity with chosen emotions. So, for example, let's suppose Jones was slumped on the sofa through disappointment: what scenarios might emerge? Now let's suppose (s)he is apathetic/helpless/awed/lonely. You might consider giving groups the same context sentence but different emotional links, then having a feedback session to compare scenarios.

- A further variation is to have children 'step in' to a scenario and explore from the inside how they/the characters would feel.

- You can gather a fund of context sentences by combing through stories. Here're a few to start you off...

  They shook hands on the promise they'd made, though only Jay was smiling.

  By the time they found him, it was far too late.

  That one tiny detail made today different from all other days.

  She closed the lid and realised there was no going back.

  In the fading light he saw only the tip of its tail as it vanished.

  Those few words made them feel like they'd never felt before.

GROUPING	Any
TIME	15-20 minutes
EQUIPMENT	None needed
SKILLS DEVELOPED	Questioning, deduction, inference and speculation
AGE	7+

Ideas Box

In many companies employees are encouraged to come up with ideas for improving the efficiency of the organisation or its products. All ideas are welcomed, valued and considered. The best ideas are implemented and the originator rewarded.

I am in no way suggesting that schools should or could be considered as businesses, nor children as consumers (for as Postman and Weingartner maintain, knowledge is a quest, not a commodity). On the other hand, creative ideas and innovations are to be encouraged (aren't they?). An Ideas Box allows children to express their thoughts while maintaining anonymity if they wish.

A mechanism I found works well is an Official Ideas Slip. These slips are numbered and made available from a central point. When a child collects one, the number of the slip is checked off against his name. This will allow him to be rewarded if the idea is viable, or spoken to if the suggestion is inappropriate.

The Ideas Box might be a receptacle for any suggestions relating to school life, and may be whole-school or just classroom based. Alternatively, specific 'challenges' might be issued. A challenge board beside the box could be regularly updated... How can we improve the efficiency of the dinner-sitting system? How can we best keep parents in touch and up-to-date with the life of the school? How can we make best use of the open area next to the Science Block?...

Naturally it needs to be made clear from the outset that the Ideas Box is not there for people to whinge or criticise or insult. Nor should it be a token gesture. Rather, it represents an ethos which celebrates creative thinking, equality, individual contribution and co-operation throughout the school.

Flicker Book

Flicker books were all the rage when I was a boy. Making one was the first thing we did when the new rough books were given out at the start of term. If you've never heard of flicker books (in which case your education is not complete):

Basic activity

Use the bottom right-hand corner of the pages in a notebook, and begin at the back. The aim is to draw a short action sequence frame by frame, altering each frame slightly. When you flick through afterwards, the figures and objects appear to move.

My favourite sequence was a stick-man who walked along the high-diving board, prepared himself, and then jumped. As he dropped towards the water, someone pulled the plug in the pool and the level quickly fell. By the time he reached the bottom, the pool was completely drained. Splat.

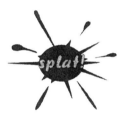

Extension activities/variations

Less frivolous uses for flicker books might be for learning

- spelling rules
- word lists
- sentence construction
- scientific principles (orbits, eclipses, the moon's phases come immediately to mind)
- changing facial expression and body posture

When flicker books are used, say, for word lists, then obviously there is no sequence of movement when the pages are flicked. But what does happen is that the eye registers the fleetingly glimpsed words and the information is absorbed nonconsciously, without conscious intellectual effort.

NOTE
The phenomenon of nonconscious learning and the educational uses of subliminal information (information which enters the mind below the threshold of conscious awareness) is an important one. See Alistair Smith's book *Accelerated Learning In Practice* for more detail.

The benefits of having children make flicker books are twofold. They are exposed to the information when they flick the pages, but they will also have concentrated and worked hard to construct the book in the first place. It goes without saying that most children can't resist the temptation of flicking through their books many times during their construction!

GROUPING Individual work

TIME A series of 10-15 minute slots

EQUIPMENT Notebooks

SKILLS DEVELOPED Reviewing information, concentration, nonconscious learning

AGE 7+

Concentric Circles

This device is useful for 'unfolding' the ingredients of a story: for deconstruction and analysis during shared text work. Beyond that, and in terms of developing children's emotional resourcefulness, once they have become familiar with patterns and themes in narratives, you can move on to the analogy of 'the life story'. Life too is a kind of narrative, with characters and events, sub-plots, 'chapters', sequences, motifs, patterns and themes.

NOTE The life story analogy is especially applicable when used with other techniques such as *Future Diary* (p.136) and *Letters To Myself* (p.129).

Basic activity

Select a story that the children know. Draw a series of four (or more, if you feel that's necessary) large concentric circles on the whiteboard. Explain that small 'bits' of the story will be listed in the middle, while larger ideas will fit into the outer circles.

The actual function of the circles will vary depending on the story you're studying. One suggested pattern might be:

1) plot and character details
2) scenes and sequences of action
3) motifs (regular features within that genre or category of story)
4) broad themes (which you'd find repeated through many stories)

The worked example shown will hopefully clarify the idea.

Extension activities/variations

There are, as I've suggested, many benefits in using *Concentric Circles* with fictional stories as a precursor to looking at real lives. The same procedure applies. Draw four (or more) circles and, using either your own / the children's real experiences or a character from fiction, work outwards, moving from the minutiae of life to large-scale structure. So:

1) day-to-day events
2) regular or repeated events, patterns, motifs
3) the 'ages of man', stereotyped ideas arising from that notion
4) major life themes

Sidebar

GROUPING
Whole class / large group

TIME
30 minutes

EQUIPMENT
None needed

SKILLS DEVELOPED
Brainstorming and review, understanding of the concept of themes and patterns (in stories and in real life)

AGE
Top primary

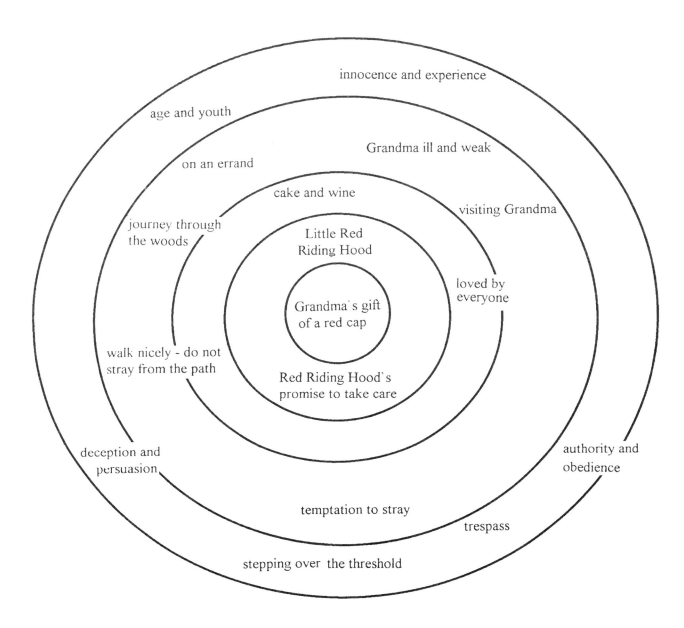

innocence and experience

age and youth

Grandma ill and weak

on an errand

cake and wine

visiting Grandma

journey through
the woods

Little Red
Riding Hood

loved by
everyone

Grandma`s gift
of a red cap

walk nicely - do not
stray from the path

Red Riding Hood`s
promise to take care

deception and
persuasion

authority and
obedience

temptation to stray

trespass

stepping over the threshold

Memo Mime

GROUPING Whole class

TIME 15-20 minute sessions (+ preparatory work)

EQUIPMENT None needed

SKILLS DEVELOPED Recollection and review of information, preprocessing & anticipation, co-operative development of ideas, social skills

AGE 7+

An end-of-term treat for my class would be to play charades. Children took it in turns to mime an occupation, animal, machine, or whatever, and the rest of us would try to guess what it was. The same 'game' can be played to review and revise information and link ideas together creatively. The aim here is not so much just to guess what the answer is, as to explore ideas in more depth and detail, and to review course content in another way, a way that's very different from conventional revision.

An added benefit of *Memo Mime* is that children gain a powerful kinaesthetic element to their learning and revising: they literally embody the knowledge.

Some preparatory work might need to be done if the mime is an elaborate one.

Basic activity

Mimes can be individual efforts or any combination of groups.

Let's say a group wanted to mime the formation of the Solar System and its current structure. Over a dozen children would be needed; one for the sun, one for each of the nine known planets, one or two representing other features, such as comets or major moons, and perhaps one child guiding the mime and adding details and refinements.

In this example, you might like to work beforehand with the group to help them prepare. Watching astronomical videos, studying books, discussing ideas, and rehearsal of the mime would all be necessary before presenting it to the class.

The mime might be performed once for the other children to 'guess the answer'. Then run it a couple of times more to point out further details, introduce new ideas and information, and ask questions.

 Videotaping the session creates a resource for use with other groups.

Theme Cards

Themes run through stories and through our own lives. Sometimes we are attracted to a certain kind of story or character because, at whatever level, we identify something in them that is also a part of ourselves. I empathise with shy, unsure and unconfident characters – especially children – because that's how I used to be, and there's some part of me still feeling like that. And I love science fiction because it opens up new worlds and possibilities; it sprays out ideas; it anticipates, and in so doing, gives me time to consider alternative strategies and outcomes.

Theme cards work well with adults and (perhaps in a less sophisticated form) with children.

Basic activity

When working with children, approach the idea by asking them what's important in their lives, or the kinds of things they keep thinking about, or the kinds of feelings they often have. Responses may focus on negative aspects. This is acceptable if the child is already resourceful enough to deal with these issues; otherwise, concentrate on the positive elements of the child's life.

Using this 'raw material' you can make up a theme card. It may include pictures, symbols, sayings, insights, whatever. Occasional review keeps the theme in mind (i.e., directs the subconscious to actualise the theme) and leads to further understandings.

See also *Resource Cards* (p.78) and a variation on *Theme Cards in Imagine That...*

GROUPING	Pairs or small groups, then larger groups or whole class for feedback
TIME	10 minutes for activity plus time afterwards for feedback
EQUIPMENT	File cards
SKILLS DEVELOPED	Observation, visual acuity, discussion
AGE	Across the range

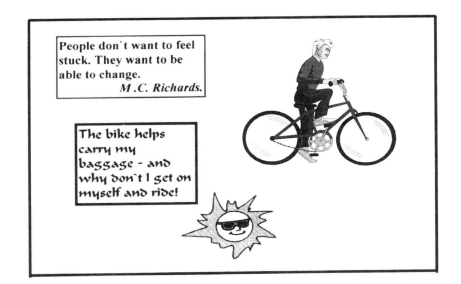

People don`t want to feel stuck. They want to be able to change.
M .C. Richards.

The bike helps carry my baggage - and why don`t I get on myself and ride!

Many Endings

This is a technique that can be used in a range of contexts: to challenge linear or limited thinking or passively held beliefs; as a goal-setting device; and as a story-mapping game.

It's easy for any of us to 'buy into' patterns of thinking which often harden into limiting beliefs. If you find yourself confronted, for example, with an 'I can't' barrier (in a child or yourself!) respond by saying 'I can't, because...' - put an ending on it.

Basic activity

You're not asking for any soul-searching here, or for an analytical assessment of the issue. Encourage the child simply to come up with an idea, which can be evaluated later. Keep up a gentle encouragement for the child to generate a number of endings to the sentence. So:

> *Child:* I can't, because it's too hard.
>
> *Teacher:* OK, now put another ending on it. I can't, because -
>
> *Child:* I can't, because I don't understand what to do.
>
> *Teacher:* All right. Now put another ending on it – I can't, because -
>
> *Child:* I can't, because I'm scared of getting it wrong.

And so on. This is a powerful way of allowing people to identify and admit areas of difficulty. If you're working with yourself, you have to be prepared to 'let stuff out' and have the sense of responsibility (response-ability) to act on your intuitions. If you're working with someone else, observe her reactions closely. If she begins to get distressed, terminate the work or switch seamlessly to another technique.

Alternative activities/ variations

Many Endings work can be combined with other procedures such as *Positive Reframe* (p.95) and *Stepping Stars* (p.138).

If you're working in the context of story-making, *Many Endings* is a useful way of overcoming 'stuckness'. At a sentence level, if a child can't think of what to write next, talk it through for a couple of minutes:

> *Teacher:* Right, so your characters arrive at the edge of the forest. And then they... put an ending on it. And then they...
>
> *Child:* And then they walk into the forest.
>
> *Teacher:* Good. Now put another ending on it. They arrive at the edge of the forest, and then they...
>
> *Child:* And then they have an argument.
>
> *Teacher:* Another ending...
>
> *Child:* They arrive at the edge of the forest and then they split up to explore...

GROUPING	One-to-one, teacher and pupil
TIME	Open-ended
EQUIPMENT	None needed
SKILLS DEVELOPED	'Ongoing' self-intelligence strategy
AGE	7+

You can incorporate these ideas into a 'Story Tree', where each branch represents a further possibility for developing the narrative. The same tree template can be used with *Many Endings* as a goal-setting device (see also *Stepping Stars*, p.138):

I will improve my creative writing by sitting down regularly to do it.

Put another ending on it – I will improve my creative writing by ...

I will improve my creative writing by editing after I've written

... and so on.

Incorporate your thinking into a tree template. This allows you to see at a glance all of the possibilities for improvement or change, and invites you to explore particular ideas in more detail along finer branches...

After I've written I will review and edit my work.

Put another ending on it -

After I've written I will edit for no more than ten minutes.

Put another ending on it -

After I've written I will detach from thinking editorially and just let other ideas come to me...

This process, like many others in the book, highlights the important principles that

● We are all more resourceful than we may realise at first.

● We find out by looking in.

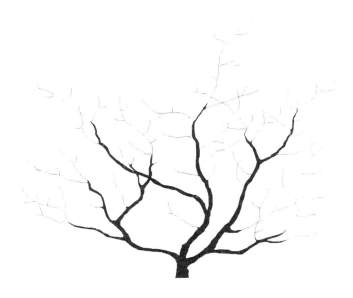

Parallel Path

This visualisation / brainstorming technique combines elements of *What If, Positive Intentions* and *Many Endings*, insofar as it encourages exploration of 'what might have been' with a view to discovering 'what could be'.

We all experience (and maybe suffer from) the 'if only' syndrome from time to time, wondering what life might have been like if we'd made different decisions at the time. *Parallel Path* allows us to 'daydream systematically' in this way and encourages us to use what we find out from and about ourselves more beneficially.

Basic activity

Begin with a life-decision you once made and map out where it's led you.
So: After college I decided to enter teaching in this country instead of travelling abroad.

Set out what seems to be the logical progression of events, like a flagged path. (Read upwards, from the bottom of the page.)

	Writing career grows slowly but surely
Left teaching to do more writing	
	Reached mid-career, time for a review!
Felt a sense of 'staleness and stuckness'	
	Wife's career kept us in one location
Sense of being settled and safe	
	Wife's business established
Realisation that I have not pursued the career path	
	Wife starts small business
Initial writing successes	
	Start of career for wife and self
Marriage and mortgage	

START

Side panel

GROUPING
One-to-one, teacher and pupil

TIME
Open-ended

EQUIPMENT
None needed

SKILLS DEVELOPED
'Ongoing' self-intelligence strategy

AGE
7+

Draw a parallel path based on how life might have progressed had you decided otherwise. So in my case, if I'd gone abroad and done VSO or similar...

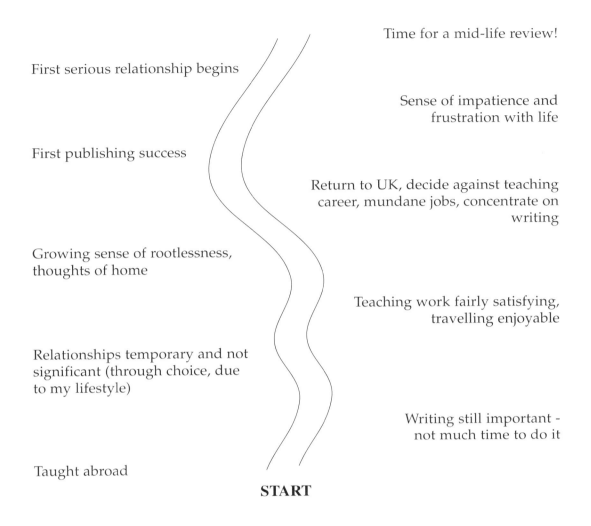

Time for a mid-life review!

First serious relationship begins

Sense of impatience and frustration with life

First publishing success

Return to UK, decide against teaching career, mundane jobs, concentrate on writing

Growing sense of rootlessness, thoughts of home

Teaching work fairly satisfying, travelling enjoyable

Relationships temporary and not significant (through choice, due to my lifestyle)

Writing still important - not much time to do it

Taught abroad

START

The value of this exercise is not to indulge in wishful thinking or pick over missed opportunities, but rather to examine in some detail your emotional response as you review the way your life has progressed and the way it might have done if you'd made other choices. Ask yourself:

● What emotions do I experience as I review my life as it has been?
● What emotions do I experience as I review how my life might have progressed?
● What are these emotions telling me/what are the positive intentions behind these emotions?
● What are the best uses to which I can put these emotions now?
● What are the aspects of my actual life path that I'm happiest to keep?
● What are the aspects of my hypothetical life path that I would like to have as a resource?
● What do I need to know/do in order to have the most useful aspects of both life paths as resources to use in the future?

NOTE *Parallel Path* is a fairly high-level activity, which is to say it works most usefully when you or the people you're working with are familiar and experienced in noticing their own emotions and the intuitions that accompany them.

I emphasise that the primary aim of the activity is not to generate a sense of regret (although if it does – what is the best use you can make of that emotion?) but to assemble resources – ideas, insights, drives – that will enhance your life as you are living it.

Alternative activities/variations

Combine *Parallel Path* with other self-intelligence techniques as appropriate. On the following pages are few you may find effective.

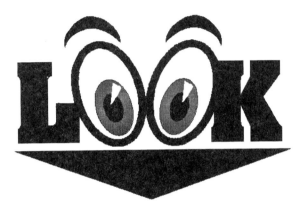

Think Radical!

When I was a young boy, usually at Saturday tea-time after the football results, Mum, Dad, my brother and I would talk about what we'd do if we won the pools. Together we conjured up wonderful scenarios, all of which took us away from the little terrace house where we lived in South Wales.

These flights of fancy were just that: houses of cards. Wishful thinking per se serves no useful purpose except that of escapism. I think of it as desiring-without-action. It's like sitting in a car and wishing it would start, without making any effort to turn the ignition key. Quite futile.

But prior to action comes thought. In order to realise my desired state I need to reflect in some detail on how to get there. Before I do that, it might prove useful for me to map out exactly what my desired state is, and what my present state is, in order to have a more informed idea of what is realistically possible.

Think Radical! is a technique that invites you to do just that. How do you know what's possible until you have defined the limits (and then maybe modified those limits) and looked beyond them?

The principle of the activity is to allow yourself the wildest and most outrageous ideas of what you can do and where you can go in your life. This is the stage where you generate the raw material on which you will work. Set no limits. If you could be whatever you wanted to be and do whatever you wanted to do, what would you be and do?

Brainstorm and enjoy it! Then set to work...

- What pleasant emotions do I experience as I think radically?
- What unpleasant emotions do I experience as I think radically?
- How can I make best use of these feelings to help guide me towards my desired state?
- How do I rate the chances of any particular scenario unfolding (on, say, a scale of 1-10, where one is inevitable and ten is highly unlikely)?
- What leads me to give these ratings to the scenarios I've considered? (At this stage you're chunking down to the components of the beliefs you carry, and may experience some startling insights.)
- At this point in my learning, what do I think is realistically possible, given my perceived strengths and limitations?
- How would the route to my desired state alter if I looked at the whole thing from a different perspective? (And you know some techniques for doing this!)
- Having worked on the issue thus far, how would I now rate the chances of the scenarios I've considered unfolding?

> **NOTE** If, by chance, you are sceptical about radical thinking, consider what purposes that scepticism serves for you. Then read some of Anthony Robbins' work such as *Awaken The Giant Within* or *Giant Steps*, both of which deliver a powerful inspirational kick.

Only by defining our limits can we anticipate going beyond them. I'm reminded of two instances pertinent to this idea.

I meet a writer friend of mine whenever I'm in London. We drink some beer, grumble about editors, talk about our ongoing projects and possible future books. I knew that my friend enjoyed reading crime fiction, and on this particular occasion he kept bringing the subject up. So I said, 'Dennis, why don't you write a crime novel then?' His reply was, ' Well my agent feels I'm too old now to begin carving a reputation in that field.' It hardly needs me to point out the limiting influence of this agent's opinion!

On another occasion I was running a stress management workshop with a group of professionals. I pointed out that stress is an inner response to external pressures. At this, several of the participants began growing angry at my suggestion that they were responsible for their own stress feelings. I told them that if they believed they were stressed because of outside forces that were beyond their control, then they were buying into the 'passive victim' scenario of stress. On the other hand, if they were willing to take responsibility for their own stress, they were in a much more powerful position, since that awareness would lead to greater understanding, which would lead to greater control. At that point, red faced and furious, one of the group blurted out, 'Well the only thing that would help my stress is if I got out of this damn job!' This was followed by a brief silence, and then he said, 'And of course I can't do that.'

... A classic 'Yes, but' barrier.

The Maybe Tree

The usefulness of the tree template has already been mentioned. In this context we combine the classic properties of a *Decision Tree* (p.192) with *Radical Thinking*.

Basic activity

Prepare a tree template on a large sheet of paper. At first, of course, you'll need only the trunk and a few stumpy main branches.

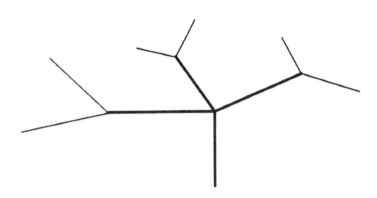

From a few basic premises or a vague sense of direction you can begin to speculate on how to move beyond your present state to various future states (of thinking/feeling/doing) which right now might be more or less well defined. Side branches represent points-of-decision. At this stage in your thinking you may not even know what decisions need to be made, let alone what you need to know in order to best make them. But don't let this stop you from exploring.

Clearly the tree template maps out different routes 'holistically': at a glance, and as you work through the scenarios, you come to see how far you can take certain possibilities for change, what's involved in getting there, what the consequences and outcomes of change might be, and how various routes of change relate to and interact with one another.

Extension activities/variations

A variation of the basic activity is to draw a whole tree: begin at the end of a branch and work backward. (See *Stepping Stars* (p.138), which is a related technique.) In effect, by starting at the end point, what you are saying is, 'OK, I know where I want to be, so how do I get there?'

Note the resemblance between this activity and other tree-template techniques like *Many Endings* (p.182) and *Story Tree* (in *Imagine That...*). In all cases you have the flexibility to speculate within the structure the template provides. In 'growing' a Maybe Tree you are consolidating your thinking on how to achieve change. And when the tree has grown – pick the fruits.

GROUPING	One-to-one, or teacher and small group
TIME	Open-ended
EQUIPMENT	Writing materials cards tree templates (optional)
SKILLS DEVELOPED	'Ongoing' self-intelligence strategy
AGE	Top primary upwards

The Upside-Down Tree

GROUPING	One-to-one, or teacher and small group
TIME	Open-ended
EQUIPMENT	Writing and drawing materials, tree templates (optional)
SKILLS DEVELOPED	'Ongoing' self-intelligence strategy
AGE	Top primary upwards

A tree template can also be used in this way to work back to possible starting points. The technique has an obvious application in story-making. Children tend to start thinking about stories at the beginning, but the 'many startings' model encourages more prolific and fruitful thinking.

Basic activity

Use any story-making game (see *Imagine That...*, for instance). Tell children that they will start thinking about their stories half-way through. This means they not only have to explore what might possibly happen, but what might have happened to bring the characters together at this point. By following the process, children will have good ideas by having lots of ideas. They will also gain insights into more logical connections between events in stories, and develop a surer sense of direction in taking the story on.

Upside-Down Tree is also useful in reviewing and understanding issues. Take a situation – a falling out of friends, for example – and make it the point from which you will look back. If the incident is a real one, at the very least the ex-friends will realise what steps they took to reach the stage of falling out (And by looking at other, hypothetical, ways a quarrel could develop, the protagonists might begin to see patterns in their behaviour which led to that outcome.)

If the situation is 'made up', a review of many beginnings will serve to forewarn children. By pointing out in some detail the steps leading to a quarrel, children will be more aware of what's happening as it happens. This reduces the chances of conflicts occurring thoughtlessly by default.

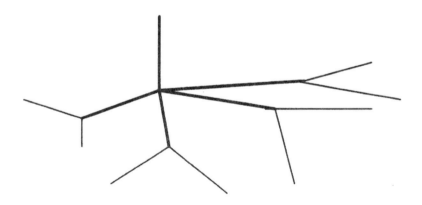

Futurescopes

Throughout history a huge amount of effort has been put into attempting to foretell the future. Whether or not this can be done remains open to question – although millions of people live by their horoscopes. (Luckily I'm not superstitious, touch wood.) What all of us can do, however, is to anticipate possible outcomes and consequences of our current circumstances and decisions, and in so doing prepare ourselves to respond more effectively as and when the time comes. We can also set outcomes for ourselves – aims, targets, goals – and work towards them with a will.

One important feature of the language of horoscopes (and other predictive devices) is its general, all-encompassing nature: 'The last few weeks have seen a balance between the light and the dark in your life, and this trend is likely to continue' can mean anything, and it prompts us to think selectively, to search around and find instances, remembered or imagined, to confirm the truth of the statement. *Futurescopes* exploits this process.

Basic activity

Write out the following generalities on cards. Pick one or two and allow ideas to come to mind about how these statements could be true for you in the future. Don't evaluate the ideas yet, since even seemingly outrageous or absurd notions might have some validity when you've explored them further.

1   Consider your needs and the environment.
2   Partnerships are likely.
3   It's time for a parting or separation.
4   Be sensitive to signals and coincidence.
5   Be strong and determined now.
6   You are about to break into new areas.
7   Things happen to limit you.
8   You move into a fertile environment.
9   Look to your defences.
10   To protect now will prevent difficulty later.
11   Possessions change their significance.
12   Joy is coming soon in new ways.
13   Openings lie ahead.
14   Soon you will reap the harvest of your efforts.
15   Be prepared to work for whatever you want.
16   This is a time of new growth.
17   Move on and see obstacles removed.
18   Don't fight, just go along with circumstances.
19   Everything is about to suffer disturbance.
20   Important messages are imminent.
21   A deliberate change of direction brings benefits.
22   Be patient, you stand on a threshold.
23   Around lies the solution to a problem.
24   Recognise the usefulness of standing still.
25   Look at the whole thing again to see anew.
26   Knowledge comes now from what was unknown.

GROUPING	Any
TIME	Open-ended
EQUIPMENT	Writing and drawing materials, tree templates (optional)
SKILLS DEVELOPED	'Ongoing' self-intelligence strategy
AGE	Top primary upwards

Run the game through a few times, you may be surprised at how much 'raw material' it generates, which you can then sift, evaluate and use.

Extension activities/variations

A variation is to use a *Decision Tree* template. Pick a number of the sayings and position them on your tree. Begin at the base of the trunk with an issue you want to learn more about and resolve, a problem you want to solve, or a goal you have just set for yourself.

Allow your thinking to follow a certain route along the branches, using the 'Futurescopes' as springboards for further ideas and prompts.

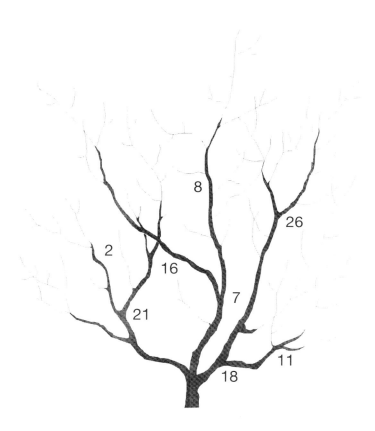

I want to feel greater self-confidence in the personal projects I undertake.

Map It

This is a story-exploration activity. The best fiction draws us in and speaks to us in profound and important ways even about experiences we've never had, or may never have. Conventional review-and-comprehension exercises focus on children's recall of events and other story components, taken in sequence. *Map* It offers a different approach.

Basic activity

On large sheets of paper – or, if you're working with the whole class, on a central display – draw the story as a map. This may be a literal geography, such as the maps you find of Middle Earth in *The Hobbit*, Pooh's Ten-Acre Wood, or Alderley Edge in Alan Garner's *The Weirdstone of Brisingamen*. In this case the map acts as an effective revision aid, allowing children to recall more easily what happened where, and to whom.

Alternatively, maps can be more symbolic and representative of characters' feelings and/or readers' emotional responses to events. (See also *Landscape Metaphor and Landscape of the Day*, pp.116-7.)

Because the maps are holistic representations, the needs and requirements of children who like to have 'the big picture' are more effectively met. Emotion-symbol maps capitalise on the emotional impact of a good book, and allow children to anchor the experience of the reading in another way.

 Story maps come in useful if you want children to write their own stories using characters and places from set texts.

GROUPING Any

TIME Open-ended

EQUIPMENT Large sheets of paper drawing materials

SKILLS DEVELOPED 'Ongoing' self-intelligence strategy

AGE Top primary upwards

Icons and Symbols

The psychologist Carl Jung maintained that many symbols are archetypal, existing across cultures as part of the collective unconscious of mankind. Personal symbols are also powerful in consolidating and expressing individual emotions and issues.

Visual symbols form the language of the subconscious, which is the fertile soil in which the roots of many of our emotions grow. The inclusion of a symbolic component, overtly or implicitly, in the stories we make and share with children allows them to address and articulate more readily how they feel and what events mean for them.

> **NOTE**
>
> The writer Tom Chetwynd has produced a rich resource in the form of a trilogy of dictionaries – *The Dictionary of Symbols, A Dictionary for Dreamers,* and *A Dictionary of Sacred Myth* (see Bibliography). These form a treasure hoard of symbols and ideas which can be used to introduce children to the notion of using metaphors as part of the language of how they feel.
>
> Once awareness of this basic idea has been raised, myths, legends, fables and fairy tales can be examined in a new light – and new stories can be created which are layered and meaningful.

tree – the leaves, trunk and roots represent conscious awareness and health, the strength and rising energy, the deeper wisdom and connectedness of an individual

trickster – that part of us which mischievously (though with positive intentions!) sets out to cause confusion and sometimes conflict inside us

dragon – the life force, the energy and essence of Nature

child – the potential for growth; energy and spontaneity; the part that childhood continues to play in adult life

hand – the whole of an individual in miniature, so that the state of the hand represents that person's overall state and life-map

fox – animal, or basic and deep-seated, intuition

clouds – forces of nature, bringing life after drought

pearl – the incorruptible product of one's life's work

flags – symbols of union

sword – the blade of rational thought which discriminates and separates and judges

dance – the patterns of energy bringing order out of confusion

monkey – a potential source of renewal through basic instincts and understandings

These are general symbols, according to Chetwynd. Individual symbols work just as well. Make up some other symbols that have a more personal meaning, or a consensus meaning across the class. Draw your symbols on pieces of card and create a story using a story map. (See also *Dice Journey* in *Imagine That...*). Enjoy the storymaking, and discuss with the children afterwards what they've learnt.

Fairy Telling

This is an extension of mapping techniques, using icons and symbols. Fairy tales have always been powerful vehicles for conveying important learnings – warnings, reminders, protections, preventions. Consider using fairy tales from this perspective, having first thought out the metaphorical significance of the stories' themes, motifs, characters, settings and events (in terms of either universal or personal symbolism).

For instance, Little Red Riding Hood (known as Little Red-Cap in Grimm's *Complete Fairy Tales*) becomes a deeper and more powerful story when the symbolic dimension is added ...

Little Red-Cap – innocence, defencelessness, wish to please

Grandmother – age, infirmity, helplessness, the primal ancestor

red velvet cap (a gift from Grandmother) - bond of love

cake and wine (for Grandmother) - nourishment, worldly goods

mother (and the errand) - reinforcing female stereotypes, rules and social mores

the woods – the world and its unknowns

the path through the forest - 'the straight and narrow', a life path, the lines that are drawn and not to be crossed

straying from the path – disobedience and its consequences, unfamiliar territory and danger

the flowers Little Red-Cap picks – temptation away from innocence

the wolf – evil, animal instincts, greed, deceit, unrestrained power not open to reason, male sexuality and aggression, the predator

'what big eyes you have', etc. - dawning realisations, worldliness

the huntsman – rightness and justice, vengeance

the wolf's skin (taken by the huntsman) - wildness tamed, just rewards

The extent to which you as a teacher would wish to draw upon the depth and layers of meaning in the old fairy tales depends upon many factors, not least the present cultural tendency to nanny children rather than raise issues so that they can be addressed and dealt with. On a personal level, however, fairy telling is still a powerful tool for learning and self-realisation.

GROUPING — Any

TIME — Open-ended

EQUIPMENT — Books of fairy-tales

SKILLS DEVELOPED — 'Ongoing' self-intelligence strategy

AGE — Top primary upwards

Beyond the Frame

GROUPING	One-to-one, teacher and pupil
TIME	Open-ended
EQUIPMENT	Writing materials; lengths of rope(optional)
SKILLS DEVELOPED	'Ongoing' self-intelligence strategy
AGE	Top primary upwards

Beliefs put a frame around our perception of the world. Those beliefs may be expansive, optimistic and outward-looking. In that case we continually and naturally reframe our world view, learning positively from experience to redefine our limits in empowering ways. On the other hand, limiting beliefs 'freeze the frame' as it were, leading to failures of both imagination and nerve when it comes to looking beyond the way we are and what we think we can achieve. 'Mindsets' are not so called for nothing, since they exist with minimal flexibility and block us from moving on.

Beyond the Frame **is an intervention which addresses this issue, responding to the assertion 'I can't' with 'What would happen if you did?' or 'What stops you?' The latter focuses on the frame itself, the former on what lies outside it.**

The activity can be paper-based, or run in an open space with rope or similar defining the boundaries of the 'frame'.

> **NOTE**
> Be aware that this activity, like others in the field of self-intelligence, can raise other issues, so you need to be prepared to work with those, or know someone who can guide you/your pairworker in the right direction.

Basic activity

● When working with this technique, explain to the individual that you are in no way forcing change, simply exploring possibilities.

● Ask your pairworker to imagine he's in the frame (paper-based) or have him actually stand inside the rope. Ask him to mention some of the beliefs about himself and the world which he feels are currently holding him back. Then focus on the frame itself and notice anything about it which adds to or reconfirms those beliefs.

I'm frightened that people will judge me negatively. Before they do this, I judge myself! ⟶

I keep putting myself down. I can't seem to take pride or draw confidence from anything I achieve. In fact, knowing I'll put myself down stops me from trying new things.
I get frustrated and angry with myself. I tell myself off and say I'm pathetic for being such a wimp – but deep down I know I'm a loser.

I used to get upset when people criticised me. I used to think things were all my fault.

- You and your pairworker will both find it easier to gather insights about the nature of the frame if you are familiar with self-intelligence work. Suggest, then, that you could draw another frame around the first, one that's just a bit bigger. When it's in place, suggest taking the old one away, and notice how things are different.

- Check first that it's OK for you both to do this. If your partner feels any hesitation or unease, ask him to notice what's causing this. He may ask 'How do I do that?' in which case you say, 'In the way that's easiest, most comfortable and most natural for you – or you can just make it up as you go along.'

- Be aware of the wisdom that you shouldn't take someone's crutch away until you've offered them a chair to fall back on. When it's all right to recreate the frame, go ahead and repeat your request for your partner to notice what's changed.

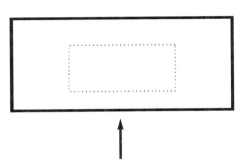

OK, I notice now that I was frightened
of being criticised as a kid, because
some of the adults I knew were just like that.
They criticised most people! That's their
problem. It's all right for me to be
pleased if I do something well. Yes, that
feels more comfortable now...

Of course, insights might not come as fully formed as this. You may get flashes of ideas, vague feelings, bits of memory, stuff that's 'on the tip of your tongue'. If this information can't be rationalised or fully understood at the time, you can either leave the activity and resume later, or do further checks that it's OK to proceed, and then do so.

Greater understanding and feelings of empowerment and confidence are likely to develop as you enlarge the frame in a series of gentle steps. When the frame has reached the optimum size for your pairworker at this time, he'll know and will tell you so.

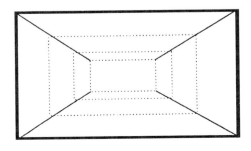

Review Board Game

GROUPING	Small group works well
TIME	Open-ended
EQUIPMENT	Materials for making board game dice question cards (optional)
SKILLS DEVELOPED	'Ongoing' self-intelligence strategy
AGE	Top primary upwards

'Work is Play' is a well-known principle for achieving high standards, and this is exemplified in *Review Board Game.* The activity is to devise a board game that allows players to progress by answering review questions based on a topic previously studied.

Basic activity

● Prepare a board of, say, 8 x 8 squares. Number the squares. The earlier squares represent the easiest questions, increasing in difficulty towards 64. You can incorporate snakes and ladders or any other shortcut devices; this allows children to leapfrog to more challenging questions, or to backtrack to easier ones.

● Prepare around one hundred questions (or, if the topic doesn't support this, use a smaller game board). You can play the game with the whole class divided into groups, or – with multiple sets of questions – different groups can play with a 'questionmaster' allocated to each group.

● Begin by asking a team one of the easier questions. If they get it right, have them roll a dice to move on that number of squares. If they get the question wrong, they must wait their turn as you give each of the other teams the opportunity to start.

● As the game proceeds, the questions become more searching. If a group gives a wrong answer, they must either drop down on to the row of squares beneath (easier questions), or roll the dice to see how many squares they backtrack. If a group lands on the equivalent of a ladder, they can choose whether to shortcut to a higher level, or opt to continue moving conventionally using dice.

You may wish to supply 'clue cards' which groups can refer to if they need to refresh their memories. The aim of the game is to allow the class to review information in a way that is challenging and enjoyable.

Memory Walk

This is a preview/review device.

Basic activity

- To preview course content, select some interesting facts, keywords and questions. Write them out clearly on large pieces of card, including any visuals as appropriate. In a large space such as the assembly hall (or rearranging your classroom as appropriate), place the cards on the floor in the form of a path. Invite children to walk slowly along the path, reading the cards as they go. You might have them do this several times over the course of, say, the week preceding the start of the coursework.

- As children follow the memory path, they may wish to add their own facts, ideas and questions. These are best written up separately for discussion when the time comes, rather than making the path overly rich in detail.

- Reinforce the work by walking with children along the memory path when the cards have been removed. Encourage children to talk about what they've learned in the card sequence: prompt questions and the use of visual keys help stimulate recall.

Extension activities/variations

Memory Path works equally well for revision.

The use of suitable music (See Colin Rose's *Accelerated Learning*) and/or *Stepping Stars* (see p.138) helps to anchor the experience. You can also incorporate side-tables or desks with items pertinent to the learning. Allow children to handle these as they stroll along the path.

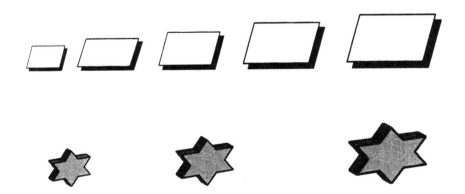

GROUPING	Small groups or pairs
TIME	Open-ended
EQUIPMENT	Large pieces of card (see instructions)
SKILLS DEVELOPED	'Ongoing' self-intelligence strategy
AGE	Top primary upwards

Grid Template

GROUPING	Any
TIME	Open-ended
EQUIPMENT	Prepared cards (see instructions) dice
SKILLS DEVELOPED	'Ongoing' self-intelligence strategy
AGE	7+

Grid templates (see examples reproduced here) are useful devices for generating ideas and organising information. A 6 x 6 grid allows for the use of dice, although the size can be varied depending upon the task to hand and the ability of the group you're working with.

Grid Template variations

For brainstorming, fill up the 36 spaces with random words. Roll a dice twice to select each word. Brainstorm links between the two or more words chosen.

For generating characters in storymaking, pick two parameters and work with the group to fill in the boxes using those parameters.

In Example 1, we chose the genre of fantasy. One parameter was good/evil, while the other was human/less human.

Example 2 focuses on landforms for settings in stories. The parameters are hot/cold and flat/rugged.

Example 3 demonstrates how a grid can be used to 'chunk down' components of a story. Print out the story chunks on cards:

● Shuffle the cards and ask children to put them in the right order.
● Shuffle the cards and have groups put them in different sequences to suggest other plot possibilities.
● Give out some of the cards and ask groups to talk about which chunks are missing.
● Give out some cards and ask children to invent their own chunks to fill the spaces.
● Mix cards from two stories to suggest further story ideas.
● Have children elaborate on the detail of one of the chunks: what was the character feeling at that time? What was the scenery like (sights, sounds, textures, smells)? What choices did the character have just then? What would have happened if (s)he had made a different choice?

Example 4 emphasises emotions. The parameters are pleasant/unpleasant and mild/intense. In this case the fine distinctions between some emotions can be illustrated, while the matrix allows a spread of emotions to be recognised at a glance.

CHARACTER LANDSCAPE IN STORYMAKING

EG – FANTASY GENRE

LESS HUMAN ⟶

INCREASINGLY EVIL

typical hero figure				friendly helpful ice dragon
	hobgoblin friend			
		elvish helper		
	skeleton warriors			
evil step-brother enemy				black force in the mountain

LOCATION PLANNER IN STORYMAKING

HOT / COLD ⟶

FLAT / MOUNTAINOUS

Desert		Meadowland			Flat snowfield
		Rolling hills			
				Craggy northern hills	
Active volcanic mountain					Mountain glaciers

Fill in spare boxes with features you'd find in these areas – waterfalls, lakes, forests, etc.
Illustrate with pictures / examples of real places. Add 'genre-related' features.
Brainstorm features and then fill in grid.

GRID TEMPLATE AS A STORY AID

Red Riding Hood decided to take some cakes to her Grandma...	She was told to take care and not to talk to strangers...
Just then the woodcutter rushed in....	Red Riding Hood arrived at her Grandma's house....

PLEASANT – UNPLEASANT →

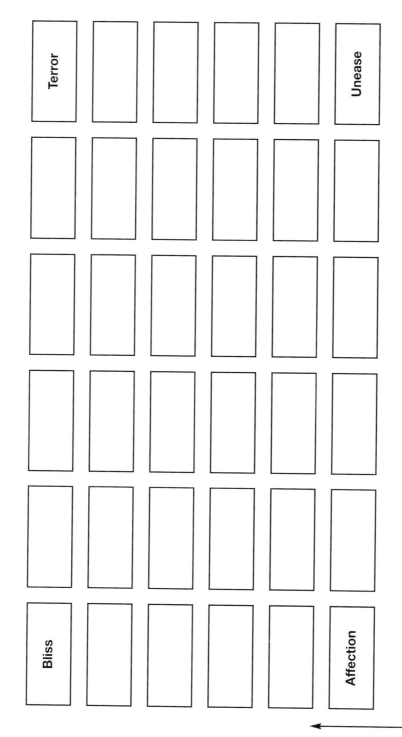

| Terror | | | | | Unease |

| Bliss | | | | | Affection |

MILD – INTENSE

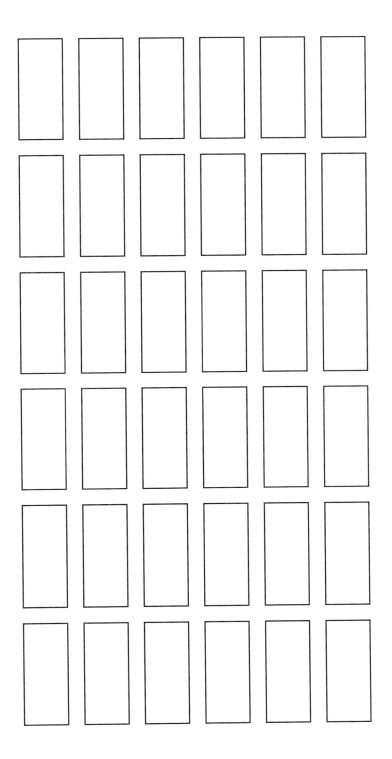

It's not necessary to
understand something
fully in order to
use it effectively

Anon

APPENDIX

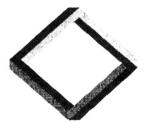

Example visualisation

Whole body deep relaxation

Children will get as much out of this sitting up as lying down, with eyes open or closed. If you or the children prefer their eyes open, have them stare at a blank surface such as the whiteboard, and let their gaze settle and remain on that spot. Allow 15 – 20 minutes. Keep your voice soft and gentle, easily flowing. Read the script smoothly and give yourself plenty of time. At the end when you do the count-out, put more pace and energy into your voice.

Just make yourself comfortable now, with your ankles uncrossed and your fingers unclenched. Settle yourself so that you can sit or lie still and peacefully for the next few minutes

Let your attention settle on your breathing. There's no need to try to breathe in any particular way, just let the breath come into your body and go out again and simply be aware of this happening, without putting any effort into it; without trying to influence it in any way. Just concentrate on the slow flow of your breathing... Let the air come and go, come and go, gently and quietly by itself. And with each breath you take, you will feel yourself becoming more and more relaxed, more deeply relaxed with each and every breath... (Pause.)

And now I want you to imagine that the air coming into your body is glowing softly with white light. Imagine this in your mind's eye... As you breathe in, allowing the air into your body perfectly effortlessly, see this gentle white light streaming down into your lungs and through your body... It is a very soothing white light that fills you with its energy. And this energy can be used to charge up your batteries, so that you will begin to feel more and more refreshed... And it will help you to become more relaxed, soothing away the stresses and strains of the day, allowing you to drift into deeper and deeper states of peacefulness: the white light can also be used to ease away aches and pains in any part of your body... Just imagine the light glowing brighter in any area of hurt, or in a spot where discomfort has gathered. Feel the white light gently soothing away the aches and pains. And it will carry on doing this all the time you are relaxing here, even as your mind wanders away to other things... So just go on imagining the light working through the whole of your body now, flowing in with your breath... So that with each and every breath you take you can become more and more relaxed... And that white light will become clearer and clearer in your mind, so that when I speak to you again you'll be able to imagine it much more clearly... And you will then be much much more relaxed... (Pause.)

And now as you continue to relax and let the air move in and out of your body without any effort at all, become more aware of your breathing out... Just let yourself notice a little more as you breathe out... And as you do this I want you to imagine a blue light streaming out through your nose and mouth as you exhale... Imagine that this blue light, once it has soaked through all of your muscles and bones and tissues, leaves your lungs and streams out of your body, carrying away the aches and pains, the stresses and strains of the day... And the blue light is now carrying them away, away, far away as you relax... And as you relax more and more, so the blue light becomes clearer and clearer in your mind... So that when I talk to you again in a few moments time you'll be much, much more relaxed than you are now... (Pause.)

Now just let your breathing happen effortlessly, easily, naturally... As you imagine that the white light and the blue light do their work, filling you with energy and peacefulness, carrying away the aches and pains and stresses and strains of the day... So that even as your mind wanders to other things the light will do its work as you drift more into relaxation, unconcerned with anything at all that's going on... (Pause.)

And as you drift and settle in this lovely state of relaxation, become aware of your toes... Notice your toes to the very tips of your toes... And you can count every single toe, letting your mind then wander to your feet ... to your heels ... to the soles of your feet ... to the tops of your feet... And as your attention touches them and moves through them, so you feel a very gentle sensation of warmth and peace following on through your toes and soles and heels and ankles as you drift and settle more and more into relaxation... (Pause.)

And move your attention along to your legs now ... moving through the bones and muscles of your lower legs to your knees... Without making any effort at all you can notice your knees, with the warmth and peace flowing and soaking through your knees, relaxing all the little tensions, and relaxing and relaxing ... as you let your mind wander along through the tops of your legs and thighs and around your hips and waist ... And the warmth and peacefulness follow your thoughts like a warm blanket wrapping you round in a delicious sensation of relaxation ... so that it feels as though the whole of your lower body is surrounded by comfort and warmth ... as you feel more and more settled and comfortable and relaxed... (Pause.)

And let your attention drift on now, moving slowly through your stomach and round and along the bottom of your spine... Feel the muscles loosening and relaxing and easing... Feel yourself becoming beautifully warm and peaceful and more and more comfortable... As your mind moves on in an easy and leisurely way round to your ribs and your chest and inside ... feeling the warmth and relaxation spreading through your body ... soothing your muscles and bones and tissues and nerves ... with every part of your stomach and chest responding gently and easily to the soothing sensation of warmth soaking through you ... becoming more settled and peaceful and more and more relaxed... (Pause.)

Move on now, drawing your attention up towards your shoulders... Let the warmth and relaxation spread to the top of your chest and out over your shoulders, so that it feels as though that light and comfortable blanket is drawn up across almost all of your body... (Pause.)

Shift your attention down to your fingers now ... to the very tips of your fingers. You can feel them tingle as your mind touches them... And allow your mind to move along your fingers, over and through every little joint and knuckle, and into your hands, and through your hands, and slowly on to your wrists... Feel all the little bones of your wrists relax as the warmth soaks through... Imagine tensions easing away as you become more and more relaxed ... letting your mind move on now, through your forearms and along the bones and muscles of your upper arms, and on to your shoulders ... so that now you feel that warm blanket pulled up gently, over your neck, and under your chin ... like a cocoon of warmth and comfort in which you can drift into deeper and more enjoyable states of relaxation... (Pause.)

Now, let that warmth soak around the back of your head... Let it move up and around your head, over your scalp, around your ears, until it seems that you are floating in this wonderful sensation of comfort and relaxation... Let the warmth move across your forehead, soothing away the tensions of your brow ... then along your jaw, over your mouth, your nose, your cheekbones ... so only your eyes are left uncovered, and your sense of relaxation is deeper now than it has ever been before... And it's getting deeper and deeper, moment by moment... Now let your attention drift softly across your eyes, so that you are entirely wrapped in this delicious sensation of warmth and comfort and relaxation... Your entire body now feeling more deeply relaxed than it has ever been before... So just go on enjoying this very pleasant state, because in a few moments, when I speak to you again, you will be even more deeply relaxed... In a few moments, when I speak to you again... (Pause.)

Your attention is floating now, very peaceful, very tranquil... Floating as your body enjoys this pleasant and beneficial state of relaxation... So let yourself go on relaxing in this way, because now I want you to turn your attention inward... I want you to imagine a sunny woodland scene... green trees in leaf, a blue sky, a light and refreshing breeze... a wonderful sunny summer's day... Nearby there is a stream... And move towards this stream and sit comfortably on the bank watching the cool, clear, sparkling waters streaming by ... and not only do you see the water ... you can see every detail in and of that water ... the stones and plants on the stream-bed, the bubbles in the water itself, every swirl and gleam and reflection of light as the stream tumbles by ... and you can hear that water clearly gurgling and bubbling and gushing along ... and you can smell the water too, a refreshing clean and natural smell that you find very pleasing... (Pause.)

And now I want you to iniagine that the stream is like your mind, forever flowing on, never still, always busy with its own thoughts and ideas and dreams that come and go like the swirling bubbles in the water... And the person sitting by the strean, watching the flow of the stream is the real you ... the one who can watch the drift and flow of thoughts and worries and tensions, and yet remain unaffected by them ... because life brings these problems to our attention and we can notice them and we can decide what to do about them without getting drawn in and carried away in the currents ... because we are always more than the endless stream of thoughts that pass through our minds ... so that we never feel trapped or carried along by the cares and worries, the tensions and the problems of life... So go on relaxing now, just let your mind's eye watch the busy waters of that little woodland stream... Go on enjoying this sensation, because in a few moments I am going to count from five to one, and as I count from five to one you will feel refreshed, happy, confident and very optimistic and pleased with what you have done and the way you feel, and looking forward to the next time you can enter this enjoyable state of relaxation... And as I count towards one you will come back to the here and now, feeling good as you bring the pleasant thoughts and feelings and ideas with you...

Five – four – three – two – one – fully here now, fully awake and looking forward to the rest of the day. Have a stretch and a yawn if you like, and when you're ready, sit up.

> **NOTE** This is such a relaxing visualisation that some children may drift off to sleep! Ask the rest of the group to sit quietly as you gently waken the others. Give the children a few minutes to reorient themselves before moving on.

Self-Intelligence Glossary

Admit – to let in or out, in the same way that a swing door works. Admission may be unthinking, insofar as you may not have considered allowing ideas through. It is a state of consent, a passive thing. The active allowance of information into consciousness from outside, or from the subconscious, is more accurately called a permission (see *permit*). Resistance to change sometimes occurs because an individual will not admit into consciousness beliefs held at a deeper level.

Consciousness – that part of us (thoughts/feelings/behaviours) which is self-aware. The conscious point-of-attention (POA) may be directed externally – the so-called state of 'normal waking consciousness' - or directed inwardly to a lesser or greater degree. Daydreaming, hypnoidal or trance states and lucid dreaming are all examples of inwardly directed POA.

Default behaviours – these are patterns of behaviour (thoughts, feelings and actions/enactments) that develop by default in an individual; i.e., without being deliberately created (consciously or subconsciously) to serve a purpose. Over time, behaviours that were deliberately created can become obsolete and, without intervention to change, can 'run on' pointlessly, like a TV set left on in an empty room. Conversely, behaviours which were originally default behaviours may come to serve purposes on a conscious and/or subconscious level. Part of the work of therapists in helping clients to construct well-formed outcomes and explore the context of problem behaviours is to ascertain whether these have arisen and continue by default.

Explicate knowledge – knowledge which is 'unfolded', realised, laid out in consciousness and fully accessible at will.

Factless knowledge – that intuitive sureness we've all experienced that something is 'just so'. An idea, intuition, insight, memory rises from the subconscious and blooms into consciousness – *and we know it's right*, without having to explain or justify it to anyone, or to verify it independently for ourselves. Such awarenesses constitute factless knowledge.

Forgetting – the subject of forgetting is large, complex and subtle. It is quite widely believed that at some level we never forget anything. And it makes sense to suppose that, at least for survival's sake, our maps of reality remain as detailed as possible. If so, then forgetting might occur for several reasons: most commonly because events or information have little conscious significance for us, and so pass beyond our awareness; or we might deliberately suppress memories; our subconscious minds might withhold information as a protective measure; or forgetting might occur through a combination of these. Quite often, memory-related problems do not mean that information has disappeared from the mind, but that it is not accessible at will, usually for good reasons and through positive intentions generated within the subconscious.

Goal – a goal has been described as 'a dream within a timescale'. It is often a predominantly abstract expression of a longer-term aspiration: 'I want to be happy', or, more negatively, 'I don't want to worry about things any more'. Note that a goal is fixed, in the same way that, say, Edinburgh is fixed on a map. But there are many ways of getting there.

Imagination – the capability of the human mind to move beyond the immediate here-and-now. Imagination may be predominantly conscious (as in daydreaming/being 'miles away'), or subconscious. In this case, dreaming represents one aspect of subconscious imagination.

Implicate knowledge – subconscious knowledge. This may be 'factless' knowledge when it rises into consciousness as intuitions, and/or may be deeply enfolded in symbolism/used in dreams that may never come into the conscious realm.

Inlook – we are used to having an outlook on life: an inlook is the way we perceive ourselves, the attitude we consciously and subconsciously adopt with regard to ourselves – our image, our health, our potentials. Because the subconscious reacts to conscious thinking, the thoughts we project or let trickle down into subconsciousness will influence our deeper mental landscape and self-image. And since 'perception is projection', the way we regard ourselves affects the way we regard the world and our place within it. Perhaps the first step in developing a deliberate inlook is to thank the subconscious for all it does on our behalf.

Inscape – a term coined by the poet Gerard Manley Hopkins to refer to the uniqueness of every created thing. Used here to mean 'inner landscape' (see also *instress, mindscape, wordscape*).

Insight – a 'looking in' that is part of the exploration-of-context which occurs within therapy and self-intelligence work. An insight may be a sudden realisation which, like a jigsaw-puzzle piece, 'falls into place' and allows one to make sense of a larger picture; or it could take the form of 'slow knowing', a more gradual understanding of context and/or the directions for change.

Instress – used by Gerard Manley Hopkins to mean the expression of anything's individual nature into the world. Read it as 'inner stress', the creative tension that impels us to be uniquely ourselves.

Intuition – read it as 'inner tuition', being taught from within. And of course, in order for the subconscious to teach most effectively, the conscious mind must be willing to learn, which requires us to *permit* and *admit*.

Map of reality – our individual total understanding of the world and our place within it, derived largely if not wholly from our life experiences, and the interpretation we place upon them. We are all, at this moment, the outcome of everything that's ever happened in our lives. Thus, our ideas, opinions, attitudes, beliefs and values have their roots in the map of reality. If we have a problem, therefore, whether we feel its source lies within or without, we can access the map of reality for guidance and advice to initiate change – and most everything is accessible, and negotiable.

Mindscape – another name for the map of reality. And, continuing that analogy, all locations on the map are connected, however distantly, to all others. This is an essentially holistic idea in line with the so-called holographic model of the brain, wherein information is somehow spread across the entire field of the brain. Neurological evidence offers some support to this model – most spectacularly perhaps in the brain's 'plasticity', or ability to reprogram itself after injury and set up alternative neural pathways serving mental and physical functions.

Nonconscious – see *subconscious*

Ongoing outcome – the continuing process of being alive! We set ourselves targets, aspire to goals, define outcomes; and yet we are always becoming, so that any 'outcome' is just a marker along the way. And our story isn't over till it's over.

Osmotic learning – information is constantly woven into the map of reality, whether or not we consciously notice and evaluate it. We learn anyway by 'soaking up' the world. This subliminal process is called osmotic learning. The subconscious will always endeavour to do its best to allow us as individuals to survive and flourish. But problematical behaviours/outcomes may arise into our conscious lives as a result of such learnings. When this happens, the problems seem to 'come from nowhere', and we may not be able to connect them to anything happening in our lives at the time. This is because the context and history which triggered the behaviours lies at a subconscious level, and may stretch back many years in time.

Permit – to decide to allow information into consciousness from the subconscious, and/or to accept ideas and suggestions from outside. In doing this, the individual accepts responsibility for the consequences of those ideas. Permission is an important concept in self-intelligence: since control (denial, resistance, etc) is often an issue. To invite the client to permit gives him/her control over the process of working towards a resolution.

Point-of-attention (POA), the spotlight of our intellectual/analytical/evaluative conscious awareness as it shines on the landscape of our minds. In hypnotic and trance states, the POA is directed more internally, rather than externally as in so-called 'normal waking consciousness'.

Quiet acknowledgement – an acceptance of ideas, from outside or within, whilst in a state of relaxed alertness/quiet consciousness.

Quiet consciousness – another, better name for the state commonly known as hypnosis or daydreaming. In hypnosis the subject is not asleep: the conscious mind, aware, alert, curious, patient and passive, can more easily admit ideas from outside and within. 'Relaxed alertness' is another useful term for the same state.

Realise – to 'make real' within conscious awareness. Once something – a memory, an idea, a belief – has been consciously realised, then interventions can be made: it can be acted upon and changed.

Recall – to 'call back' into consciousness. When memories are recalled, the information comes out of the subconscious into the mature and experienced adult consciousness.

Recognise – to 're-cog-nise', to bring back into cognition. Recognition implies conscious awareness, a precursor to decision making and action.

Represent – to 're-present' something to ourselves or to the world. Thinking of the word in this way reminds us that the world is filtered through our perception; it is translated within, so that our awareness of what's outside is textured by what goes on inside of ourselves.

Resolution – the point at which change is possible. Part of the process of change is to to define an outcome after interventions have been made – a so-called well-formed outcome. This does not just mean the absence of the problem or unwanted behaviour, but a clear impression of what life can be like in an active and positive way once the process has been completed. One can also think of resolution as 're-solution' - to solve again. This reminds us that many behaviours come into being and/or are created initially as attempts to solve problems (in line with the positive intentions principle).

State-bound behaviour – all of us are always in one of any number of mental-emotional-physical states. What happens to us – our experiences and the way these are woven into the map of reality – are connected to the state we are in at the time. We may become 'stuck' in that state and behaviour and, as it were, bound by it through time. Many of the problems that people bring to therapists are, at least in part, state-bound behaviours.

Subconscious – also called the unconscious or nonconscious aspect of our selves: the thinking/feeling/behaving that goes on largely or wholly outside or beyond the realm of our conscious awareness. It is the crew to our conscious captain, and has a complete knowledge of our bodies and, for all practical purposes, a complete knowledge of our histories. Subconscious processes can and do come into the ambit of consciousness regularly, and can also be accessed deliberately at will by using one of a vast range of techniques.

Subliminal – occurring outside the realm of our conscious awareness and attention. Huge amounts of information enter the mind, and are processed, subliminally. What we consciously think about forms just the tip of the iceberg of our minds. Thus it is well said that we know much more than we realise we know / we are much more than we realise we are.

Systematic daydreaming – when we daydream, following the drift of our thoughts, the conscious mind is passive and 'idly aware' of impressions rising up from subconscious levels. It is like an engine running in neutral, active but doing no work. Such daydreaming may lead our conscious point-of-attention on a circuitous 'free associational' route around our map of reality. Or, through interventions that are self-initiated or externally guided, specific information pertinent to a particular issue may be drawn into consciousness to be connected, analysed and realised. This process can usefully be called systematic daydreaming, and is something we all do more or less routinely. A writer plotting a novel or a client in hypnotherapy have deliberately arranged opportunities to daydream systematically in a very effective way.

Undeliberate thinking – conscious thoughts that we are not paying attention to at the time. A pop song playing in our heads that we simply allow to run on is an example of undeliberate thinking. So is any thought we fail to challenge. If I think, 'I can't do that', without reflecting on the nature of 'can't', then my thinking is undeliberate (there is no deliberation involved), but it may be accepted uncritically by the subconscious and give rise to unplanned default behaviours.

Wordscape – we express ourselves immediately through language, which represents to a greater or lesser extent how we perceive the world and ourselves. The words we use reflect in a partial way our map of reality. They are the 'surface structure' which offer clues to the richer weave of the deep structure of our minds.

BIBLIOGRAPHY

Alder, H. **The Right Brain Manager**, Piatkus 1993
Biddulph, S. **The Secret of Happy Children**, Thorsons 1993.
Bowkett, S. **Meditations for Busy People** , Thorsons 1996
        For The Moon There Is The Cloud: tales in the Zen tradition, Collins
                            Pathways Reading Scheme, Collins
                            Educational 1996 **Imagine That...**
                            (a handbook of creative learning activities
                            for the classroom), Network Educational
                            Press 1997
Buzan, T. **Use Your Head**, BBC Books 1993
Cameron-Bandler, L. and Lebeau, M. **The Emotional Hostage**, Real People
                            Press 1986
Chetwynd, T. **A Dictionary of Sacred Myth**, Mandala/Unwin 1986
        A Dictionary For Dreamers, Thorsons 1993
        A Dictionary of Symbols, Thorsons 1993
Claxton, G. **Hare Brain, Tortoise Mind**, Fourth Estate 1998
Day, J. **Creative Visualisation with Children**, Element 1994
De Bono, E. **Lateral Thinking**, Pelican 1984
        Teach Your Child How To Think, Pelican 1993
Dennison, P. and Dennison, G.E. **Brain Gym for Teachers**, Edu-Kinesthetics 1989
Dilts, R. and Epstein, T. **Dynamic Learning**, Meta Publications 1995
Faelton, S. and Diamond, D. **Stress Relief**, Ebury Press 1989
von Franz, M-L. **Shadow and Evil in Fairy Tales**, Shambala 1995
Gawain, S. **Creative Visualisation**, Bantam Books 1982
Goldberg, P. **The Intuitive Edge**, Turnstone Press 1985
Goleman, D. **Emotional Intelligence**, Bloomsbury 1996
Goleman, D., Kaufman, P. and Ray, M. **The Creative Spirit**, Dutton 1992
Greenfield, S. **The Human Brain: A Guided Tour**, Phoenix 1997
Hall, C. and E., Leech, A. **Scripted Fantasy in The Classroom**, Routledge 1990
Harp, D. **The Three-Minute Meditator**, Piatkus 1992
Hewitt, J. **Teach Yourself Relaxation** , Hodder and Stoughton 1985
Hickman, D.E. and Jacobson, S. **The Power Process: an NLP approach to writing**,
                            Anglo-American Book Company 1997
Hill, N. and Stone, W. C., **Success Through a Positive Mental Attitude,**
                            Thorsons 1984
Jacobson, S. **Solution States**, Anglo-American Book Company 1996
James, T. and Woodsmall, W. **Time Line Therapy and The Basis Of Personality**
                            Meta Publications 1988
Jung, C. **Man and His Symbols**, Picador 1978
Knight, S. **NLP at Work**, Nicholas Brealey Publishing 1997
Kohler, M. **The Secrets of Relaxation**, Pan 1973
LeBoeuf, M. **Creative Thinking**, Piatkus 1994
Lewis, B. and Pucelik, F. **Magic of NLP Demystified**, Metamorphous Press 1993
Lewis, D. **Mind Skills**, Souvenir Press 1987
Markham, U. **Visualisation**, Element 1991
Meyer, R. **The Wisdom of Fairy Tales**, Floris Books 1988
Murphy, J. **The Power of Your Subconscious Mind**, Simon and Schuster 1991
Mutke, P.H.C. **Selective Awareness**, Westwood Publishing Co. 1987
O'Connor, J. and Seymour, J. **Introducing Neuro-Linguistic Programming,**
                            Mandala 1990
O'Hanlon Hudson, P. **Making Friends with Your Unconscious Mind,**
                            The Center Press 1993

Ostrander, S., Schroeder, L. **Cosmic Memory: the Supermemory Revolution**,
Simon and Schuster 1993

Ozaniec, N. **Everyday Meditation**, Dorling Kindersley 1997

Page, M. **Visualisation**, Aquarian 1990

Pease, A. **Body Language**, Sheldon Press 1987

Porter, P.K. **Psycho-Linguistics: the Language of the Mind**,
ATG Publishing 1995

Postman, N. and Weingartner, C. **Teaching as a Subversive Activity**,
Penguin 1972

Robbins, A. **Awaken The Giant Within**, Simon and Schuster 1991
Giant Steps, Simon and Schuster 1994

Roet, B. **All In The Mind? - Think yourself better**, Optima 1987
A Safer Place To Cry, Optima 1989

Rose, C. **Accelerated Learning**, Accelerated Learning Systems Ltd. 1996

Rossi, E. L., **The Psychobiology of Mind-Body Healing (New Concepts Of
Therapeutic Hypnosis)**, Norton,1993

Schnieder, M. and Killick, J. **Writing for Self-Discovery,** Element 1998

Schutz, W. **Joy**, Pelican 1973

Scott-Macnab, J. (Ed. British Edition) **Reader's Digest Marvels and Mysteries
of the Human Mind** 1992

Smith, A. **Accelerated Learning in Practice**, Network Educational Press 1998

Thouless, R. H. **Straight and Crooked Thinking**, Pan 1953

Von Oech, R. **A Whack on the Side of the Head: How You can Be
More Creative**, Thorsons 1990

Watzlawick, P. **The Language of Change**, Norton and Co. 1993

Wilson, C. **Frankenstein's Castle,** Ashgrove Press 1988

Zipes, J. **Creative Storytelling**, Routledge 1995

INDEX

STEVE BOWKETT

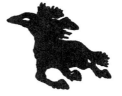

Steve taught English for 18 years in a Leicestershire High School. He is now a full-time writer and trainer, and is also a qualified hypnotherapist.

He was born and brought up in the mining valleys of South Wales, and his childhood experiences have been an important influence in the development of his fiction. Steve began writing at the age of thirteen when, purely by chance, an irate French teacher sent him to the naughty corner and told him to 'get on with something'. This gave him the opportunity to begin writing for fun.

Steve's early published work consisted of fantasy for teenagers. He has since diversified into adult and teen horror, teen romance, mainstream fiction for pre-teens, fiction and non-fiction for younger readers, educational nonfiction, and poetry for all ages.

In his spare time, Steve enjoys rock music, cooking oriental food, drinking beer and cleaning up after his three cats. " I am fond of cats," Steve maintains, "because they love me for myself and because I feed them promptly three times a day." He does not love venomous creatures, nor those that are larger than himself or have sharper teeth, quite as much.

When asked what advice he would give to an aspiring writer, Steve always replies: Have faith in yourself. Be prepared to work hard.
Ideas are like plants. Cultivate the seeds and the trees will grow.

Publications

- **Spellbinder** (teen fantasy) - Gollancz 1985 / Tellerup 1986 / Pan 1988
- **The Copy Cat Plan** – Blackwell 1986
- **Gameplayers** (teen fantasy) - Gollancz 1986 / Pan 1988
- **Dualists** (teen fantasy) - Gollancz 1987 / Pan 1989 / Praha 1993
- **Catch & Other Stories** (teen genre) - Gollancz 1988 / Pan 1990
- **Frontiersville High** (teen SF) - Gollancz 1990
- **The Community** (adult horror) - Pan 1993
- **The Bidden** (adult horror) - Pan 1994
- **A Rare Breed** (adult horror) - Pan 1996
- **Panic Station** (teen horror) - Henderson 1996 / Gallimard 1996
- **Dinosaur Day** (young fantasy) - Heinemann Banana Book 1996
- **For The Moon There Is The Cloud** (tales in the Zen tradition) - Collins, Pathways Reading scheme, 1996.
- **The World's Smallest Werewolf** – Macdonald, Shivery Storybooks 1996.

- **Meditations For Busy People** (How To Stop Worrying & Stay Calm) - HarperCollins 1996 (USA 1996 as *A Little Book Of Joy*).
- **Dreamcastle** (pre-teen SF), Orion Children's Books 1997 / Mondadori, Italy '97.
- **Dino Discoveries** (non-fiction 7+) - Henderson FunFax Dinosaur file, 1997.
- **Imagine That!** *A Handbook Of Creative Learning Activities for the Classroom*, Network Educational Press, 1997.
- **Another Girl, Another Planet** (adult SF, with Martin Day) - Virgin New Adventures, 1998.
- **Roy Kane – TV Detective** – A & C Black's Graffix series, 1998, pbk 1999.

Forthcoming books include, *Dreamcatcher* [Book 2 of Orion's *Dreamtime* series] and *Eleanor* [from the **Horror At Halloween** series scheduled autumn 1999]. Steve has also begun work on *The Wintering*, a Fantasy/SF trilogy to be published by Orion 2000-2001.

Prior to the publication of his first novel, Steve's short stories and poetry were broadcast on BBC Radio Leicester, BRMB (Birmingham) and Radio Northampton, and published in a large number of small press magazines. More recently, he has had short stories published in *Interzone*, and the small press magazines *Peeping Tom*, *Kimota* and the BFS publication *Chills*.
To date, Steve has written something over one hundred novels, several hundred short stories, over five hundred poems, plays and works of non-fiction.
Film rights for *Dualists* optioned by Walt Disney 1991-93.

Steve's freelance work as an author, therapist and trainer is extensive. He has for many years visited schools, libraries and other venue to do storytellings, give talks and run workshops. More recently he has developed Hypnotherapy and Self-Hypnosis training modules and offers INSET on Creative Thinking Skills, Literacy, Stress Management and Self Intelligence.

For more information or to contact Steve Bowkett:-

email - steve@sbowkett.freeserve.co.uk
website - http://www.sbowkett.freeserve.co.uk